Straight A's

in

Medical-Surgical Nursing

Straight A's in Medical-Surgical Nursing

LIPPINCOTT WILLIAMS & WILKINS
A **Wolters Kluwer** Company
Philadelphia • Baltimore • New York • London
Buenos Aires • Hong Kong • Sydney • Tokyo

STAFF

Executive Publisher
Judith A. Schilling McCann, RN, MSN

Senior Acquisitions Editor
Elizabeth Nieginski

Editorial Director
David Moreau

Clinical Director
Joan M. Robinson, RN, MSN

Senior Art Director
Arlene Putterman

Editorial Project Manager
Tracy S. Diehl

Clinical Project Manager
Jana L. Sciarra, RN, MSN, CRNP

Clinical Editor
Marcy Caplin, RN, MSN

Copy Editors
Kimberly Bilotta (supervisor), Tom DeZego, Amy Furman, Dona Hightower Perkins, Dorothy P. Terry

Designers
ON-TRAK graphics, inc. (project manager), Lynn Foulk

Digital Composition Services
Diane Paluba (manager), Joyce Rossi Biletz, Donna S. Morris

Manufacturing
Patricia K. Dorshaw (director), Beth Janae Orr

Editorial Assistants
Megan L. Aldinger, Tara L. Carter-Bell, Arlene Claffee, Linda K. Ruhf

Indexer
Karen C. Comerford

The clinical treatments described and recommended in this publication are based on research and consultation with nursing, medical, and legal authorities. To the best of our knowledge, these procedures reflect currently accepted practice. Nevertheless, they can't be considered absolute and universal recommendations. For individual applications, all recommendations must be considered in light of the patient's clinical condition and, before administration of new or infrequently used drugs, in light of the latest package-insert information. The authors and publisher disclaim any responsibility for any adverse effects resulting from the suggested procedures, from any undetected errors, or from the reader's misunderstanding of the text.

STRMS – D N
05 04 03 10 9 8 7 6 5 4 3 2 1

Library of Congress Cataloging-in-Publication Data

Straight A's. Medical-surgical nursing.
p. ; cm.
Includes bibliographical references and index.
1. Nursing—Outlines, syllabi, etc. 2. Nursing—Examinations, questions, etc. 3. Surgical nursing—Outlines, syllabi, etc. 4. Surgical nursing—Examinations, questions, etc.
[DNLM: 1. Nursing Care. WY 100 S896 2004] I. Title: Medical-surgical nursing. II. Lippincott Williams & Wilkins.
RT52.S77 2004
610.73'076—dc22
ISBN 1-58255-284-3 (alk. paper) 2003015977

Contents

Advisory board

Ivy Alexander, PhD, CANP
Assistant Professor, Yale University
New Haven, Conn.

Susan E. Appling, RN, MS, CRNP
Assistant Professor, Johns Hopkins University School of Nursing
Baltimore

Paul M. Arnstein, PhD, APRN-BC, FNP-C
Assistant Professor, Boston College

Bobbie Berkowitz, PhD, CNAA, FAAN
Chair and Professor, Psychosocial and Community Health
University of Washington
Seattle

Michael A. Carter, BSN, MNSc, DNSc, FAAN, APRN-BC
University Distinguished Professor, University of Tennessee
Memphis

Karla Jones, RN, MSN
Nursing Faculty, Treasure Valley Community College
Ontario, Ore.

Manon Lemonde, RN, PhD
Associate Professor, University of Ontario Institute of Technology
Oshawa, Ontario, Canada

Sheila Sparks Ralph, DNSc, RN, FAAN
Director and Professor, Division of Nursing and Respiratory Care
Shenandoah University
Winchester, Va.

Kristine Anne Scordo, PhD, RN, CS, ACNP
Director, Acute Care Nurse, Practitioner Program, Wright State University
Dayton, Ohio

Contributors and consultants

Elizabeth A. Archer, RN, EdD(C)
Assistant Professor
Baptist College of Health Sciences
Memphis

Roseanne Baughman, RN, MSN, CRNP
Nurse Practitioner – Internal Medicine
Central Bucks Internal Medicine
Doylestown, Pa.

Cheryl L. Brady, RN, MSN
Adjunct Faculty
Youngstown (Ohio) State University

Michelle M. Byrne, RN, MS, PhD, CNOR
Clinical Faculty
North Georgia College & State University
Dahlonega

Marcy Caplin, RN, MSN
Instructor
Kent (Ohio) State University College of Nursing

Kathleen Clark, RN, MSN, APN,BC CNRN,
Instructor, Department of Nursing
Thomas Jefferson University
Philadelphia

Litta Dennis, RN, BSN, MS, CNA
Part-time Instructor, LPN Program & Health Careers
Illinois Central College
East Peoria

Tina Dietrich, RN, BSN
Consultant
Harleysville, Pa.

Shelba Durston, RN, MSN, CCRN
Staff Nurse V
San Joaquin General Hospital
French Camp, Calif.
Adjunct Faculty
San Joaquin Delta College
Stockton, Calif.

Ellie Z. Franges, MSN, CNRN
Clinical Nurse Specialist — Neuroscience
St. Luke's Hospital & Health Network
Bethlehem, Pa.

Joyce Lyne Heise, RN, MSN, EdD
Professor of Nursing
Kent State University
East Liverpool, Ohio

Bobbie L. Hunter, RN, MSN, FNP
Nursing Instructor — Program Manager
Practical Nursing Department
Columbus (Ga.) Technical College

René A. Jackson, RN, BSN
RN Special Procedures
Charlotte Regional Medical Center
Punta Gorda, Fla.

Dawna Martich, RN, MSN
Clinical Trainer
American Healthways
Pittsburgh

Lisa A. Salamon, RNC, MSN, CNS, ET
Clinical Nurse Specialist
Cleveland Clinic Foundation

How to use this book

Straight A's is a multivolume study guide series developed especially for nursing students. Each volume provides essential course material in a unique two-column design. The easy-to-read interior outline format offers a succinct review of key facts as presented in leading textboks on the subject. The bulleted exterior columns provide only the most crucial information, allowing for quick, efficient review right before an important quiz or test.

Special features appear in every chapter to make information accessible and easy to remember. **Learning objectives** encourage the student to evaluate knowledge before and after study. **Chapter overview** highlights the chapter's major concepts. Within the outlined text, color is used to highlight critical information and key points. Key points may include cardinal signs and symptoms, current theories, important steps in a nursing procedure, critical assessment findings, crucial nursing interventions, or successful therapies and treatments. **NCLEX checks** at the end of each chapter offer additional opportunities to review material and assess knowledge gained before moving on to new information.

Other features appear throughout the book to facilitate learning. **Time-out for teaching** highlights key areas to address when teaching patients. **Go with the flow** charts promote critical thinking. Finally, a brand-new Windows-based software program (see CD-ROM on inside back cover) poses more than 250 multiple-choice and alternate-format NCLEX-style questions in random or sequential order to assess your knowledge.

The *Straight A's* volumes are designed as learning tools, not as primary information sources. When read conscientiously as a supplement to class attendance and textbook reading, *Straight A's* can enhance understanding and help improve test scores and final grades.

Foreword

Whether in hospitals, long-term care facilities, or even the patient's home, nurses are on the front line of patient care. While medical-surgical nursing remains one of the most demanding practices for professional nursing, it's also one of the most exciting and challenging for today's nurses.

Medical-surgical nursing offers diverse practice opportunities in rapidly changing health care settings. Innovations in biomedical sciences and technologies, improved disease prevention and management, and changes in health care financing and delivery systems — coupled with a growing nursing shortage — often require medical-surgical nurses to care for more acutely ill patients in less time, with fewer personnel.

Consequently, as experts in health promotion and restoration in acute, subacute, and rehabilitative care, medical-surgical nurses are essential for enhanced quality of life and enhanced quality of health services.

Straight A's in Medical-Surgical Nursing offers a comprehensive foundation for providing nursing care to patients and their families. Organized by body system, this book provides detailed information on a wide range of health problems, making it an excellent clinical reference for undergraduate nursing students. Students and faculty will find theory and practice standards presented in an easy-to-read bulleted outline format.

Straight A's in Medical-Surgical Nursing provides highlighted points that summarize major disorders, pathophysiology, clinical manifestations, assessment, diagnostic testing, and interventions. The pathology of diseases is described in flow charts; diagnostic tests and treatments are detailed in graphics and tables; strategies to promote learning retention are provided through teaching tips and NCLEX quizzes.

In addition to the simple outline format in the main text, this book offers students the option of going straight to the most critical information. The outer columns of *Straight A's in Medical-Surgical Nursing* feature key points every med-surg nursing student should study right before a quiz or exam.

This time-saving study tool is complemented by a free CD-ROM enclosed in the book. The more than 250 questions on the CD give students an extra chance to improve their knowledge of medical-surgical nursing, and it's great practice for the NCLEX exam!

The nursing diagnoses, interventions, and outcomes in this book form standards for practice that ultimately enhance the student's clinical expertise and professionalism when caring for patients.

Recognizing the vast need for nurses to know how to treat patients in various settings, this text provides succinct information for managing patients across the spectrum of care — from patient and family education and preoperative precautions to collaborative care and home management.

Written by medical-surgical nursing experts, *Straight A's in Medical-Surgical Nursing* promotes continuous development among students by providing current standards of medical-surgical nursing practice.

Sally J. Reel, RN, PhD, APRN,BC, FNP
Clinical Professor and Coordinator, Nurse Practitioner Programs
University of Arizona College of Nursing
Tucson

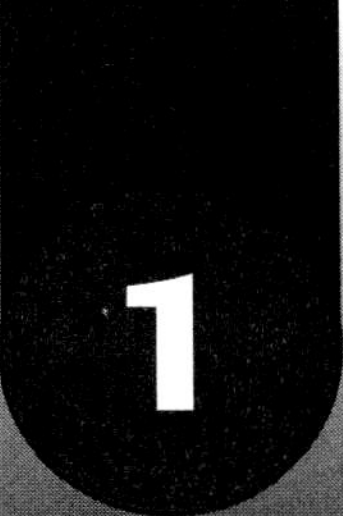

Cardiovascular system

LEARNING OBJECTIVES

After studying this chapter, you should be able to:

- Describe the psychosocial impact of cardiovascular disorders.
- Differentiate between modifiable and nonmodifiable risk factors in the development of a cardiovascular disorder.
- List three probable and three possible nursing diagnoses for a patient with any cardiovascular disorder.
- Identify nursing interventions for a patient with a cardiovascular disorder.
- Write three teaching goals for a patient with a cardiovascular disorder.

CHAPTER OVERVIEW

Caring for the patient with a cardiovascular disorder requires a thorough understanding of cardiovascular anatomy and physiology as well as hemodynamic function. A comprehensive assessment is essential for planning and implementing appropriate patient care. The assessment includes a complete history, physical examination, diagnostic testing, identification of modifiable and nonmodifiable risk factors, and information related to the psychosocial impact of the disorder on the patient.

Nursing diagnoses focus primarily on ineffective tissue perfusion and decreased cardiac output. Nursing interventions are designed to decrease the cardiac workload and increase blood supply, thereby improving tissue perfusion.

Patient teaching — a crucial nursing activity — involves information about medical follow-up, medication regimens, signs and symptoms of possible complications, and reduction of modifiable risk factors through weight control, activity and diet restrictions, stress management, and smoking cessation.

3 layers of the heart's wall

- Epicardium (visceral pericardium)
- Myocardium
- Endocardium

4 valves of the heart

- Tricuspid (atrioventricular valve)
- Mitral (atrioventricular valve)
- Pulmonic (semilunar valve)
- Aortic (semilunar valve)

2 main arteries

- Left coronary artery
- Right coronary artery

Circulation through the heart

- Inferior and superior venae cavae to right atrium
- Through tricuspid valve to right ventricle
- Through pulmonic valve to pulmonary artery
- To lungs
- Through pulmonary veins to left atrium
- Through mitral valve to left ventricle
- Through aortic valve to aorta
- To systemic circulation

ANATOMY AND PHYSIOLOGY REVIEW

Cardiac structures

- The heart is a muscular organ composed of two atria and two ventricles
- It's surrounded by a pericardial sac that consists of two layers
  - Visceral (inner) layer
  - Parietal (outer) layer
- The heart wall has three layers
  - Epicardium (visceral pericardium)
  - Myocardium
  - Endocardium
- The heart has four valves
  - Tricuspid (atrioventricular valve)
  - Mitral (atrioventricular valve)
  - Pulmonic (semilunar valve)
  - Aortic (semilunar valve)

Myocardial blood supply

- The left coronary artery branches into the left anterior descending (LAD) artery and the circumflex artery
  - The LAD artery supplies blood to the anterior wall of the left ventricle, the anterior ventricular septum, and the bundle branches
  - The circumflex artery provides blood to the lateral and posterior portions of the left ventricle
- The right coronary artery (RCA) fills the groove between the atria and ventricles and gives rise to the acute marginal artery, ending as the posterior descending artery
  - The RCA sends blood to the sinus and atrioventricular nodes and to the right atrium
  - The posterior descending artery supplies the posterior and inferior wall of the left ventricle and the posterior portion of the right ventricle
- Coronary arteries receive blood primarily during ventricular relaxation (diastole)
- Blood is pumped out to the systemic circulation during contraction of the ventricles (systole)

Circulation

- From the inferior and superior venae cavae to the right atrium
- Through the tricuspid valve to the right ventricle
- Through the pulmonic valve to the pulmonary artery, to the lungs where blood is oxygenated, through the pulmonary veins to the left atrium
- Through the mitral valve to the left ventricle
- Through the aortic valve to the aorta and the systemic circulation

Normal cardiac conduction

Each electrical impulse travels from the sinoatrial node (1) through the intra-atrial tracts (2), producing atrial contraction. The impulse slows momentarily as it passes through the atrioventricular junction (3) to the bundle of His (4). It then descends the left and right bundle branches (5) and reaches the Purkinje fibers (6), stimulating ventricular contraction.

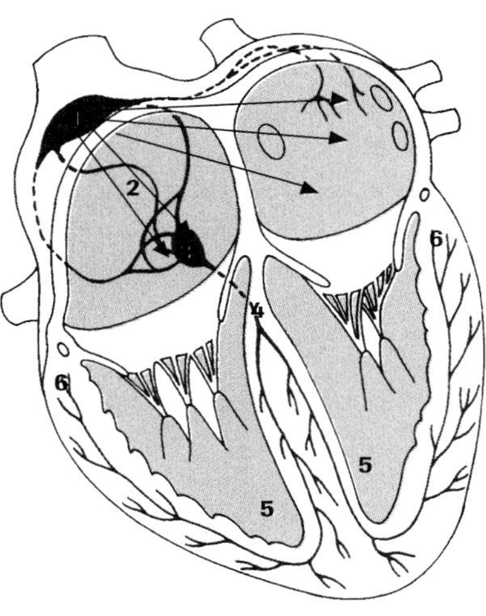

Components of the cardiac conduction system

- Sinoatrial node
- Intra-atrial tracts
- Atrioventricular junction
- Bundle of His
- Right and left bundle branches
- Purkinje fibers

Electrical conduction

- The heart contains specialized muscle fibers that generate and conduct their own electrical impulses spontaneously
- The sinoatrial (SA) node, internodal tracts, atrioventricular (AV) node, bundle of His, right and left bundle branches, and Purkinje fibers make up the system that conducts electrical impulses and coordinates chamber contraction (see *Normal cardiac conduction*)
- Impulses follow a right-to-left, top-to-bottom path
- A normal electrical impulse is initiated at the SA node, the heart's intrinsic pacemaker
- Once generated, the normal impulse must move forward through the conduction system to the ventricles
- Numerous events occur almost simultaneously in the following order after initiation of the impulse at the SA node
  - Atrial depolarization
  - Atrial contraction
  - Impulse transmission to the AV node
  - Impulse transmission to the bundle of His, bundle branches, and Purkinje fibers
  - Ventricular depolarization
  - Ventricular contraction
  - Ventricular repolarization

Electrical conduction

- Heart's muscle fibers generate and conduct electrical impulses
- Impulses follow a right-to-left, top-to-bottom path
- Initiated at the sinoatrial node
- Impulse moves through the conduction system to the ventricles

Cardiac function

- Cardiac output (CO) is the total amount of blood ejected per minute
- Stroke volume (SV) is the amount of blood ejected with each beat

- Cardiac output equals stroke volume times heart rate (HR) (CO = SV × HR)
- Alterations in cardiac output affect every body system
- Ejection fraction is the percent of left ventricular end-diastolic volume ejected during systole (60% to 70% normal)

Cardiac function

- Cardiac output is the total amount of blood ejected per minute.
- Stroke volume is the amount of blood ejected with each beat.
- Cardiac output = stroke volume × heart rate.

Blood vessels

- Arteries are three-layered vessels (intima, media, adventitia) that carry oxygenated blood from the heart to the tissues
- Arterioles are small-resistance vessels that feed into capillaries
- Capillaries join arterioles to venules (larger, lower-pressured vessels than arterioles), where nutrients and wastes are exchanged
- Venules join capillaries to veins
- Veins are large-capacity, low-pressure vessels that return unoxygenated blood to the heart

Characteristics of arteries

- Three-layered vessels
- Carry oxygenated blood from the heart to the tissues

PHYSICAL ASSESSMENT FINDINGS

History

- Dyspnea
- Paroxysmal nocturnal dyspnea
- Orthopnea
- Chest pain (see *Patterns of cardiac pain*)
- Fatigue and weakness
- Cough
- Syncope
- Palpitations
- Leg pain

Key assessment findings

- Dyspnea
- Chest pain
- Syncope
- Pulse and blood pressure changes
- Edema
- Arrhythmias

Physical examination

- Blood pressure changes
- Pulse changes including rate, rhythm, and quality
- Skin color and temperature
- Abnormal heart sounds
- Edema
- Arrhythmias
- Jugular vein distention
- Respiratory distress
- Vascular bruits
- Point of maximal impulse alterations
- Pruritus

Electrocardiography

- Noninvasive test
- Graphical representation of the heart's electrical activity
- Intervention: interpret ECG for changes

DIAGNOSTIC TESTS AND PROCEDURES

Electrocardiography (ECG)

- Definition and purpose
  - Noninvasive test of the heart
  - Graphical representation of the heart's electrical activity

Patterns of cardiac pain

PERICARDITIS

Onset and duration
- Sudden onset; continuous pain lasting for days; residual soreness

Location and radiation
- Substernal pain to left of midline; radiation to back or subclavicular area

Quality and intensity
- Mild ache to severe pain, deep or superficial; "stabbing," "knifelike"

Signs and symptoms
- Precordial friction rub; increased pain with movement, inspiration, laughing, coughing; decreased pain with sitting or leaning forward (sitting up pulls the heart away from the diaphragm)

Precipitating factors
- Myocardial infarction or upper respiratory tract infection; invasive cardiac trauma

ANGINA

Onset and duration
- Gradual or sudden onset; pain usually lasts less than 15 minutes and not more than 30 minutes (average: 3 minutes)

Location and radiation
- Substernal or anterior chest pain, not sharply localized; radiation to back, neck, arms, jaws, upper abdomen, or fingers

Quality and intensity
- Mild-to-moderate pressure; deep sensation; varied pattern of attacks; "tightness," "squeezing," "crushing," "pressure"

Signs and symptoms
- Dyspnea; diaphoresis; nausea; urge to void; belching; apprehension

Precipitating factors
- Exertion; stress; eating; cold or hot and humid weather

MYOCARDIAL INFARCTION

Onset and duration
- Sudden onset; pain lasts 30 minutes to 2 hours; waxes and wanes; residual soreness 1 to 3 days

Location and radiation
- Substernal, midline, or anterior chest pain; radiation to jaws, neck, back, shoulders, or one or both arms

Quality and intensity
- Persistent, severe pressure; deep sensation; "crushing," "squeezing," "heavy," "oppressive"

Signs and symptoms
- Nausea; vomiting; apprehension; dyspnea; diaphoresis; increased or decreased blood pressure; gallop heart sound; "sensation of impending doom"

Precipitating factors
- Occurrence at rest or during physical exertion or emotional stress

- Nursing interventions
  - Determine the patient's ability to lie still
  - Reassure the patient that electrical shock won't occur
  - Interpret ECG for changes, such as life-threatening arrhythmias

Ambulatory electrocardiography (Holter monitoring)

- Definition and purpose
  - Noninvasive test of the heart

Patterns of cardiac pain

- Pericarditis: sudden onset of mild ache to severe pain, deep or superficial; "stabbing," "knifelike"; continuous pain lasting for several days; residual soreness
- Angina: gradual or sudden onset of mild-to-moderate pressure; deep sensation; varied pattern of attacks; "tightness," "squeezing," "crushing," "pressure"; pain usually lasts less than 15 minutes and not more than 30 minutes (average: 3 minutes)
- Myocardial infarction: sudden onset of persistent, severe pressure; deep sensation; "crushing," "squeezing," "heavy," "oppressive"; pain lasts 30 minutes to 2 hours; waxes and wanes; residual soreness 1 to 3 days

Ambulatory electrocardiography

- Noninvasive test
- Records the heart's electrical activity and cardiac events for 24 hours
- Intervention: advise the patient on activity limitations while wearing monitor

Cardiac catheterization

- Invasive, fluoroscopic procedure
- Examines intracardiac structures, pressures, oxygenation, and cardiac output
- Intervention: note the patient's allergies before testing

Coronary arteriography

- Invasive, fluoroscopic procedure
- Examines the coronary artery
- Intervention: note the patient's allergies before the test and monitor his vital signs

  - Recording of the heart's electrical activity and cardiac events for 24 hours
- Nursing interventions
  - Instruct the patient to keep an activity diary
  - Advise the patient not to bathe, shower, operate machinery, or use a microwave oven or an electric shaver while wearing the monitor

Cardiac catheterization

- Definition and purpose
  - Fluoroscopic procedure using a radiopaque dye
  - Examination of the intracardiac structures, pressures, oxygenation, and cardiac output after the dye is injected
- Nursing interventions before the procedure
  - Withhold the patient's food and fluids after midnight
  - Take baseline vital signs and palpate peripheral pulses
  - Place obtained written informed consent in the patient's chart
  - Inform the patient about possible nausea, chest pain, flushing of the face, or throat irritation from the injection of radiopaque dye
  - **Note the patient's allergies to seafood, iodine, or radiopaque dyes**
  - Shave and scrub the insertion site, as ordered
  - Mark peripheral pulses with an "X"
  - Administer sedation, as prescribed
  - Remove all jewelry and prosthetic devices
  - Ensure patent I.V. access
- Nursing interventions after the procedure
  - Monitor vital signs, peripheral pulses, and the insertion site for bleeding
  - Maintain a pressure dressing and bed rest for 4 to 8 hours, or as ordered
  - Increase fluid intake unless contraindicated
  - Allay the patient's anxiety
  - **Monitor for complaints of chest pain, a possible sign of myocardial infarction (MI)—a serious complication of cardiac catheterization—and report immediately**
  - Keep affected leg extended
  - Assess peripheral pulses in both legs and compare to baseline
  - Monitor urinary output
  - Monitor for delayed reaction to radiopaque dye

Coronary arteriography

- Definition and purpose
  - Fluoroscopic procedure using a radiopaque dye
  - Examination of the coronary arteries
- Nursing interventions before the procedure
  - Note the patient's allergies to iodine, seafood, or radiopaque dyes
  - Monitor the patient's vital signs
  - Allay the patient's anxiety

- Inform the patient about possible flushing of the face or throat irritation from the injection
- Nursing interventions after the procedure
  - Check the insertion site for bleeding
  - Assess peripheral pulses
  - Maintain a pressure dressing and bed rest

Digital subtraction angiography

- Definition and purpose
  - Invasive procedure using a computer system and fluoroscopy with an image intensifier
  - Complete visualization of the arterial blood supply to a specific area, especially the carotid and cerebral arteries
- Nursing interventions before the procedure
  - Place obtained written informed consent in the patient's chart
  - Monitor the patient's vital signs
  - Remove all jewelry in the area to be imaged
  - Perform a baseline neurological examination before cerebral angiography
  - Administer sedation, as ordered
- Nursing interventions after the procedure
  - Check the insertion site for bleeding
  - Instruct the patient to drink at least 1 L of fluid
  - Monitor for delayed reaction to radiopaque dye

Echocardiography

- Definition and purpose
  - Noninvasive examination of the heart
  - Uses echoes from sound waves to visualize intracardiac structures and direction of blood flow
- Nursing interventions
  - Determine the patient's ability to lie still
  - Explain the procedure

Exercise testing (stress)

- Definition and purpose
  - Noninvasive test of the heart
  - Study of the heart's electrical activity and ischemic events during prescribed levels of exercise
- Nursing interventions
  - Withhold food and fluids, especially those that contain caffeine, for 1 hour before the test
  - Instruct the patient to wear loose-fitting clothing and supportive shoes
  - Explain the procedure

Nuclear cardiology

- Definition and purpose
  - Visual examination of the heart using radioisotopes
  - Imaging of myocardial perfusion and contractility after I.V. injection of isotopes

Digital subtraction angiography

- Invasive, fluoroscopic procedure
- Allows for complete visualization of the arterial blood supply to a specific area (especially the carotid and cerebral arteries)
- Intervention: perform a baseline neurological examination before cerebral angiography

Echocardiography

- Noninvasive test
- Uses echoes from sound waves to visualize intracardiac structures and direction of blood flow
- Intervention: determine the patient's ability to lie still

Exercise testing

- Noninvasive test
- Study of the heart's electrical activity and ischemic events during prescribed levels of exercise
- Intervention: withhold food and fluids for 1 hour before the test

Nuclear cardiology

- Noninvasive test
- Allows for visual examination of the heart
- Intervention: determine the patient's ability to lie still

- Nursing interventions
  - Explain the procedure
  - Allay the patient's anxiety
  - Determine the patient's ability to lie still during the procedure

Hemodynamic monitoring

- Invasive procedure involving catheter placed in pulmonary artery
- Allows for examination of intracardiac pressures and cardiac output
- Intervention: monitor the pressure tracings and record readings

Hemodynamic monitoring (single procedure or continuous monitoring)

- Definition and purpose
  - Procedure using a balloon-tipped, flow-directed catheter (pulmonary artery catheter)
  - Examination of intracardiac pressures and cardiac output
- Nursing interventions before the procedure
  - Place obtained written informed consent in the patient's chart
  - Explain the procedure and its purpose to the patient
- Nursing interventions after the procedure
  - Check the insertion site for signs of infection
  - Monitor the pressure tracings and record readings (see *Putting hemodynamic monitoring to use*)

Chest X-ray

- Noninvasive test
- Provides radiographic picture of the heart and lungs
- Intervention: ensure that the patient removes jewelry before test

Chest X-ray

- Definition and purpose
  - Noninvasive examination of the heart and lungs
  - Radiographic picture of the heart and lungs
- Nursing interventions
  - Determine the patient's ability to hold his breath
  - Ensure that the patient removes jewelry

Blood tests

- Blood chemistries:
  - Sodium, potassium, magnesium, calcium, phosphorus
  - Glucose
  - Cholesterol, triglycerides
  - Uric acid
  - Bicarbonate
  - BUN, creatinine
  - CK, CK isoenzymes, troponin I, troponin T
  - Bilirubin, AST, alanine aminotransferase
- Hematologic studies:
  - RBCs
  - WBCs
  - ESR
  - PT
  - PTT
  - Platelets
  - Hemoglobin
  - HCT

Blood chemistries

- Definition and purpose
  - Laboratory test of a blood sample
  - Analysis for sodium, potassium, magnesium, calcium, glucose, phosphorus, cholesterol, triglycerides, uric acid, bicarbonate, creatine, blood urea nitrogen (BUN), bilirubin, creatine kinase (CK), CK isoenzymes, lactate dehydrogenase (LD), LD isoenzymes, troponin I, troponin T, aspartate aminotransferase (AST), and alanine aminotransferase
- Nursing interventions
  - Note any drugs that may alter test results
  - Restrict the patient's exercise before the blood sample is drawn
  - Withhold I.M. injections or note the time of the injection on the laboratory slip (alter CK levels)
  - Withhold food and fluids, as ordered
  - Assess the venipuncture site for bleeding

Hematologic studies

- Definition and purpose
  - Laboratory test of a blood sample
  - Analysis for red blood cells (RBCs), white blood cells (WBCs), erythrocyte sedimentation rate (ESR), prothrombin time (PT), partial thromboplastin time (PTT), platelets, hemoglobin, and hematocrit (HCT)

Putting hemodynamic monitoring to use

Hemodynamic monitoring provides information on intracardiac pressures and cardiac output. To understand intracardiac pressures, picture the cardiovascular system as a continuous loop with constantly changing pressure gradients that keep the blood moving.

RIGHT ATRIAL PRESSURE (RAP), OR CENTRAL VENOUS PRESSURE (CVP)

The RAP reflects right atrial, or right heart, function and end-diastolic pressure.

- **Normal:** 1 to 6 mm Hg (1.34 to 8 cm H_2O). (To convert mm Hg to cm H_2O, multiply mm Hg by 1.34)
- **Elevated value suggests:** right-sided heart failure, volume overload, tricuspid valve stenosis or insufficiency, constrictive pericarditis, pulmonary hypertension, cardiac tamponade, or right ventricular infarction.
- **Low value suggests:** reduced circulating blood volume.

RIGHT VENTRICULAR PRESSURE (RVP)

Right ventricular (RV) systolic pressure normally equals pulmonary artery systolic pressure; RV end-diastolic pressure, which equals right atrial pressure, reflects RV function.

- **Normal**: systolic, 15 to 25 mm Hg; diastolic, 0 to 8 mm Hg.
- **Elevated value suggests:** mitral stenosis or insufficiency; pulmonary disease; hypoxemia; constrictive pericarditis; chronic heart failure; atrial and ventricular septal defects; and patent ductus arteriosus.

PULMONARY ARTERY PRESSURE (PAP)

Pulmonary artery systolic pressure reflects right ventricular function and pulmonary circulation pressures. Pulmonary artery diastolic pressure reflects left ventricular pressures, specifically left ventricular end-diastolic pressure.

- **Normal:** Systolic, 15 to 25 mm Hg; diastolic, 8 to 15 mm Hg; mean, 10 to 20 mm Hg.
- **Elevated value suggests:** left-sided heart failure, increased pulmonary blood flow (left or right shunting, as in atrial or ventricular septal defects), and any condition causing increased pulmonary arteriolar resistance.

PULMONARY ARTERY WEDGE PRESSURE (PAWP)

PAWP reflects left atrial and left ventricular pressures unless the patient has mitral stenosis. Changes in PAWP reflect changes in left ventricular filling pressure. The heart momentarily relaxes during diastole as it fills with blood from the pulmonary veins; this permits the pulmonary vasculature, left atrium, and left ventricle to act as a single chamber.

- **Normal**: mean pressure, 6 to 12 mm Hg.
- **Elevated value suggests:** left-sided heart failure, mitral stenosis or insufficiency, and pericardial tamponade.
- **Low value suggests:** hypovolemia.

LEFT ATRIAL PRESSURE

This value reflects left ventricular end-diastolic pressure in patients without mitral valve disease.

- **Normal:** 6 to 12 mm Hg.

CARDIAC OUTPUT

Cardiac output is the amount of blood ejected by the heart each minute.

- **Normal:** 4 to 8 L; varies with a patient's weight, height, and body surface area. Adjusting the cardiac output to the patient's size yields a measurement called the *cardiac index.*

What hemodynamic monitoring measures

- Right atrial pressure (RAP) or central venous pressure (CVP)
- Right ventricular pressure (RVP)
- Pulmonary artery pressure (PAP)
- Pulmonary artery wedge pressure (PAWP)
- Left atrial pressure
- Cardiac output

Normal values in hemodynamic monitoring

- RAP or CVP – 1 to 6 mm Hg (1.34 to 8 cm H_2O)
- RVP – systolic: 15 to 25 mm Hg; diastolic: 0 to 8 mm Hg
- PAP – systolic: 15 to 25 mm Hg; diastolic: 8 to 15 mm Hg; mean: 10 to 20 mm Hg
- PAWP – mean pressure: 6 to 12 mm Hg
- Left atrial pressure – 6 to 12 mm Hg
- Cardiac output – 4 to 8 L

- Nursing interventions
  - Note any drugs that might alter test results before the procedure
  - Assess the venipuncture site for bleeding after the procedure

Arterial blood gas (ABG) analysis

- Definition and purpose
  - Test of arterial blood
  - Assessment of tissue oxygenation, ventilation, and acid-base status
- Nursing interventions before the procedure
  - Document the patient's temperature
  - Note whether the patient needs supplemental oxygen or mechanical ventilation
  - Perform Allen's test prior to obtaining the sample before attempting a radial puncture
  - Avoid using a limb with an arteriovenous shunt
- Nursing interventions after the procedure
  - Check the site for bleeding
  - Maintain a pressure dressing
  - Check peripheral pulses in the affected limb

ABG analysis

- Assesses: tissue oxygenation, ventilation, and acid-base status
- Test of arterial blood
- Interventions:
- Note whether the patient needs supplemental oxygen or mechanical ventilation
- Perform Allen's test prior to obtaining sample

Doppler ultrasound

- Definition and purpose
  - Noninvasive procedure that transforms echoes from sound waves into audible sounds
  - Examination of blood flow in peripheral circulation
- Nursing interventions
  - Determine the patient's ability to lie still
  - Explain the procedure

Doppler ultrasound

- Noninvasive test
- Allows for examination of blood flow in peripheral circulation
- Intervention: determine the patient's ability to lie still

Venogram

- Definition and purpose
  - Visualization of the veins after I.V. injection of a dye
  - Diagnosis of deep vein thrombosis or incompetent valves
- Nursing interventions before the procedure
  - Withhold food and fluids after midnight
  - Record the patient's baseline vital signs and peripheral pulses
  - Place obtained written informed consent in the patient's chart
  - **Note the patient's allergies to seafood, iodine, or radiopaque dyes**
  - Inform the patient about possible flushing of the face or throat irritation from the injection
  - Ensure the patient is adequately hydrated
- Nursing interventions after the procedure
  - Check the injection site for bleeding and hematoma
  - Force fluids unless contraindicated
  - Evaluate for signs of delayed reaction to radiopaque dye
  - Assess vital signs and compare to baseline

Venogram

- Invasive test involving injection of a dye
- Allows for visualization of the veins
- Intervention: note the patient's allergies before the test

- **Pulse oximetry**
  - Definition and purpose
    - Noninvasive procedure using infrared light to measure arterial oxygen saturation in the blood
    - Continuous measurement of oxygen saturation assists in pulmonary assessment of patient and weaning patient from a ventilator
  - Nursing interventions
    - Avoid placing the sensor on an extremity that has impeded blood flow
    - Protect the sensor from bright light
    - Attach the monitoring sensor to a fingertip, ear lobe, or toe.
    - **Consider using the earlobe if the patient has artificial nails, nail tips, or nail polish, as these may interfere with light transmission. (Some sensors can accurately read through these as long as polish is removed, but this isn't recommended)**

PSYCHOSOCIAL IMPACT OF CARDIOVASCULAR DISORDERS

- **Developmental impact**
  - Fear of rejection
  - Lowered self-esteem
  - Fear of dying
  - Role conflict
- **Economic impact**
  - Disruption or loss of employment
  - Cost of hospitalization, medications, and special diets
- **Occupational and recreational impact**
  - Restrictions in work activity
  - Changes in leisure activity
  - Restrictions in physical activity (walking, climbing stairs)
  - Restrictions in activity related to environmental temperature; for example, hot or cold weather may interfere with the patient's ability to take walks or go outside
- **Social impact**
  - Changes in dietary habits such as dining out
  - Changes in sexual function
  - Changes in role performance, including work and family roles
  - Social isolation

RISK FACTORS

- **Modifiable risk factors** (impact of cardiovascular disorders can be reduced by altering these)
  - Smoking
  - Hypertension

Pulse oximetry

- Noninvasive test
- Measures arterial oxygen saturation in the blood
- Intervention: avoid placing the pulse oximetry sensor on an extremity that has impeded blood flow

Key psychosocial impact of a cardiovascular disorder

- Fear of dying
- Financial issues related to loss of wages and medical costs
- Restrictions in activity
- Changes in role performance

Modifiable risk factors

- Smoking
- Hypertension
- Hypercholesterolemia
- Obesity
- Physical inactivity
- Emotional stress

- Hypercholesterolemia
- Obesity
- Physical inactivity
- Emotional stress

Nonmodifiable risk factors

- Gender
- Family history of cardiovascular illness
- Childhood history of cardiovascular illness
- Ethnicity
- Race
- Age

NURSING DIAGNOSES

Probable nursing diagnoses

- Decreased cardiac output
- Chronic pain
- Ineffective tissue perfusion: Cardiopulmonary
- Ineffective tissue perfusion: Peripheral
- Ineffective tissue perfusion: Cerebral
- Risk for peripheral neurovascular dysfunction

Possible nursing diagnoses

- Excess fluid volume
- Activity intolerance
- Fear
- Anxiety
- Ineffective coping
- Disabled family coping
- Situational low self-esteem
- Ineffective role performance
- Disturbed body image
- Sexual dysfunction
- Noncompliance
- Chronic low self-esteem
- Risk for situational low self-esteem
- Fatigue

CARDIAC SURGERY

Description

- Coronary artery bypass graft (CABG) — surgical revascularization of the coronary arteries using the saphenous veins or the internal mammary artery to bypass an obstruction caused by atherosclerosis
- Valve replacement — surgical replacement of stenotic or incompetent valves with a mechanical or bioprosthetic valve, such as Starr-Edwards "ball-in-cage" valves, porcine valves, or Bjork-Shiley "tilting disk" valves

Nonmodifiable risk factors

- Gender
- Family history of cardiovascular illness
- Childhood history of cardiovascular illness
- Ethnicity
- Race
- Age

Cardiovascular nursing diagnoses

- Decreased cardiac output
- Chronic pain
- Ineffective tissue perfusion: Cardiopulmonary
- Ineffective tissue perfusion: Peripheral
- Ineffective tissue perfusion: Cerebral
- Risk for peripheral neurovascular dysfunction

CABG defined

- The surgical revascularization of the coronary arteries using the saphenous veins or the internal mammary artery
- Revascularization bypasses obstructions caused by atherosclerosis.

- Valvular annuloplasty—surgical repair or reconstruction of the leaflets and annulus of the valve
- Mitral valve commissurotomy—surgical opening of the fused portion of the mitral valve leaflets, using a dilator
- Valvuloplasty—surgical repair or reconstruction of the valve
- Percutaneous transluminal valvuloplasty—dilation of calcified and stenotic valvular leaflets, using a balloon catheter
- Percutaneous transluminal coronary angioplasty—dilation of a coronary artery using a balloon-tipped catheter to compress plaque against the vessel wall (see *Relieving occlusions with angioplasty,* page 14)

Preoperative nursing interventions

- Complete patient and family preoperative teaching
  - Determine the patient's understanding of the procedure
  - Describe the operating room, postanesthesia care unit (PACU), and preoperative and postoperative routines
  - Demonstrate postoperative turning, coughing, deep breathing, splinting, and range-of-motion (ROM) exercises
  - Explain the postoperative need for drainage tubes, surgical dressings, oxygen therapy, I.V. therapy, and pain control
- Allay the patient's and family's anxiety about surgery
- Document the patient's history and physical assessment data base
- Obtain baseline hemodynamic variables, ECG readings, and ABG studies
- Complete a preoperative checklist
- Administer preoperative medications

Postoperative nursing interventions

- Assess cardiac, respiratory, and neurologic status
- Assess pain and administer analgesics, as prescribed
- Administer oxygen and maintain an endotracheal (ET) tube to the ventilator
- Monitor vital signs, intake and output (I/O), laboratory studies, ECG, hemodynamic variables, daily weight, and pulse oximetry
- Monitor and maintain the water-seal chest drainage system for mediastinal and pleural chest tubes
- Monitor and maintain the position and patency of drainage tubes and catheters, such as a nasogastric (NG) tube, indwelling urinary catheter, and wound drainage and chest tubes
- Administer I.V. fluids and transfusion therapy, as prescribed
- Inspect and change the surgical dressing, as ordered
- Keep the patient in semi-Fowler's position
- Provide incentive spirometry after extubation or ET suction
- Reinforce turning, coughing, and deep breathing, and splinting of the incision
- Administer antiarrhythmics, anticoagulants, vasopressors, beta adrenergic blockers, diuretics, or cardiac glycosides, as prescribed
- Monitor the patient for arrhythmias
- Check peripheral circulation: color, temperature, pulses, and complaints of abnormal sensations, such as numbness or tingling

Cardiac surgery preoperative teaching

- Demonstrate postoperative turning, coughing, and deep breathing; splinting; and ROM exercises.
- Explain the postoperative need for drainage tubes, surgical dressings, oxygen therapy, I.V. therapy, and pain control.

Cardiac surgery postoperative monitoring parameters

- Vital signs
- I/O
- Laboratory studies
- ECG
- Hemodynamic variables
- Daily weight
- Pulse oximetry
- Water-seal chest drainage system for chest tubes
- Position and patency of drainage tubes and catheters

Facts about angioplasty

- Invasive procedure to open an occluded artery without surgery
- Performed under fluoroscopy by a physician
- A balloon catheter is guided through the occlusion
- The balloon is inflated to flatten plaque and dilate the artery's diameter

Relieving occlusions with angioplasty

Percutaneous transluminal coronary angioplasty can open an occluded coronary artery without opening the chest—an important advantage over bypass surgery. Initially, coronary angiography must confirm the presence and location of the arterial occlusion. Next, the physician threads a guide catheter through the patient's femoral artery into the coronary artery under fluoroscopic guidance, as shown at right.

When angiography shows the guide catheter positioned at the occlusion site, the physician carefully inserts a smaller double-lumen balloon catheter through the guide catheter and directs the balloon through the occlusion (lower left).

A marked pressure gradient will be obvious.

The physician alternately inflates and deflates the balloon until an angiogram verifies successful arterial dilation (lower right) and the pressure gradient has decreased.

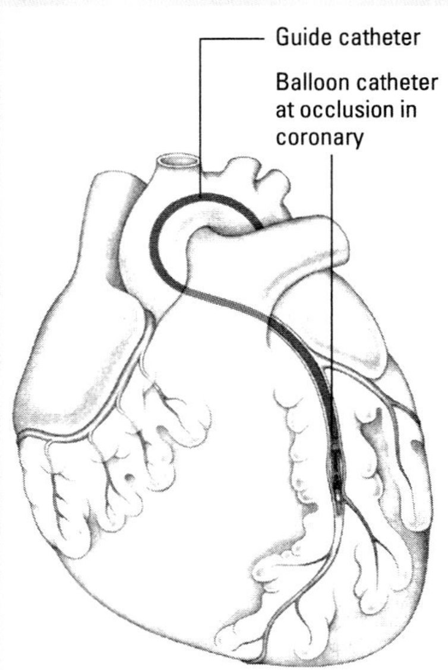

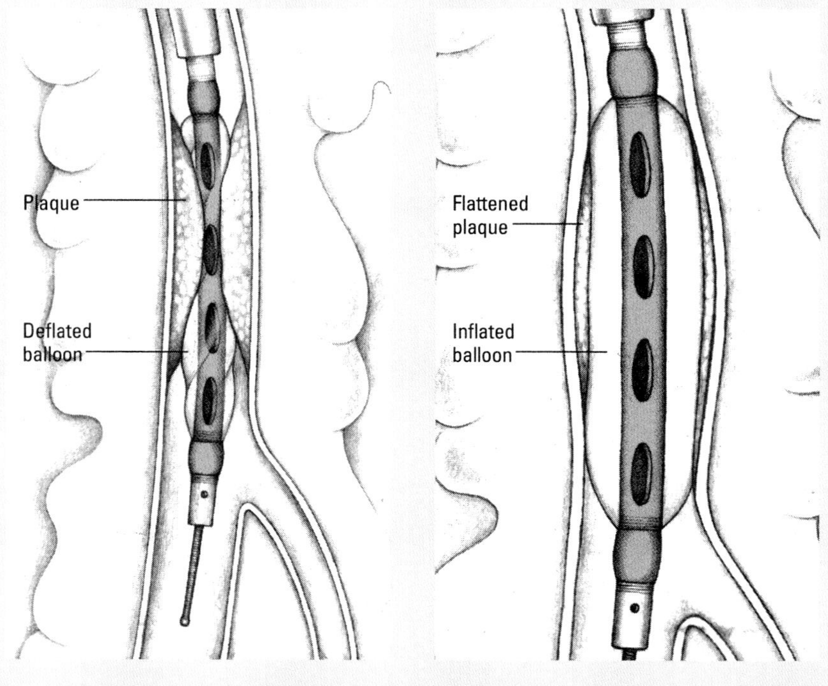

- Insulate epicardial pacing wires; have temporary pacemaker available
- Administer antibiotics, as prescribed
- Assess for return of peristalsis
- Provide the prescribed diet, as tolerated
- Assist the patient with active and passive ROM and isometric exercises, as tolerated
- Allay the patient's anxiety
- Encourage the patient to express feelings about changes in body image or a fear of dying
- Provide information about support groups such as Mended Hearts
- Individualize home care instructions
  - Avoid driving and heavy lifting for 6 weeks
  - Complete incision care daily
  - Elevate the leg with the saphenous graft when seated
  - Wear antiembolism stockings
  - Follow a low-sodium, low-fat diet

Possible surgical complications

- Bleeding from the mediastinal tube
- MI
- Decreased cardiac output
- Arrhythmias
- Cardiac tamponade
- Heart block
- Embolism
- Valve malfunction

PACEMAKER THERAPY

Description

- Electronic device that stimulates the heart to contract when the intrinsic pacemaker or conduction system fails

Types of pacemakers

- Demand (synchronous, non-competitive) — pacemaker fires when inherent heart rate falls below predetermined set rate
- Fixed rate (asynchronous, competitive) — pacemaker fires at a constant, preset rate
- Temporary — pulse generator is attached to pacemaker wires that are inserted temporarily
  - Transvenous
  - Epicardial
  - Transcutaneous
- Permanent — pulse generator implanted in subcutaneous tissue in right or left pectoral area or abdomen

Key steps in cardiac surgery postoperative care

- Assess cardiac, respiratory, and neurologic status.
- Assess pain and administer analgesics, as prescribed.
- Inspect and change the surgical dressing, as ordered.
- Provide incentive spirometry after extubation or ET suction.
- Check peripheral circulation: color, temperature, pulses, and complaints of abnormal sensations, such as numbness or tingling.

Understanding the pacemaker

- An electronic device
- Stimulates the heart to contract when the intrinsic pacemaker or conduction system fails

Types of pacemakers

- Demand (synchronous, non-competitive)
- Fixed rate (asynchronous, competitive)
- Temporary
- Permanent

Components of a pacemaker

- Pulse generator: power source
- Lead: insulated wire that transmits electrical impulses from pulse generator to the heart

Key steps before pacemaker insertion

- Obtain a baseline of heart rhythm and rate and peripheral circulation.
- Complete patient and family preoperative teaching.

Key steps after pacemaker insertion

- Obtain a 12-lead ECG as ordered.
- Protect control settings if temporary pacer.
- Monitor vital signs and cardiac rhythm.

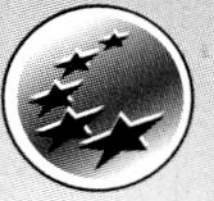

TOP 3

Home care instructions after pacemaker insertion

1. Recognize signs of pacemaker malfunction.
2. Carry a pacemaker identification card at all times.
3. Check pulse daily.

Pacemaker components

- Pulse generator — power source of pacemaker, which is controlled electronically
  - Plutonium — lasts 20+ years
  - Lithium — lasts 10 years
  - Mercury-zinc — lasts 3 to 4 years
- Lead — insulated wire implanted in the heart and connected to pulse generator to transmit electrical impulses from the pulse generator to the heart
- Controls
  - Sensitivity
  - Rate
  - Output

Classification system — International Pacemaker Code (see *Pacemaker codes*)

Preoperative nursing interventions

- Complete patient and family preoperative teaching
  - Determine the patient's understanding of the procedure
  - Describe the operating room, PACU, and preoperative and postoperative routines
  - Demonstrate postoperative turning, coughing, deep breathing, splinting, and ROM exercises
  - Explain the postoperative need for surgical dressings, oxygen therapy, I.V. therapy, and pain control
- Complete a preoperative checklist
- Administer preoperative medications, as prescribed
- Allay the patient's and family's anxiety about surgery
- Document the patient's history and physical assessment data base
- Obtain a baseline assessment of heart rhythm and rate and peripheral circulation
- Administer antibiotics, as prescribed

Postoperative nursing interventions

- Assess cardiac status: heart sounds, rhythm
- Assess pain and administer analgesics as prescribed
- Monitor vital signs, I/O, neurovascular checks, and pulse oximetry
- Obtain a 12-lead ECG as ordered
- Protect control settings if temporary pacer
- Change dressing as ordered
- Monitor insertion site for signs of infection
- Immobilize upper extremity if used for insertion of temporary pacer
- Individualize home care instructions
  - Recognize signs of pacemaker malfunction
  - Carry a pacemaker identification card at all times
  - Perform active ROM to upper extremity on side of insertion
  - Check pulse daily
  - Avoid physical contact sports
  - Recognize signs of electrical interference

Pacemaker codes

CHAMBER PACED	CHAMBER SENSED	RESPONSE TO SENSING	PROGRAMMABLE FUNCTIONS AND RATE MODULATION	ANTITACHY-ARRHYTHMIA FUNCTIONS
V (ventricle)	V (ventricle)	T (triggers pacing)	P (programmable rate, output, or both)	P (pacing)
A (atrium)	A (atrium)	I (inhibits pacing)	M (multiprogrammable rate, output, sensitivity)	S (shock)
D (dual, A + V)	D (dual, A + V)	D (dual, T + I)	C (communicating functions, such as telemetry)	D (dual, P + S)
O (none)	O (none)	O (none)	R (rate modulation) O (none)	O (none)

  - Know the rate and battery life of pacemaker
  - Use of an implantable-cardioverter-defibrillator, if inserted

Possible surgical complications
- Pneumothorax
- Perforation of heart
- Infection
- Breakage of a lead
- Migration of a lead

Pacemaker codes

Usually three letters
- 1st letter: chamber paced
- 2nd letter: chamber sensed
- 3rd letter: response to sensing
- 4th and 5th letter: optional

Abdominal aneurysm resection

- Surgical removal of a portion of weakened arterial wall
- End-to-end anastomosis to a prosthetic graft

ABDOMINAL ANEURYSM RESECTION

Description
- Surgical removal of a portion of weakened arterial wall with an end-to-end anastomosis to a prosthetic graft

Preoperative nursing interventions
- Complete patient and family preoperative teaching
  - Determine the patient's understanding of the procedure
  - Describe the operating room, PACU, and preoperative and postoperative routines
  - Demonstrate postoperative turning, coughing, deep breathing, splinting, and ROM exercises
  - Explain the postoperative need for drainage tubes, surgical dressings, oxygen therapy, I.V. therapy, and pain control
- Complete a preoperative checklist
- Administer preoperative medications, as prescribed
- Allay the patient's and family's anxiety about surgery
- Document the patient's history and physical assessment data base
- Assess renal status and urine output

Key steps before abdominal aneurysm resection

- Complete patient and family teaching.
- Demonstrate turning, coughing, deep breathing, splinting, and ROM exercises.

Key steps in assessing abdominal aneurysm resections

- Assess cardiac, respiratory, and neurologic status.
- Monitor vital signs, I/O, CVP, laboratory studies, ECG, hemodynamic variables, and pulse oximetry.
- Assess for scrotal and retroperitoneal bleeding.
- Measure and record the patient's abdominal girth.
- Assess for return of peristalsis.

Key home care instructions after abdominal aneurysm repair

- Avoid lifting, bending, and driving for 6 weeks or as the physician allows.
- Monitor blood pressure daily.
- Identify ways to reduce stress.
- Complete incision care daily.

Vascular grafting highlights

- Surgical revascularization of an artery
- Uses a graft
- Bypasses or resects the diseased segment
- Types include femoropopliteal, aortofemoral, aortoiliac, femorofemoral, and axillofemoral

Postoperative nursing interventions

- Assess cardiac, respiratory, and neurologic status
- Assess fluid balance
- Assess pain and administer analgesics, as prescribed
- Administer I.V. fluids and transfusion therapy, as prescribed
- Administer oxygen and maintain an ET tube to the ventilator
- Provide incentive spirometry after extubation or ET suction
- Reinforce turning, coughing, and deep breathing, and splinting of the incision
- Monitor vital signs, I/O, central venous pressure (CVP), laboratory studies, ECG, hemodynamic variables, and pulse oximetry
- Monitor and maintain the position and patency of NG tubes and indwelling urinary catheters
- Administer antibiotics, as prescribed
- Assess for scrotal and retroperitoneal bleeding
- Check peripheral circulation: color, temperature, complaints of abnormal sensation, and pulses in extremities
- Inspect and change the surgical dressing, as directed
- Keep the patient flat; set up a turning schedule, turning from side to side regularly
- Assist the patient with active and passive ROM and isometric exercises, as tolerated
- Assess for return of peristalsis
- Provide the prescribed diet, as tolerated
- **Measure and record the patient's abdominal girth**
- Allay the patient's anxiety
- Individualize home care instructions
  - Avoid lifting, bending, and driving for 6 weeks or as the physician allows
  - Monitor blood pressure daily
  - Identify ways to reduce stress
  - Complete incision care daily

Possible surgical complications

- Renal failure
- Atelectasis
- Graft hemorrhage
- Retroperitoneal rupture

VASCULAR GRAFTING

Description

- Surgical revascularization of an artery
- Uses a synthetic or autogenous graft
- Bypasses or resects the diseased segment

Types of revascularization

- Femoropopliteal
- Aortofemoral

- Aortoiliac
- Femorofemoral
- Axillofemoral

Preoperative nursing interventions

- Complete patient and family preoperative teaching
  - Determine the patient's understanding of the procedure
  - Describe the operating room, PACU, and preoperative and postoperative routines
  - Demonstrate postoperative turning, coughing, deep breathing, splinting, and ROM exercises
  - Explain the postoperative need for drainage tubes, surgical dressings, oxygen therapy, I.V. therapy, and pain control
- Complete a preoperative checklist
- Administer preoperative medications, as prescribed
- Allay the patient's and family's anxiety about surgery
- Document the patient's history and physical assessment data base
- Obtain a baseline assessment of peripheral circulation
- Administer antibiotics, as prescribed

Postoperative nursing interventions

- Assess cardiac and neurovascular status
- Assess pain and administer analgesics, as prescribed
- Administer I.V. fluids and transfusion therapy, as prescribed
- Monitor vital signs, I/O, laboratory studies, neurovascular checks, and pulse oximetry
- Monitor and maintain the position and patency of NG tubes and indwelling urinary catheters
- Administer anticoagulants, as prescribed
- Inspect and change the surgical dressing, as directed
- **Keep the patient in semi-Fowler's position; avoid positioning on or flexion of the graft site**
- Provide a bed cradle
- Check peripheral circulation: temperature, color, pulses, and complaints of abnormal sensations in extremities distal to the graft site
- Measure and record the patient's ankle, calf, and thigh circumferences
- Provide incentive spirometry
- Reinforce turning, coughing, and deep breathing and splinting of the incision
- Assess for return of peristalsis
- Provide the prescribed diet, as tolerated
- Measure and record the patient's abdominal girth
- Assist the patient with active and passive ROM and isometric exercises, as tolerated
- Allay the patient's anxiety
- Encourage the patient to express feelings about changes in body image
- Increase ambulation, as tolerated
- Individualize home care instructions

Key steps before vascular grafting

- Demonstrate turning, coughing, deep breathing, splinting, and ROM exercises.
- Explain all drainage tubes, dressings, therapies, and pain control.

Key steps after vascular grafting

- Assess cardiac and neurovascular status.
- Keep the patient in semi-Fowler's position; avoid positioning on or flexion of the graft site.
- Check peripheral circulation: temperature, color, pulses, and complaints of abnormal sensations in extremities distal to the graft site.
- Measure and record the patient's ankle, calf, and thigh circumferences.
- Increase ambulation, as tolerated.

Key home care instructions after vascular grafting

- Avoid pressure or flexion of the graft site.
- Avoid wearing constrictive clothing.
- Complete incision care daily.
- Check pulses distal to the graft site daily.
- Adhere to long-term anticoagulant therapy.
- Provide proper foot care daily.

Classifying hypertension

- Normal: less than 120 mm Hg/ less than 80 mm Hg
- Prehypertension: 120 to 139 mm Hg/80 to 89 mm Hg
- Stage 1: 140 to 159 mm Hg/ 90 to 99 mm Hg
- Stage 2: greater than or equal to 160 mm Hg/greater than or equal to 100 mm Hg

Calculating blood pressure

- Blood pressure = cardiac output × peripheral resistance

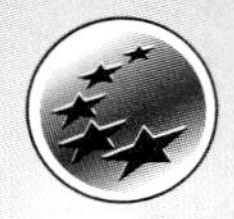

TOP 2

Assessment findings in hypertension

1. Asymptomatic
2. Elevated blood pressure

  - Avoid pressure or flexion of the graft site
  - Avoid wearing constrictive clothing
  - Complete incision care daily
  - Check pulses distal to the graft site daily
  - Adhere to long-term anticoagulant therapy
  - Provide proper foot care daily

Possible surgical complications

- Thrombosis
- Embolism
- Graft rejection
- Hemorrhage

HYPERTENSION

Definition

- High blood pressure
- Classifications based on the 7th Report of the Joint National Committee on Prevention, Detection, Evaluation, and Treatment of High Blood Pressure (2003):
  - Normal: less than 120 mm Hg/less than 80 mm Hg
  - Prehypertension: 120 to 139 mm Hg/80 to 89 mm Hg
  - Stage 1: 140 to 159 mm Hg/90 to 99 mm Hg
  - Stage 2: greater than or equal to 160 mm Hg/greater than or equal to 100 mm Hg

Causes

- Primary hypertension — unknown etiology
- Secondary hypertension
  - Renal disease
  - Pheochromocytoma
  - Cushing's disease

Pathophysiology

- Blood pressure = Cardiac output × peripheral resistance
- Narrowing of the arterioles, which increases peripheral resistance
- Increased force needed to circulate blood, which elevates blood pressure (see *Understanding blood pressure regulation*)

Assessment findings

- Asymptomatic
- Elevated blood pressure
- Headache
- Vision disturbances
- Left ventricular hypertrophy
- Renal failure
- Dizziness
- Papilledema
- Heart failure
- Cerebral ischemia

Understanding blood pressure regulation

Hypertension may result from a disturbance in one of these intrinsic mechanisms.

RENIN-ANGIOTENSIN SYSTEM

The renin-angiotensin system acts to increase blood pressure through these mechanisms:

- sodium depletion, reduced blood pressure, and dehydration stimulate renin release
- renin reacts with angiotensin, a liver enzyme, and converts it to angiotensin I, which increases preload and afterload
- angiotensin I converts to angiotensin II in the lungs; angiotensin II is a potent vasoconstrictor that targets the arterioles
- circulating angiotensin II works to increase preload and afterload by stimulating the adrenal cortex to secrete aldosterone; this increases blood volume by conserving sodium and water.

AUTOREGULATION

Several intrinsic mechanisms work to change an artery's diameter to maintain tissue and organ perfusion despite fluctuations in systemic blood pressure. These mechanisms include stress relaxation and capillary fluid shifts.

- In stress relaxation, blood vessels gradually dilate when blood pressure rises to reduce peripheral resistance.
- In capillary fluid shift, plasma moves between vessels and extravascular spaces to maintain intravascular volume.

SYMPATHETIC NERVOUS SYSTEM

When blood pressure drops, baroreceptors in the aortic arch and carotid sinuses decrease their inhibition of the medulla's vasomotor center. The consequent increases in sympathetic stimulation of the heart by norepinephrine increases cardiac output by strengthening the contractile force, raising the heart rate, and augmenting peripheral resistance by vasoconstriction. Stress can also stimulate the sympathetic nervous system to increase cardiac output and peripheral vascular resistance.

ANTIDIURETIC HORMONE

The release of antidiuretic hormone can regulate hypotension by increasing reabsorption of water by the kidney. With reabsorption, blood plasma volume increases, thus raising blood pressure.

Diagnostic test findings

- Blood pressure: sustained readings greater than 140/90 mm Hg
- ECG: left ventricular hypertrophy
- Chest X-ray: cardiomegaly
- Ophthalmoscopic examination: retinal changes, such as severe vasoconstriction, papilledema, and retinopathy
- Blood chemistry: elevated sodium, BUN, creatinine, and cholesterol levels

Medical management

- Diet: low-sodium, low-calorie, low-cholesterol, and low-fat; restrict alcohol and caffeine
- I.V. therapy: saline lock
- Activity: as tolerated
- Monitoring: vital signs, ECG, and I/O

Intrinsic blood pressure regulators

- Renin-angiotensin system
- Autoregulation
- Sympathetic nervous system
- Antidiuretic hormone

Most important diagnostic finding for hypertension

- Sustained blood pressure readings greater than 140/90 mm Hg

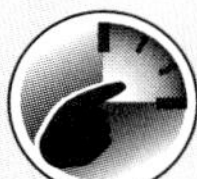

TIME-OUT FOR TEACHING

Patients with cardiovascular disorders

Be sure to include these topics when teaching patients with cardiovascular disorders.

- Smoking cessation
- Regular exercise
- Optimal weight maintenance
- Medication therapy, including the action, adverse effects, and scheduling
- Dietary recommendations and restrictions
- Stress reduction
- Rest and activity patterns
- Frequent blood pressure monitoring
- Risk factor modification

Medications to manage hypertension

- Diuretics
- Antihypertensives
- Vasodilators
- Calcium channel blockers
- Beta-adrenergic blockers
- ACE inhibitors
- Angiotensin II antagonists

Key steps in monitoring hypertension

- Assess cardiovascular status.
- Monitor and record vital signs, I/O, laboratory studies, and daily weight.
- Take an average of two or more blood pressure readings rather than relying on one single abnormal reading.

Main complications of hypertension

- Stroke
- Renal failure
- Hypertensive crisis

- Laboratory studies: sodium, potassium, and cholesterol
- Thiazide diuretics: chlorothiazide (Diuril), hydrochlorothiazide (HydroDIURIL)
- Loop diuretics: furosemide (Lasix), bumetanide (Bumex)
- Aldosterone receptor blocker: spironolactone (Aldactone)
- Antihypertensives: methyldopa (Aldomet), hydralazine (Apresoline), prazosin (Minipress), doxazosin (Cardura)
- Vasodilator: nitroprusside (Nipride)
- Calcium channel blockers: nifedipine (Procardia), verapamil (Calan), diltiazem (Cardizem), nicardipine (Cardene)
- Beta-adrenergic blockers: propranolol (Inderal), metoprolol (Lopressor), carteolol (Cartrol), penbutolol (Levatol)
- Angiotensin-converting enzyme (ACE) inhibitors: captopril (Capoten), enalapril (Vasotec), lisinopril (Prinivil)
- Angiotensin II antagonists: candesartan (Atacand), irbesartan (Avapro), losartan (Cozaar), valsartan (Diovan)

Nursing interventions

- Maintain the patient's prescribed diet
- Assess cardiovascular status
- Monitor and record vital signs, I/O, laboratory studies, and daily weight
- Administer medications, as prescribed
- Encourage the patient to express feelings about daily stress
- Maintain a quiet environment
- Provide information about the American Heart Association
- **Take an average of two or more blood pressure readings rather than relying on one single abnormal reading**
- Individualize home care instructions (for more information about teaching, see *Patients with cardiovascular disorders*)
  - Take blood pressure daily
  - Start an exercise program

Complications

- Stroke
- Vision changes

- Renal failure
- Heart failure
- Hypertensive crisis

Possible surgical interventions

- None

CORONARY ARTERY DISEASE (CAD)

Definitions

- Arteriosclerosis — loss of elasticity of the arteries' intimal layer (sometimes called hardening of the arteries)
- Atherosclerosis — accumulation in the arteries of fatty plaque made of lipids

Causes

- Aging
- Stress
- Genetics
- Depletion of estrogen after menopause
- High-fat, high-cholesterol diet
- Use of cigarettes, tobacco, and alcohol
- Hypertension
- Diabetes mellitus
- Overweight or obesity
- Inactivity

Pathophysiology

- Narrowing or obstruction of the coronary arteries by an embolus, vasospasm, or accumulated plaque (see *Atherosclerotic plaque development*, page 24)
- Decreased perfusion and inadequate myocardial oxygen supply

Assessment findings

- Hypertension
- Angina
- MI
- Heart failure

Diagnostic test findings

- ECG or Holter monitoring: ST depression, T-wave inversion
- Stress test: elevated ST segment, multiple premature ventricular contractions on ECG, chest pain
- Coronary arteriography: plaque formation
- Blood chemistry: increased cholesterol (decreased high-density lipoproteins, increased low-density lipoproteins)
- Cardiac enzymes and proteins: monitor for increase in CK, CK-MB, LD, LD isoenzymes, troponin I, and troponin T

Key facts on CAD

- Arteriosclerosis: loss of elasticity in the artery wall
- Atherosclerosis: accumulation of fatty plaque in the arteries

How CAD happens

- Narrowing or obstruction of the coronary arteries
- Decreased perfusion
- Inadequate myocardial oxygen supply

Cardiac enzymes and proteins to monitor CAD

- CK
- CK-MB
- LD
- LD isoenzymes
- Troponin I
- Troponin T

Atherosclerotic plaque development

- Stiffening and loss of dilatory response leads to fatty deposits in the vessel.
- Fibrous plaque and lipids progressively narrow the lumen and impede blood flow to the myocardium.
- Plaque continues to grow, and in advanced stages, may become a calcified lesion that may rupture.

Key steps in medically managing CAD

- Low-calorie, low-sodium, low-cholesterol, and low-fat diet; increased dietary fiber
- Weight reduction
- Percutaneous transluminal coronary angioplasty
- Antilipemic agents
- Nitrates
- Beta-adrenergic blockers
- Calcium channel blockers
- Analgesics
- Antianxiety agents

Atherosclerotic plaque development

The illustrations below show how plaque develops in coronary arteries, eventually leading to calcification and rupture of lesions if left untreated.

1. The coronary arteries are made of three layers: intima (the innermost layer, media (the middle layer), and adventitia (the outermost layer).

Adventitia
Media
Intima
Lumen

2. Stiffening and loss of dilatory response leads to fatty deposits in the vessel.

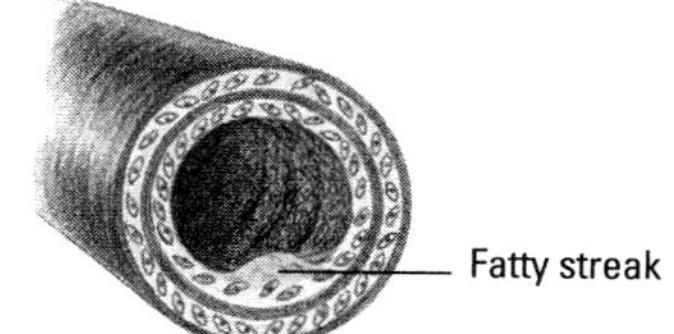

3. Fibrous plaque and lipids progressively narrow the lumen and impede blood flow to the myocardium.

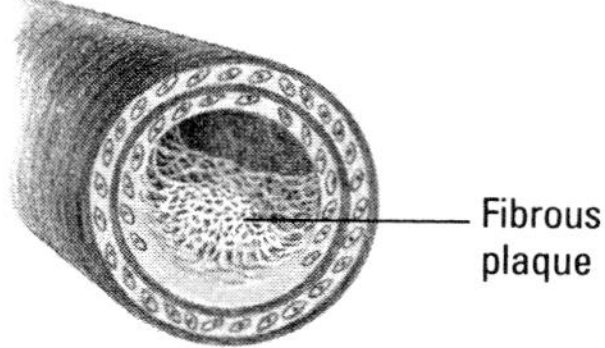

4. The plaque continues to grow and, in advanced stages, may become a complicated calcified lesion that may rupture.

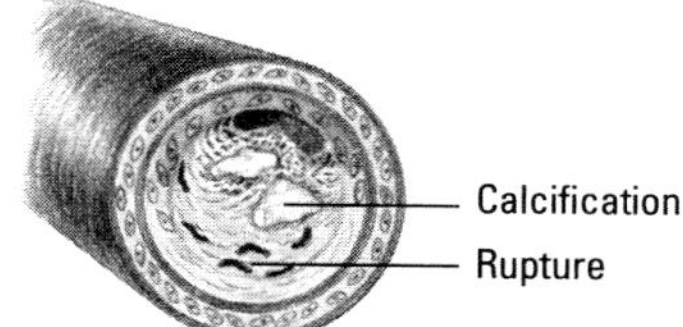

Medical management

- Diet: low-calorie, low-sodium, low-cholesterol, and low-fat; increased dietary fiber
- I.V. therapy: saline lock
- Oxygen therapy
- Monitoring: vital signs, CVP, ECG, hemodynamic variables, I/O, and neurovascular checks
- Laboratory studies: sodium, potassium, cholesterol, CK, LD, AST, CK isoenzymes, LD isoenzymes, troponin I, and ABGs
- Weight reduction
- Arterial line for blood pressure monitoring
- Intra-aortic balloon pump
- Thrombolytic therapy: streptokinase (Streptase)
- Percutaneous transluminal coronary angioplasty
- Indwelling urinary catheter
- Antilipemic agents: cholestyramine (Questran), lovastatin (Mevacor), nicotinic acid (Niacin), gemfibrozil (Lopid), colestipol (Colestid)
- Nitrates: nitroglycerin (Nitro-Bid), isosorbide dinitrate (Isordil)
- Beta-adrenergic blockers: propranolol (Inderal), nadolol (Corgard)

- Calcium channel blockers: nifedipine (Procardia), verapamil (Calan), diltiazem (Cardizem)
- Analgesic: morphine (I.V.)
- Antianxiety agent: diazepam (Valium)
- Laser angioplasty
- Atherectomy

Nursing interventions

- Maintain the patient's prescribed diet
- Administer oxygen and medications, as prescribed
- Assess cardiovascular status
- Monitor and record vital signs, hemodynamic variables, I/O, ECG, and laboratory studies
- Obtain ECG during anginal episodes
- Encourage the patient to express anxiety, fears, or concerns
- Provide information about the American Heart Association
- Individualize home care instructions
  - Adhere to activity limitations
  - Limit daily alcohol intake to 2 oz
  - Limit dietary fat intake

Complications

- Angina
- MI
- Heart failure
- Arrhythmias

Possible surgical intervention

- CABG

Key nursing interventions for a patient with CAD

- Assess cardiovascular status.
- Monitor and record vital signs, hemodynamic variables, I/O, ECG, and laboratory studies.
- Obtain ECG during anginal episodes.

Limitations for a patient with CAD

- Limit dietary fat intake.
- Limit activity (as necessary).
- Limit daily alcohol intake to 2 oz.

ANGINA

Definition

- Angina is chest pain caused by inadequate myocardial oxygen supply
  - Classical effort (exertional angina, chronic stable angina) — consistent symptoms with pain relieved by rest
  - Unstable or acute angina — increase in severity, duration, and frequency of pain which is eventually relieved by nitroglycerin
  - Prinzmetal or variant angina — pain that occurs at rest
  - Microvascular angina — impairment of vasodilator reserve causes angina-like chest pain in a patient with normal coronary arteries
- Complaints of chest pain have increased significance in a patient with a peripheral vascular problem

Causes

- Atherosclerosis
- Vasospasm
- Aortic stenosis
- Activity or disease that increases metabolic demands

Key facts about angina

- Chest pain caused by inadequate myocardial oxygen supply
- Complaints of chest pain are more significant in patients with a peripheral vascular problem
- Four types: classical effort (exertional angina, chronic stable angina), unstable or acute angina, Prinzmetal or variant angina, and microvascular angina

Pathophysiology
- Narrowing of the coronary arteries, which results from plaque accumulation in the intimal lining
- Obstruction of blood flow, which diminishes myocardial oxygen supply

Assessment findings
- Substernal, crushing, compressing pain
  - May radiate to the arms
  - Usually lasts 3 to 5 minutes
  - Usually occurs after exertion, emotional excitement, or exposure to cold but also can develop when the patient is at rest
- Dyspnea
- Palpitations
- Epigastric distress
- Tachycardia
- Diaphoresis
- Anxiety

Diagnostic test findings
- ECG: ST depression, T-wave inversion during acute pain
- Stress test: abnormal ECG, chest pain
- Coronary arteriography: plaque accumulation
- Blood chemistry: increased cholesterol
- Cardiac enzymes: within normal limits, depending on severity and type of angina
- Holter monitoring: ST depression, T-wave inversion

Medical management
- Diet: low-calorie, low-sodium, and low-cholesterol
- I.V. therapy: saline lock
- Oxygen therapy
- Position: semi-Fowler's
- Monitoring: vital signs, ECG, hemodynamic variables, I/O, and neurovascular checks
- Laboratory studies: ABGs, sodium, potassium, CK with isoenzymes, LD with isoenzymes, troponin I, troponin T, and AST
- Percutaneous transluminal coronary angioplasty
- Arterial line for blood pressure monitoring
- Nitrates: nitroglycerin (Nitrostat), isosorbide dinitrate (Isordil)
- Beta-adrenergic blockers: propranolol (Inderal), nadolol (Corgard), atenolol (Tenormin), metoprolol (Lopressor)
- Calcium channel blockers: verapamil (Calan), diltiazem (Cardizem), nifedipine (Procardia), nicardipine (Cardene)
- ACE inhibitors: captopril (Capoten), enalapril (Vasotec), lisinopril (Prinivil), quinapril (Accupril)
- Cardiac glycoside: digoxin (Lanoxin)
- Antiarrhythmics: lidocaine, procainamide (Pronestyl), adenosine (Adenocard)
- Analgesics: morphine, meperidine (Demerol)

Pathophysiology of angina
- Plaque accumulation causes narrowing of the coronary arteries
- Obstruction of blood flow diminishes myocardial oxygen supply

Key assessment findings of anginal pain
- Substernal, crushing, compressing pain:
  - may radiate to the arms
  - usually lasts 3 to 5 minutes
  - usually occurs after exertion, emotional excitement, or exposure to cold but also can develop when the patient is at rest.

Key ECG findings during acute anginal pain
- ST depression
- T-wave inversion

Nursing interventions

- Maintain the patient's prescribed diet (low-fat, low-sodium, and low-cholesterol)
- Administer oxygen and medications, as prescribed
- Assess cardiovascular status
- Monitor and record vital signs, hemodynamic variables, I/O, and laboratory studies
- Assess for chest pain
- Encourage the patient to express anxiety, fears, or concerns
- Advise the patient to rest if pain begins
- Obtain an ECG reading during an acute attack
- Keep the patient in semi-Fowler's position
- Provide information about the American Heart Association
- Individualize home care instructions
  - Discard nitroglycerin tablets after 6 months
  - Know the difference between angina and MI
  - Avoid activities or situations that cause angina, such as exertion, heavy meals, emotional upsets, and exposure to cold
  - Seek medical attention if pain lasts longer than 20 minutes

Complications

- Arrhythmias
- Heart failure
- MI

Possible surgical intervention

- CABG

MYOCARDIAL INFARCTION

Definition

- Death of a portion of the myocardial muscle cells caused by a lack of oxygen from inadequate perfusion

Causes

- Atherosclerosis
- Inadequate perfusion to meet metabolic demands
- Embolism or thrombus
- Coronary artery spasm

Pathophysiology

- Narrowing and eventual obstruction of the coronary arteries from plaque accumulation
- Death of the myocardial cells from inadequate perfusion and oxygenation

Assessment findings

- **Crushing, burning, tightness, or squeezing substernal pain**
  - May radiate to the jaw, back, arms, neck, ears, or shoulders
  - Lasts longer than anginal pain, usually longer than 30 minutes
  - Is unrelieved by rest or nitroglycerin

Key nursing interventions for a patient with angina

- Assess cardiovascular status.
- Assess for chest pain.
- Obtain an ECG reading during an acute attack.
- Administer oxygen and medications, as prescribed.

Key tips for a patient with angina

- Avoid activities or situations that cause angina, such as exertion, heavy meals, emotional upsets, and exposure to cold.
- Seek medical attention if pain lasts longer than 20 minutes.

Characteristics of myocardial infarction

- Plaque accumulation narrows and obstructs the coronary arteries
- Lack of oxygen causes death of a portion of the myocardial muscle cells

Key MI symptoms

- Crushing, burning, tightness, or squeezing substernal pain:
  - may radiate to the jaw, back, arms, neck, ears, or shoulders
  - lasts longer than anginal pain, usually longer than 30 minutes
  - is unrelieved by rest or nitroglycerin
  - may not be present (asymptomatic or "silent" MI).

Blood chemistry findings in MI

- Increased CK, LD, lipids
- Positive CK-MB fraction
- Flipped LD_1 (LD_1 levels exceed LD_2 levels, the reversal of their normal patterns)
- Elevated myoglobin, troponin I, and troponin T

Key medications used to manage MI

- Antiarrhythmics
- Antiplatelet agents
- Anticoagulants
- Analgesics
- Antihypertensives
- ACE inhibitors
- Nitrates
- Beta-adrenergic blockers
- Calcium channel blockers

  - May not be present (asymptomatic or "silent" MI)
- Atypical signs of MI: nausea, vomiting, and diaphoresis
- Dyspnea, tachypnea, crackles, and frothy sputum
- Nausea and vomiting
- Anxiety
- Restlessness, confusion, agitation
- Denial
- Diaphoresis
- Pallor
- Arrhythmias
- Elevated temperature
- Decreased urinary output

Diagnostic test findings

- ECG: enlarged Q wave, elevated ST segment, T-wave inversion (see *Pinpointing MI*)
- Blood chemistry: increased CK, LD, lipids; positive CK-MB fraction; flipped LD_1 (LD_1 levels exceed LD_2 levels, the reversal of their normal patterns), and elevated myoglobin, troponin I, and troponin T
- Hematology: increased WBC count

Medical management

- Diet: low-calorie, low-cholesterol, low-fat
- Oxygen at 2 to 4 L via nasal cannula
- Antiarrhythmics: quinidine gluconate (Quinaglute), lidocaine (Xylocaine), procainamide (Pronestyl)
- Antiplatelet agents: aspirin; ticlopidine (Ticlid) if unable to tolerate aspirin
- Anticoagulant: heparin
- Analgesics: morphine, meperidine (Demerol)
- Electrolyte replacement: magnesium sulfate
- Antihypertensives: hydralazine (Apresoline), methyldopa (Aldomet)
- ACE inhibitors: captopril (Capoten), enalaprilat (Vasotec)
- Nitrates: nitroglycerin (I.V.), sublingual, translingual
- Beta-adrenergic blockers: propranolol (Inderal), atenolol (Tenormin); beta-adrenergic blockers are contraindicated if the patient also has heart failure, hypotension, or bronchospasm
- Calcium channel blockers: verapamil (Calan), diltiazem (Cardizem), nifedipine (Procardia), nicardipine (Cardene)
- Intra-aortic balloon pump
- Left ventricular assist device
- Thrombolytic therapy: anistreplase (Eminase), anisoylated plasminogen-streptokinase activator complex, streptokinase (Streptase)
- Monitoring: vital signs, I/O, ECG, and hemodynamic variables
- Oxygen therapy
- Laboratory studies: ABGs, CK, CK isoenzymes, LD, LD isoenzymes, myoglobin, troponin I, troponin T, PTT, WBC, sodium, potassium, and glucose
- Position: semi-Fowler's

Pinpointing MI

Myocardial infarction has a central area of necrosis surrounded by a zone of injury that may recover if revascularization occurs. This zone of injury is surrounded by an outer ring of reversible ischemia. Characteristic electrocardiographic changes are associated with each zone.

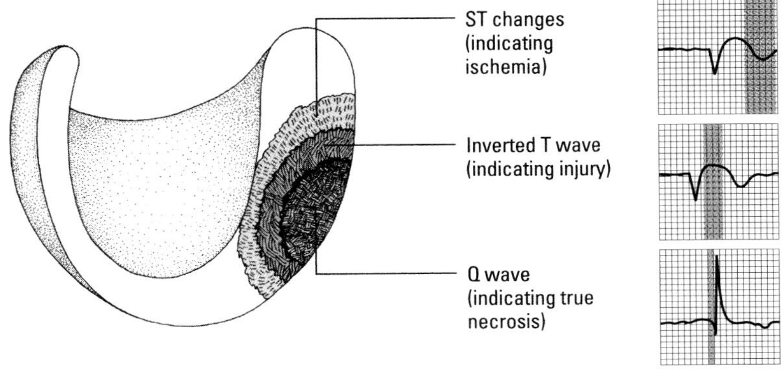

- I.V. therapy: saline lock
- Percutaneous transluminal coronary angioplasty
- Arterial line for blood pressure monitoring
- Laser angioplasty
- Vascular stents
- Atherectomy

Nursing interventions

- Maintain the patient's prescribed diet
- Assess cardiovascular and respiratory status
- Monitor and record vital signs, I/O, hemodynamic variables, laboratory studies, and ECG results
- Maintain bed rest
- Administer oxygen and medications, as prescribed
- Obtain an ECG reading during acute pain
- Allay the patient's anxiety
- Keep the patient in semi-Fowler's position
- Provide information about the American Heart Association
- Individualize home care instructions
  - Participate in a cardiac rehabilitation program
  - Maintain a low-cholesterol, low-fat, low-sodium diet
  - Know the difference between the pain of angina and MI
  - Alternate rest periods with activity

Complications

- Arrhythmias
- Cardiogenic shock

MI changes and zones

- ST changes (indicate ischemia)
- Inverted T wave (indicates injury)
- Q wave (indicates true necrosis)

Key nursing interventions for a patient with MI

- Assess cardiovascular and respiratory status.
- Monitor and record vital signs, I/O, hemodynamic variables, laboratory studies, and ECG results.
- Obtain an ECG reading during acute pain.
- Administer oxygen and medications, as prescribed.

Key home care instructions for MI

- Participate in a cardiac rehabilitation program.
- Know the difference between the pain of angina and MI.
- Maintain a low-cholesterol, low-fat, low-sodium diet.

- Heart failure
- Papillary muscle rupture
- Pericarditis
- Thromboembolism

Possible surgical intervention
- CABG

HEART FAILURE: LEFT-SIDED

Definition
- Failure of the left side of the heart to pump enough blood to meet metabolic demands

Causes
- Atherosclerosis
- Fluid overload
- MI
- Valvular stenosis
- Valvular insufficiency
- Hypertension
- Cardiac conduction defects
- Cardiomyopathy
- Infection
- Immune and connective disorder
- Endocrine imbalance

Pathophysiology
- Decreased myocardial contractility or increased myocardial workload, either of which increases left ventricular pressure and left atrial pressure and reduces cardiac output
- Impaired oxygenation and respiratory manifestations of fluid overload

Assessment findings
- Dyspnea
- Paroxysmal nocturnal dyspnea
- Crackles, wheezes, rhonchi
- Cough
- Hemoptysis
- Gallop rhythm: S_3, S_4
- Arrhythmias
- Fatigue
- Anxiety
- Orthopnea
- Tachycardia
- Tachypnea
- Diaphoresis

Key facts about left-sided heart failure

- Myocardial contractility or increased myocardial workload increases left ventricular pressure and left atrial pressure.
- Cardiac output is reduced.
- The left side of the heart fails to pump enough blood to meet metabolic demands.

Key causes of left-sided heart failure

- Atherosclerosis
- Fluid overload
- MI
- Valvular stenosis

Key signs and symptoms of left-sided heart failure

- Dyspnea
- Gallop rhythm: S_3, S_4
- Crackles, wheezes, rhonchi

Diagnostic test findings

- Chest X-ray: increased pulmonary congestion, left ventricular hypertrophy
- Echocardiography: increased size of cardiac chambers and decreased wall motion
- Hemodynamic monitoring: increased pulmonary artery wedge pressure (PAWP), CVP, and pulmonary artery pressure (PAP), and decreased cardiac output
- ABGs: hypoxemia, hypercapnia
- ECG: left ventricular hypertrophy, ST-T wave changes
- Blood chemistry: decreased potassium, sodium; increased BUN, creatinine, decreased myoglobin
- Urinalysis: proteinuria, RBCs, casts

Medical management

- Diet: low-sodium; limit fluids
- I.V. therapy: electrolyte replacement, saline lock
- Oxygen therapy
- Position: semi-Fowler's
- Activity: bed rest, active ROM and isometric exercises
- Monitoring: vital signs, I/O, ECG, and hemodynamic variables
- Laboratory studies: ABGs, sodium, potassium, BUN, and creatinine, cardiac enzymes
- Indwelling urinary catheter
- Intra-aortic balloon pump
- Left ventricular assist device
- Analgesic: morphine (I.V.)
- Diuretics: furosemide (Lasix), bumetanide (Bumex), metolazone (Zaroxolyn), spironolactone (Aldactone), acetazolamide (Diamox)
- Vasodilator: nitroprusside (Nipride)
- Cardiac inotropes: dopamine (Intropin), dobutamine (Dobutrex)
- Cardiac glycoside: digoxin (Lanoxin)
- Nitrates: isosorbide dinitrate (Isordil), nitroglycerin (Nitro-Bid)
- ACE inhibitors: captopril (Capoten), enalapril (Vasotec), lisinopril (Prinivil)
- Phosphodiesterase inhibitor: inamrinone (Inocor)
- Specialized bed: active or static, low air loss (KinAir, Flexicair)

Nursing interventions

- Maintain the patient's prescribed diet
- Restrict oral fluids
- Administer I.V. fluids, oxygen, and medications, as prescribed
- Provide suctioning, turning, coughing, and deep breathing
- Assess cardiovascular and respiratory status
- Weigh the patient daily
- Keep the patient in semi-Fowler's position
- Monitor and record vital signs, CVP, hemodynamic variables, I/O, and laboratory studies
- Assess peripheral edema
- Encourage the patient to express his feelings such as a fear of dying

Chest X-ray findings in left-sided heart failure

- Increased pulmonary congestion
- Left ventricular hypertrophy

Key steps in the medical management of left-sided heart failure

- Low-sodium diet; limit fluids
- Semi-Fowler's position
- Monitoring: vital signs, I/O, ECG, and hemodynamic variables
- Analgesics
- Diuretics
- Vasodilators
- Cardiac inotropes
- Cardiac glycosides
- Nitrates
- ACE inhibitors
- Phosphodiesterase inhibitors

Key nursing interventions for left-sided heart failure

- Administer medications, as prescribed.
- Restrict oral fluids.
- Weigh the patient daily.
- Monitor vital signs, I/O, and laboratory studies.

- Provide information about the American Heart Association
- Individualize home care instructions
  - Limit sodium intake
  - Supplement the diet with foods high in potassium
  - Recognize the signs and symptoms of fluid overload

Key home care instructions for left-sided heart failure

- Supplement the diet with foods high in potassium.
- Recognize the signs and symptoms of fluid overload.

Complications

- Digoxin toxicity
- Fluid overload
- Cardiogenic shock
- Pulmonary edema
- Hypokalemia

Possible surgical interventions

- None

HEART FAILURE: RIGHT-SIDED

Characteristics of right-sided heart failure

- Increased pressure from left-sided heart failure, increased pressure from venous congestion, and increased resistance in lungs
- Right side of the heart fails to pump enough blood to meet metabolic demands

Definition

- Failure of the right side of the heart to pump enough blood to meet metabolic demands

Causes

- Atherosclerosis
- Left-sided heart failure
- Chronic obstructive pulmonary disease
- Valvular stenosis
- Valvular insufficiency
- Pulmonary hypertension

Main causes of right-sided heart failure

- Atherosclerosis
- Left-sided heart failure

Pathophysiology

- Increased pressure from left-sided heart failure
- Increased venous congestion in the systemic circulation with fluid overload
- Increased resistance in lungs

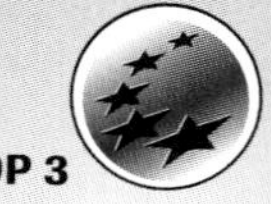

TOP 3 Assessment findings in right-sided heart failure

1. Jugular vein distention
2. Dependent edema, peripheral edema
3. Weight gain

Assessment findings

- Jugular vein distention
- Anorexia
- Nausea, vomiting
- Abdominal distention
- Ascites
- Hepatomegaly
- Dependent edema, peripheral edema
- Weight gain
- Signs of left-sided heart failure
- Gallop rhythm: S_3, S_4
- Tachycardia
- Fatigue
- Nocturia

Diagnostic test findings

- Chest X-ray: pulmonary congestion, cardiomegaly, pleural effusions
- Echocardiogram: increased size of chambers, decrease in wall motion
- Hemodynamic monitoring: increased PAWP, PAP, CVP; decreased cardiac output
- ABGs: hypoxemia
- ECG: left and right ventricular hypertrophy
- Blood chemistry: decreased sodium, potassium; increased BUN, creatinine

Medical management

- Diet: low-sodium; limit fluids
- I.V. therapy: electrolyte replacement, saline lock
- Oxygen therapy
- Position: semi-Fowler's
- Activity: bed rest, active ROM and isometric exercises
- Monitoring: vital signs, I/O, ECG, and hemodynamic variables
- Laboratory studies: ABGs, sodium, potassium, BUN, and creatinine
- Indwelling urinary catheter
- Intra-aortic balloon pump
- Thoracentesis
- Paracentesis
- Analgesic: morphine (I.V.)
- Diuretics: furosemide (Lasix), bumetanide (Bumex), metolazone (Zaroxolyn), spironolactone (Aldactone), acetazolamide (Diamox)
- Vasodilator: nitroprusside (Nipride)
- Cardiac inotropes: dopamine (Intropin), dobutamine (Dobutrex)
- Cardiac glycoside: digoxin (Lanoxin)
- Nitrates: isosorbide dinitrate (Isordil), nitroglycerin (Nitro-Bid)

Nursing interventions

- Maintain the patient's prescribed diet (low-sodium, low-cholesterol, no caffeine)
- Restrict oral fluids
- Administer I.V. fluids, oxygen, and medications, as prescribed
- Provide suctioning, turning, coughing, and deep breathing
- Assess cardiovascular and respiratory status
- Assess peripheral edema
- Keep the patient in semi-Fowler's position
- Monitor and record vital signs, I/O, hemodynamic variables, and laboratory studies
- Weigh the patient daily
- Encourage the patient to express his feelings such as a fear of dying
- Measure and record the patient's abdominal girth
- Individualize home care instructions
  - Elevate the legs when seated
  - Limit sodium intake
  - Supplement the diet with foods high in potassium
  - Recognize the signs and symptoms of fluid overload

Chest X-ray findings in right-sided heart failure

- Pulmonary congestion
- Cardiomegaly
- Pleural effusions

Key steps in the medical management of right-sided heart failure

- Low-sodium diet; limit fluids
- Oxygen therapy
- Semi-Fowler's position
- Vital signs, I/O, ECG, and hemodynamic variables monitoring
- Analgesics
- Diuretics
- Vasodilators
- Cardiac inotropes
- Cardiac glycosides
- Nitrates

Key nursing interventions for a patient with right-sided heart failure

- Restrict oral fluids.
- Assess peripheral edema.
- Keep the patient in semi-Fowler's position.
- Monitor and record vital signs, I/O, hemodynamic variables, and laboratory studies.
- Weight the patient daily.
- Measure and record the patient's abdominal girth.

Characteristics of acute pulmonary edema

- Complication of left-sided heart failure
- Edema results from heart's inability to pump adequately
- Results in impaired oxygenation and hypoxia

TOP 3 Causes of pulmonary edema

1. Heart failure
2. Atherosclerosis
3. Valvular disease

Key assessment findings in acute pulmonary edema

- Dyspnea
- Paroxysmal cough
- Blood-tinged, frothy sputum
- Orthopnea
- Tachypnea
- Restlessness

Complications
- Digoxin toxicity
- Fluid overload
- Cardiogenic shock
- Pulmonary edema
- Hypokalemia
- Hypernatremia

Possible surgical interventions
- None

ACUTE PULMONARY EDEMA

Definition
- Complication of left-sided heart failure; results in increased pressure in the capillaries of the lungs and acute transudation of fluid

Causes
- Atherosclerosis
- MI
- Myocarditis
- Valvular disease
- Smoke inhalation
- Drug overdose: heroin, barbiturates, morphine
- Overload of I.V. fluids
- Heart failure
- Acute respiratory distress syndrome

Pathophysiology
- PAWP exceeds intravascular osmotic pressure
- Alveolar and interstitial edema result from the heart's failure to pump adequately
- Impaired oxygenation and hypoxia result

Assessment findings
- Dyspnea
- Paroxysmal cough
- Blood-tinged, frothy sputum
- Orthopnea
- Tachypnea
- Agitation
- Anxiety
- Restlessness
- Intense fear
- Chest pain
- Syncope
- Tachycardia
- Cold, clammy skin
- Diaphoresis

- Gallop rhythm: S_3, S_4
- Jugular vein distention

Diagnostic test findings

- Chest X-ray: interstitial edema
- ABGs: respiratory alkalosis or acidosis
- ECG: tachycardia, ventricular enlargement
- Hemodynamic monitoring: increased PAWP, CVP, PAP; decreased cardiac output

Medical management

- Diet: low-sodium; limit fluids
- I.V. therapy: electrolyte replacement, saline lock
- Oxygen therapy
- Intubation and mechanical ventilation
- Tourniquets: rotating
- Position: high Fowler's
- Activity: bed rest; active ROM and isometric exercises
- Monitoring: vital signs, I/O, ECG, and hemodynamic variables
- Laboratory studies: sodium, potassium, ABGs, BUN, and creatinine
- Indwelling urinary catheter
- ET tube suctioning
- Analgesic: morphine (I.V.)
- Diuretics: furosemide (Lasix), bumetanide (Bumex), metolazone (Zaroxolyn)
- Vasodilator: nitroprusside (Nipride)
- Cardiac inotropes: dopamine (Intropin), dobutamine (Dobutrex)
- Cardiac glycoside: digoxin (Lanoxin)
- Nitrates: isosorbide dinitrate (Isordil), nitroglycerin (Nitro-Bid)
- Bronchodilator: aminophylline (Somophyllin)
- Pulse oximetry

Nursing interventions

- Withhold food and fluids, as directed
- Administer I.V. fluids, oxygen, and medications, as prescribed
- Provide suctioning, turning, coughing, and deep breathing
- Assess cardiovascular and respiratory status
- Keep the patient in high Fowler's position
- Monitor and record vital signs, I/O, hemodynamic variables, laboratory studies, and daily weight
- Allay the patient's anxiety
- Encourage the patient to express his feelings such as a fear of suffocation
- Note the color, amount, and consistency of sputum
- Apply rotating tourniquets
- Individualize home care instructions
  - Weigh daily
  - Recognize the signs of fluid overload
  - Sleep with the head of the bed elevated
  - Recognize the signs and symptoms of respiratory distress
  - Supplement the diet with foods high in potassium

Key steps in managing acute pulmonary edema

- Low-sodium diet; limit fluids
- Oxygen therapy
- High Fowler's position
- Vital signs, I/O, ECG, and hemodynamic variables monitoring
- Analgesics
- Vasodilators
- Cardiac inotropes
- Cardiac glycosides
- Nitrates
- Bronchodilators
- Pulse oximetry

Key nursing interventions for a patient with acute pulmonary edema

- Assess cardiovascular and respiratory status.
- Withhold food and fluids, as directed.
- Provide suctioning, turning, coughing, and deep breathing.
- Keep the patient in high Fowler's position.
- Allay the patient's anxiety.
- Note the color, amount, and consistency of sputum.

Key home care instructions for acute pulmonary edema

- Recognize the signs of fluid overload and respiratory distress.
- Sleep with the head of the bed elevated.

- **Complications**
  - Digoxin toxicity
  - Fluid overload
  - Pulmonary embolism
  - Hypokalemia
  - Hypernatremia
- **Possible surgical interventions**
  - None

CARDIOGENIC SHOCK

- **Definition**
  - Failure of the heart to pump adequately, thereby reducing cardiac output and compromising tissue perfusion
- **Causes**
  - MI
  - Myocarditis
  - Advanced heart block
  - Heart failure
  - Metabolic abnormalities
  - Cardiac tamponade
  - Pulmonary embolus
- **Pathophysiology**
  - Decreased stroke volume and cardiac output; increased left ventricular volume, increased peripheral resistance due to increased sympathetic nervous system activity (see *What happens in cardiogenic shock*)
  - Compensatory increases in heart rate and contractility, which raise the demand for myocardial oxygen
  - Imbalance between oxygen supply and demand, which increases myocardial ischemia and further compromises the heart's pumping action
- **Assessment findings**
  - Hypotension (systolic pressure of less than 90 mm Hg)
  - Oliguria (urine output of less than 30 ml/hour)
  - Cold, clammy, pale skin
  - Tachycardia
  - Restlessness
  - Hypoxia
  - Tachypnea
  - Anxiety
  - Arrhythmias
  - Disorientation and confusion
- **Diagnostic test findings**
  - ABGs: metabolic acidosis, hypoxemia
  - ECG: MI (enlarged Q wave, ST elevation)
  - Blood chemistry: increased BUN, creatinine, hyperglycemia, hypernatremia, hypokalemia

Characteristics of cardiogenic shock

- Decreased stroke volume and cardiac output cause compensatory changes in heart rate and contractility
- Imbalance between oxygen supply and demand causes failure of the heart to pump adequately
- Cardiac output is reduced and tissue perfusion is compromised

Most common cause of cardiogenic shock

- Myocardial infarction

Key assessment findings in cardiogenic shock

- Hypotension (systolic pressure of less than 90 mm Hg)
- Oliguria (urine output of less than 30 ml/hour)
- Cold, clammy, pale skin
- Tachycardia
- Restlessness

Key test findings in cardiogenic shock

- ABGs: metabolic acidosis, hypoxemia
- ECG: MI (enlarged Q wave, ST elevation)

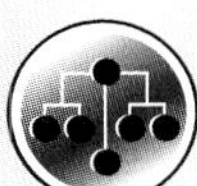

GO WITH THE FLOW

What happens in cardiogenic shock

When the myocardium can't contract sufficiently to maintain adequate cardiac output, stroke volume decreases and the heart can't eject an adequate volume of blood with each contraction. The blood backs up behind the weakened left ventricle, increasing preload and causing pulmonary congestion. In addition, to compensate for the drop in stroke volume, the heart rate increases in an attempt to maintain cardiac output. As a result of the diminished stroke volume, coronary artery perfusion and collateral blood flow decrease. All of these mechanisms increase the workload of the heart and enhance left-sided heart failure. The result is myocardial hypoxia, further decreased cardiac output, and a triggering of compensatory mechanisms to prevent decompensation and death.

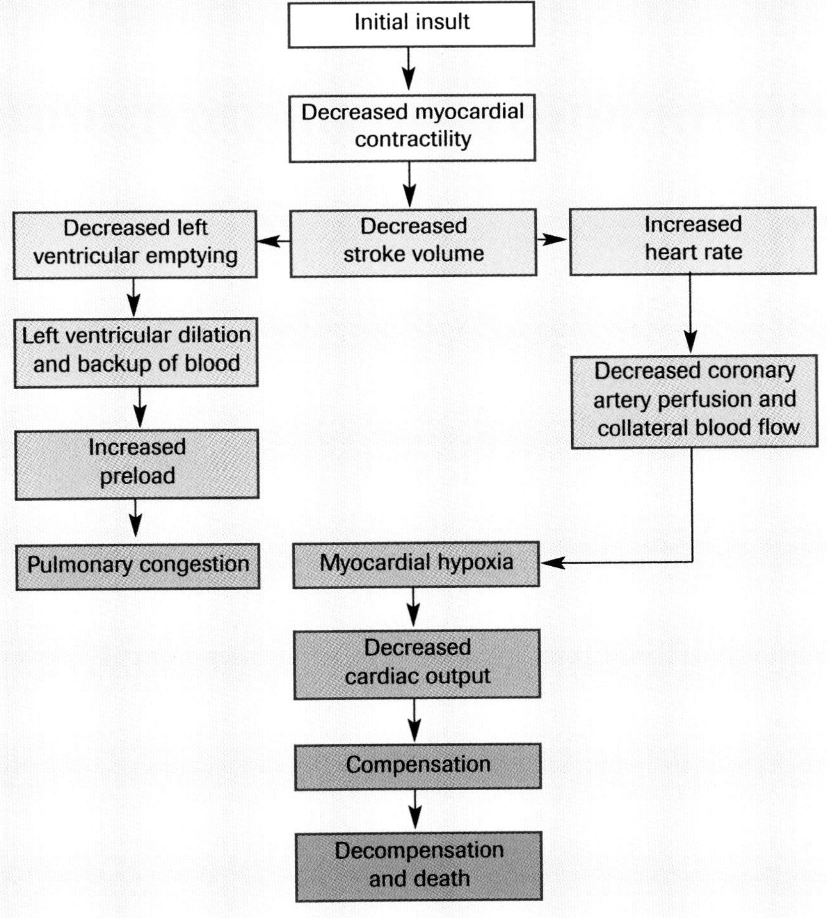

Cardiogenic shock

- Decreased myocardial contractility results in inadequate cardiac output
- Stroke volume decreases, leading to an increased heart rate and decreased left ventricular emptying
- Preload increases and coronary artery perfusion and collateral blood flow decrease
- Pulmonary congestion and myocardial hypoxia result
- Compensatory mechanisms are triggered to prevent decompensation and death

- Hemodynamic monitoring: decreased stroke volume, mixed venous oxygen saturation, and cardiac output; increased PAWP, CVP, PAP, and systemic vascular resistance

Key ways to manage cardiogenic shock

- Oxygen therapy
- Semi-Fowler's position
- Intra-aortic balloon pump
- Diuretics
- Vasodilators
- Cardiac inotropes
- Cardiac glycosides
- Vasopressors
- Adrenergic agents

Key nursing interventions for a patient with cardiogenic shock

- Administer I.V. fluids, oxygen, and medications, as prescribed.
- Assess cardiovascular status, respiratory status, and fluid balance.
- Monitor and record vital signs, I/O, hemodynamic variables, level of consciousness, and laboratory studies.

Medical management

- Diet: withhold food and fluids
- I.V. therapy: electrolyte replacement, saline lock
- Oxygen therapy
- Intubation and mechanical ventilation
- Position: semi-Fowler's
- Activity: bed rest; passive ROM and isometric exercises
- Monitoring: vital signs, I/O, ECG, hemodynamic variables, and level of consciousness
- Laboratory studies: potassium, sodium, BUN, creatinine, and ABGs
- Indwelling urinary catheter
- ET tube suctioning
- Intra-aortic balloon pump
- Left ventricular assist device
- Percutaneous transluminal coronary angioplasty
- Diuretics: furosemide (Lasix), bumetanide (Bumex), metolazone (Zaroxolyn)
- Vasodilator: nitroprusside (Nipride)
- Cardiac inotropes: dopamine (Intropin), dobutamine (Dobutrex), inamrinone (Inocor)
- Cardiac glycoside: digoxin (Lanoxin)
- Vasopressor: norepinephrine (Levophed)
- Adrenergic agent: epinephrine (Adrenalin)
- Hemopump
- Pulse oximetry
- Correction of electrolyte imbalances
- Thrombolytic therapy

Nursing interventions

- Withhold food and fluids, as directed
- Administer I.V. fluids, oxygen, and medications, as prescribed
- Provide suctioning, turning, coughing, and deep breathing
- Assess cardiovascular status, respiratory status, and fluid balance
- Keep the patient in semi-Fowler's position
- Monitor and record vital signs, I/O, hemodynamic variables, level of consciousness, and laboratory studies
- Encourage the patient to express his feelings such as a fear of dying
- Allay the patient's anxiety
- Individualize home care instructions
  - Recognize the signs and symptoms of fluid overload
  - Adhere to activity limitations
  - Alternate rest periods with activity
  - Maintain low-fat, low-sodium diet

Complications

- Arrhythmias
- Cardiac arrest
- Infection

- **Possible surgical interventions**
  - CABG
  - Heart transplantation

MITRAL STENOSIS

- **Definition**
  - Narrowing of the mitral valve opening
- **Causes**
  - Rheumatic endocarditis
  - Congenital
- **Pathophysiology**
  - Thickening and calcification of valvular tissue, thereby narrowing the mitral valve opening and limiting blood flow from the left atrium to the left ventricle
  - Increased pressure in the left atrium, leading to pulmonary hypertension and left atrial hypertrophy
  - Right ventricular failure, producing pulmonary congestion
- **Assessment findings**
  - Fatigue
  - Low cardiac output
  - Dyspnea on exertion
  - Right-sided heart failure
  - Cough
  - Peripheral edema
  - Atrial fibrillation
  - Orthopnea
  - Jugular vein distention
  - Tachycardia
  - Paroxysmal nocturnal dyspnea
  - Hemoptysis
  - Murmurs, clicks
- **Diagnostic test findings**
  - Chest X-ray: enlargement of the left atrium and right ventricle; pulmonary congestion
  - Echocardiogram: thickening of the mitral valve and left atrial enlargement
  - Cardiac catheterization: increased left atrial pressure, PAWP; decreased cardiac output
  - Angiography: mitral stenosis
- **Medical management**
  - Diet: low-sodium; limit fluids
  - I.V. therapy: saline lock
  - Oxygen therapy
  - Position: semi-Fowler's
  - Activity: bed rest; active ROM and isometric exercises

Key facts about mitral stenosis

- Thickening and calcification of valvular tissue
- Increased pressure in the left atrium
- Pulmonary hypertension and left atrial hypertrophy
- Right ventricular failure
- Narrowing of the mitral valve opening results

Key assessment findings in mitral stenosis

- Fatigue
- Dyspnea on exertion
- Peripheral edema
- Orthopnea

Key test findings in mitral stenosis

- Chest X-ray: enlargement of the left atrium and right ventricle; pulmonary congestion
- Echocardiogram: thickening of the mitral valve and left atrial enlargement

Key steps in managing mitral stenosis

- Low-sodium diet; fluid restrictions
- Semi-Fowler's position
- Cardiac glycosides
- Nitrates
- Diuretics
- Antiarrhythmics
- Anticoagulants
- Antibiotics

Key nursing interventions for a patient with mitral stenosis

- Administer I.V. fluids, oxygen, and medications, as prescribed.
- Assess cardiovascular and respiratory response.
- Monitor and record vital signs, I/O, hemodynamic variables, laboratory studies, and ECG readings.

Home care checklist for mitral stenosis

- Recognize the signs and symptoms of heart failure.
- Adhere to activity limitations.
- Monitor for infection, avoid exposure to people with infections, and seek treatment if infection develops.
- Test stools for occult blood.

Key facts about mitral insufficiency

- An incomplete closure of the mitral valve
- Caused by increased left atrial pressure, pulmonary hypertension, and left atrial hypertrophy

- Monitoring: vital signs, I/O, ECG, and hemodynamic variables
- Laboratory studies: sodium, potassium, PT, PTT, and ABGs
- Indwelling urinary catheter
- Cardiac glycoside: digoxin (Lanoxin)
- Nitrates: isosorbide dinitrate (Isordil), nitroglycerin (Nitro-Bid)
- Diuretics: furosemide (Lasix), bumetanide (Bumex)
- Antiarrhythmics: quinidine (Cardioquin), procainamide (Pronestyl)
- Anticoagulants: warfarin (Coumadin)
- Antibiotics: penicillin G potassium (Pentids)
- Percutaneous transluminal valvuloplasty

Nursing interventions

- Maintain the patient's prescribed diet; restrict oral fluids
- Administer I.V. fluids, oxygen, and medications, as prescribed
- Assess cardiovascular and respiratory status
- Keep the patient in semi-Fowler's position
- Monitor and record vital signs, I/O, hemodynamic variables, laboratory studies, and ECG readings
- Encourage the patient to express his feelings such as a fear of dying
- Assess pain
- Allay the patient's anxiety
- Assess peripheral edema
- Individualize home care instructions
  - Recognize the signs and symptoms of heart failure
  - Adhere to activity limitations; alternate rest periods with activity
  - Monitor for infection, avoid exposure to people with infections, and seek treatment if infection develops
  - Test stools for occult blood

Complications

- Thrombosis
- Embolism
- Heart failure
- Atrial fibrillation

Possible surgical interventions

- Valve replacement
- Open mitral commissurotomy

MITRAL INSUFFICIENCY

Definition

- Incomplete closure of the mitral valve

Causes

- Congenital defect
- Rheumatic fever
- Trauma
- Papillary muscle dysfunction
- Bacterial endocarditis

Pathophysiology
- Valvular incompetence
- Backflow of blood to the left atrium
- Increased left atrial pressure, pulmonary hypertension, and left atrial hypertrophy

Assessment findings
- Shortness of breath
- Cough
- Fatigue
- Dyspnea on exertion
- Peripheral edema
- Atrial fibrillation
- Angina pectoris
- Orthopnea
- Hemoptysis
- Murmurs and clicks
- S_3

Diagnostic test findings
- Chest X-ray: enlargement of the left atrium and the left ventricle
- ECG: atrial fibrillation, left atrial hypertension, and left ventricular hypertrophy
- Echocardiogram: enlargement of the left atrium, abnormal movement of the mitral valve
- Cardiac catheterization: increased left atrial and left ventricular pressure
- Cardiac angiography: insufficiency

Medical management
- Diet: low-sodium; limit fluids
- I.V. therapy: saline lock
- Oxygen therapy
- Position: semi-Fowler's
- Monitoring: vital signs, I/O, ECG, and hemodynamic variables
- Laboratory studies: sodium, potassium, BUN, creatinine, and ABGs
- Indwelling urinary catheter
- Cardiac glycoside: digoxin (Lanoxin)
- Nitrates: isosorbide (Isordil), nitroglycerin (Nitro-Bid)
- Diuretics: furosemide (Lasix), bumetanide (Bumex)
- Antiarrhythmics: quinidine (Cardioquin), procainamide (Pronestyl)
- Anticoagulants: warfarin (Coumadin)

Nursing interventions
- Maintain the patient's prescribed diet; limit oral fluids
- Administer I.V. fluids, oxygen, and medications, as prescribed
- Assess cardiovascular and respiratory status
- Keep the patient in semi-Fowler's position
- Monitor and record vital signs, I/O, hemodynamic variables, laboratory studies, and ECG readings
- Encourage the patient to express feelings such as a fear of dying

Key assessment findings in mitral insufficiency
- Fatigue
- Dyspnea on exertion
- Peripheral edema
- Angina pectoris
- Orthopnea

Key test findings in mitral insufficiency
- Echocardiogram: enlarged left atrium, abnormal movement of the mitral valve
- Cardiac catheterization: increased left atrial pressure and increased left ventricular pressure

Key steps in managing mitral insufficiency
- Low-sodium diet; fluid restrictions
- Semi-Fowler's position
- Vital signs, I/O, ECG, and hemodynamic variables monitoring
- Cardiac glycosides
- Nitrates
- Diuretics
- Antiarrhythmics
- Anticoagulants

Key nursing interventions for a patient with mitral insufficiency

- Maintain the patient's prescribed diet; limit oral fluids.
- Keep the patient in semi-Fowler's position.
- Assess peripheral edema.

- Assess pain
- Assess peripheral edema
- Allay the patient's anxiety
- Provide information about the American Heart Association
- Individualize home care instructions
  - Test stools for occult blood
  - Adhere to activity limitations; alternate rest periods with activity
  - Monitor for infection, avoid exposure to people with infections, and seek treatment if infection develops

Complications
- Embolism
- Thrombosis
- Heart failure
- Ruptured papillary muscle

Possible surgical interventions
- Mitral valve replacement
- Valvuloplasty

AORTIC STENOSIS

Aortic stenosis defined

- Narrowing of the aortic valve
- Lower cardiac output causes increased congestion in the lungs, resulting in right-sided heart failure

Definition
- Narrowing of the aortic valve

Causes
- Syphilis
- Rheumatic fever
- Atherosclerosis
- Congenital malformations

Pathophysiology
- Fibrosis and calcification of valvular tissue, which narrows the valve opening and limits blood flow
- Increased left ventricular pressure, which causes hypertrophy of the left ventricle and lowers cardiac output
- Increased congestion in the lungs, which results in right-sided heart failure

Key assessment findings in aortic stenosis

- Angina pectoris
- Pulmonary hypertension
- Left-sided heart failure
- Orthopnea

Assessment findings
- Angina pectoris
- Syncope
- Pulmonary hypertension
- Left-sided heart failure
- Fatigue
- Orthopnea
- Paroxysmal nocturnal dyspnea
- Murmurs and clicks

Diagnostic test findings
- Chest X-ray: aortic valve calcification, left ventricular enlargement

- ECG: left bundle branch block, first-degree heart block, left ventricular hypertrophy
- Echocardiogram: thickened left ventricular wall, thickened aortic valve that moves abnormally
- Cardiac catheterization: increased left ventricular pressure

Medical management
- Diet: low-sodium; limit fluids
- I.V. therapy: saline lock
- Monitoring: vital signs, I/O, ECG, and hemodynamic variables
- Laboratory studies: sodium, potassium, BUN, creatinine, and ABGs
- Cardiac glycoside: digoxin (Lanoxin)
- Nitrates: isosorbide (Isordil), nitroglycerin (Nitro-Bid)
- Diuretics: furosemide (Lasix), bumetanide (Bumex)
- Percutaneous transluminal valvuloplasty

Nursing interventions
- Maintain the patient's prescribed diet; limit fluids
- Assess cardiovascular and respiratory status
- Monitor and record vital signs, I/O, hemodynamic variables, laboratory studies, and ECG readings
- Administer I.V. therapy and medications, as prescribed
- Encourage the patient to express his feelings such as a fear of dying
- Assess pain
- Allay the patient's anxiety
- Provide information about the American Heart Association
- Individualize home care instructions
  - Recognize the signs and symptoms of heart failure
  - Adhere to activity limitations; alternate rest periods with activity
  - Follow dietary restrictions and recommendations

Complications
- Heart failure
- Pulmonary edema

Possible surgical interventions
- Aortic valve replacement
- Commissurotomy

AORTIC INSUFFICIENCY

Definition
- Incomplete closure of the aortic valve

Causes
- Rheumatic fever
- Infective endocarditis
- Syphilis
- Atherosclerosis
- Congenital defect

Key diagnostic findings in aortic stenosis

- ECG: left bundle branch block, first-degree heart block, left ventricular hypertrophy
- Echocardiogram: thickened left ventricular wall, thickened aortic valve that moves abnormally

Key steps in managing aortic stenosis

- Low-sodium diet; fluid restrictions
- Monitoring laboratory studies
- Cardiac glycosides
- Nitrates
- Diuretics
- Percutaneous transluminal valvuloplasty

Key nursing interventions for a patient with aortic stenosis

- Maintain the patient's prescribed diet; limit fluids.
- Assess cardiovascular and respiratory status.
- Monitor and record vital signs, I/O, hemodynamic variables, laboratory studies, and ECG reading.

Aortic insufficiency defined

- Retrograde flow of blood from the aorta to the left ventricle
- An incomplete closure of the aortic valve

Key assessment findings in aortic insufficiency

- Signs of left-sided heart failure
- Dyspnea on exertion
- Dizziness
- Angina pectoris

Key test findings in aortic insufficiency

- Chest X-ray: enlarged left ventricle, aortic valve calcification
- Echocardiogram: left ventricular enlargement, abnormal valve movement

Key steps in managing aortic insufficiency

- Low-sodium diet; limit fluids
- Antibiotics
- Cardiac glycosides
- Nitrates
- Diuretics
- Vasodilators
- ACE inhibitors

Key nursing interventions for a patient with aortic insufficiency

- Maintain the patient's prescribed diet; restrict oral fluids.
- Administer I.V. fluids and medications, as necessary.
- Assess cardiovascular and respiratory status.
- Monitor and record vital signs, I/O, hemodynamic variables, and laboratory studies.

Pathophysiology

- Retrograde flow of blood from the aorta to the left ventricle
- Left ventricular hypertrophy

Assessment findings

- Signs of left-sided heart failure
- Dyspnea on exertion
- Dizziness
- Neck pain
- Orthopnea
- Angina pectoris
- Tachycardia
- Paroxysmal nocturnal dyspnea
- Murmurs and clicks

Diagnostic test findings

- Chest X-ray: enlarged left ventricle, aortic valve calcification
- ECG: left ventricular hypertrophy, sinus tachycardia
- Echocardiogram: left ventricular enlargement, abnormal valve movement
- Cardiac catheterization: increased left atrial and left ventricular pressures, insufficiency

Medical management

- Diet: low-sodium; limit fluids
- I.V. therapy: saline lock
- Monitoring: vital signs, I/O, ECG, and hemodynamic variables
- Laboratory studies: ABGs, sodium, potassium, BUN, and creatinine
- Indwelling urinary catheter
- Antibiotic: penicillin G potassium (Pentids)
- Cardiac glycoside: digoxin (Lanoxin)
- Nitrates: isosorbide (Isordil), nitroglycerin (Nitro-Bid)
- Diuretics: furosemide (Lasix), bumetanide (Bumex)
- Vasodilators: hydralazine (Apresoline), nifedipine (Procardia)
- ACE inhibitors: captopril (Capoten), enalapril (Vasotec), lisinopril (Prinivil)

Nursing interventions

- Maintain the patient's prescribed diet; restrict oral fluids
- Administer I.V. fluids and medications, as prescribed
- Assess cardiovascular and respiratory status
- Monitor and record vital signs, I/O, hemodynamic variables, and laboratory studies
- Assess pain
- Encourage the patient to express his feelings such as a fear of dying
- Allay the patient's anxiety
- Provide information about the American Heart Association
- Individualize home care instructions
  - Recognize the signs and symptoms of heart failure
  - Adhere to activity limitations; alternate rest periods with activity
  - Monitor for infection

Complications
- Heart failure
- Thrombosis
- Embolism
- Infection

Possible surgical interventions
- Valvuloplasty
- Valve replacement

PERIPHERAL VASCULAR DISEASE (PVD)

Definition
- Chronic inadequate blood flow in the lower extremities

Types
- Arteriosclerosis obliterans — sclerosis of arterioles resulting in thickening of the walls and occlusion
- Raynaud's phenomenon — intermittent vasoconstriction and ischemia of fingers and toes accompanied by pallor and cyanosis
- Buerger's disease (thromboangiitis obliterans) — inflammation of blood vessels resulting in occlusion of the vessel

Causes
- Atherosclerosis
- Vasospasm
- Inflammation

Pathophysiology
- Arterial thickening and loss of elasticity, narrowing the diameter of the artery
- Decreased perfusion and blood clot formation, causing arterial blockage and ischemia (common sites are the femoral, popliteal, and iliac arteries and the aorta)

Assessment findings
- Intermittent claudication
- Pain in extremities at rest
- Trophic changes: thickened nails, absence of hair, and taut, shiny skin
- Diminished or absent pulses in extremities (a unilateral finding has greater significance than bilateral findings) (*see Managing diminished or absent pulse*, pages 46 and 47)
- Temperature changes in extremities
- Color changes in extremities: rubor, cyanosis, pallor
- Ulcerations in extremities

Diagnostic test findings
- Arteriography: location of obstructing plaque
- Doppler studies: decreased blood flow and arterial pressure
- Blood chemistry: increased lipids

(Text continues on page 48.)

Facts about PVD

- Chronic inadequate blood flow in the lower extremities
- Three types: arteriosclerosis obliterans, Raynaud's phenomenon, and Buerger's disease (thromboangiitis obliterans)
- Caused by arterial thickening and loss of elasticity
- Decreased perfusion and blood clot formation occurs, causing arterial blockage and ischemia

Key assessment findings in PVD

- Intermittent claudication
- Pain in extremities at rest
- Trophic changes: thickened nails, absence of hair, and taut, shiny skin
- Diminished or absent pulses in extremities (a unilateral finding has greater significance than bilateral findings)
- Temperature changes in extremities
- Color changes in extremities: rubor, cyanosis, pallor
- Ulcerations in extremities

Key test findings in PVD

- Arteriography: location of obstruction
- Doppler studies: decreased blood flow and arterial pressure

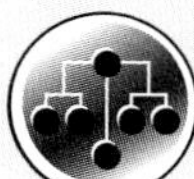

GO WITH THE FLOW

Managing diminished or absent pulse

A diminished or absent pulse can result from several life-threatening disorders. Your assessment and interventions will vary depending on whether the diminished or absent pulse is localized to one extremity or generalized. They will also depend on associated signs and symptoms. Use the decision tree here to help you establish priorities for managing this problem.

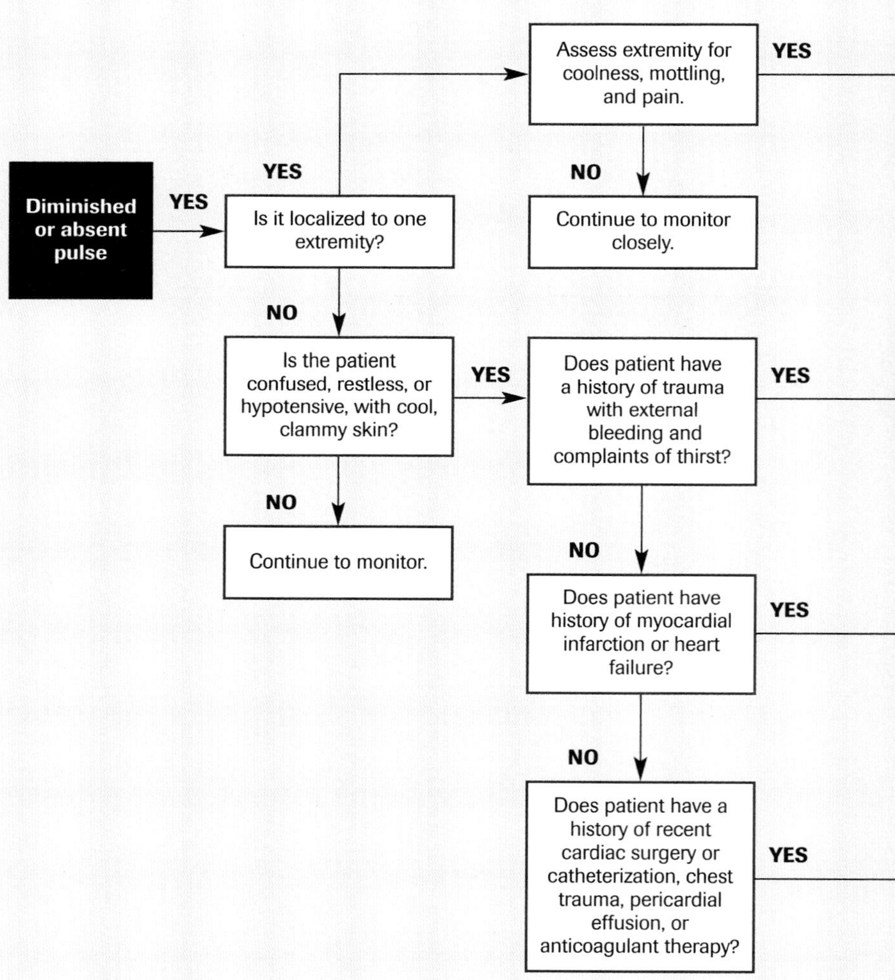

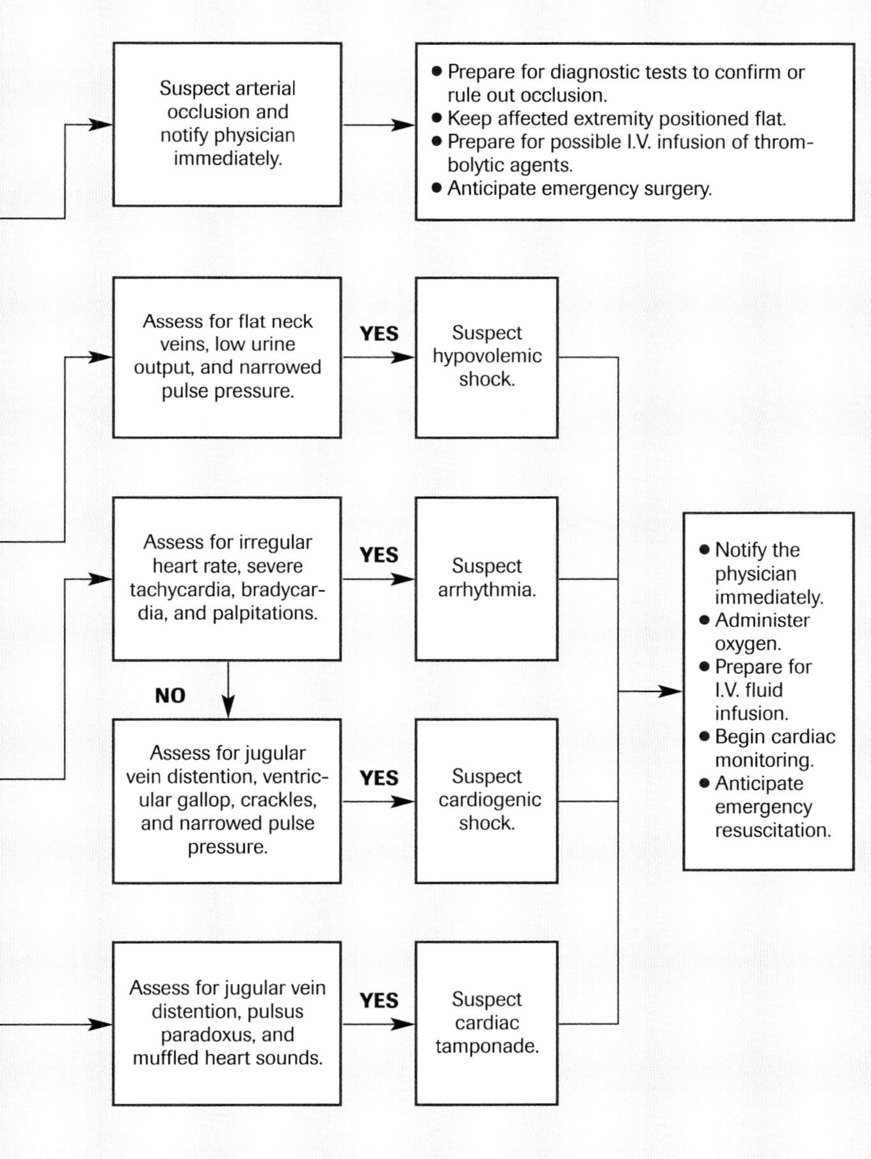
Suspect arterial occlusion and notify physician immediately.
• Prepare for diagnostic tests to confirm or rule out occlusion.
• Keep affected extremity positioned flat.
• Prepare for possible I.V. infusion of thrombolytic agents.
• Anticipate emergency surgery.
Assess for flat neck veins, low urine output, and narrowed pulse pressure.
YES
Suspect hypovolemic shock.
Assess for irregular heart rate, severe tachycardia, bradycardia, and palpitations.
YES
Suspect arrhythmia.
NO
Assess for jugular vein distention, ventricular gallop, crackles, and narrowed pulse pressure.
YES
Suspect cardiogenic shock.
Assess for jugular vein distention, pulsus paradoxus, and muffled heart sounds.
YES
Suspect cardiac tamponade.
• Notify the physician immediately.
• Administer oxygen.
• Prepare for I.V. fluid infusion.
• Begin cardiac monitoring.
• Anticipate emergency resuscitation.

Key steps in managing PVD medically

- Active ROM and isometric exercises, as tolerated
- Antiplatelet agents
- Vasodilators
- Anticoagulants
- Antilipemics

Assessing peripheral circulation in patients with PVD

- Pulses
- Color
- Temperature
- Complaints of abnormal sensations such as numbness or tingling

Key home care instructions for PVD

- Recognize the symptoms of decreased peripheral circulation.
- Monitor for skin breakdown.
- Care for the feet daily.
- Avoid activities or situations that will exacerbate the condition, such as temperature extremes, prolonged standing, constrictive clothing, or crossing the legs at the knee when seated.

Medical management

- Diet: low-fat, low-calorie
- Activity: active ROM and isometric exercises, as tolerated
- Monitoring: vital signs, I/O, and neurovascular checks
- Laboratory studies: serum lipids, PTT, and PT
- Bed cradle
- Antiplatelet agent: aspirin
- Vasodilator: pentoxifylline (Trental)
- Anticoagulant: warfarin (Coumadin)
- Antilipemics: cholestyramine (Questran), lovastatin (Mevacor)
- Percutaneous transluminal coronary angioplasty
- Laser angioplasty
- Vascular stents
- Thrombolytic therapy: streptokinase (Streptase)

Nursing interventions

- Maintain the patient's prescribed diet
- Assess cardiovascular status
- Monitor and record vital signs, I/O, and laboratory studies
- Administer medications, as prescribed
- Encourage the patient to express his feelings about changes in body image
- Check peripheral circulation: pulses, color, temperature, and complaints of abnormal sensations, such as numbness or tingling
- Encourage walking and other leg exercises
- Provide daily foot care
- Individualize home care instructions
  - Recognize the symptoms of decreased peripheral circulation
  - Monitor for skin breakdown
  - Care for the feet daily
  - Avoid activities or situations that will exacerbate the condition, such as temperature extremes, prolonged standing, constrictive clothing, or crossing the legs at the knee when seated

Complications

- Gangrene
- Septicemia
- Pressure sores
- Acute vascular occlusion

Possible surgical interventions

- Bypass grafting
- Endarterectomy
- Sympathectomy
- Amputation
- Embolectomy

THROMBOPHLEBITIS

Definition
- Inflammation of the venous wall, resulting in clot formation

Causes
- Venous stasis (from varicose veins, pregnancy, heart failure, prolonged bed rest)
- Hypercoagulability (from cancer, blood dyscrasias, oral contraceptives)
- Injury to the venous wall (from I.V. injections, fractures, antibiotics)

Pathophysiology
- Massing of RBCs in a fibrin network
- Obstruction by enlarged thrombus, leading to venous insufficiency (common sites are deep veins and superficial veins)

Assessment findings
- Superficial veins: red, warm skin that's tender to touch
- Deep veins
  - Major venous trunks: edema, positive Homans' sign, tender to touch, cramping pain, cyanosis, venous distention
  - Small veins: tenderness, induration over muscle, minimal to no distention

Diagnostic test findings
- Venography: venous-filling defects
- Ultrasound: decreased blood flow
- Phlebography: venous-filling defects
- Hematology: increased WBC count

Medical management
- Position: elevation of the affected extremity
- Activity: bed rest; active and passive ROM and isometric exercises
- Monitoring: vital signs and neurovascular checks
- Laboratory studies: WBC, PT, and PTT
- Antiembolism stockings; warm, moist compresses
- Anticoagulants: warfarin (Coumadin), heparin (Lipo-Hepin)
- Thrombolytic agent: streptokinase (Streptase)
- Anti-inflammatory agent: aspirin

Nursing interventions
- Assess cardiovascular status
- Keep the patient in bed and elevate the affected extremity
- Monitor and record vital signs, neurovascular checks, and laboratory studies
- Administer medications, as prescribed
- Assess for Homans' sign
- Assess for bleeding
- Apply warm, moist compresses
- Measure and record the circumference of thighs and calves
- Individualize home care instructions
  - Recognize the signs and symptoms of bleeding

Characteristics of thrombophlebitis
- Massing of RBCs in a fibrin network
- Obstruction by enlarged thrombus
- Result is inflammation of the venous wall, resulting in clot formation

Key assessment findings in thrombophlebitis
- Superficial veins: red, warm skin that's tender to touch
- Deep veins:
- Major venous trunks: edema, positive Homans' sign, tender to touch, cramping pain, cyanosis, venous distention
- Small veins: tenderness, induration over muscle, minimal to no distention

Diagnostic test findings in thrombophlebitis
- Venography: venous-filling defects
- Ultrasound: decreased blood flow
- Phlebography: venous-filling defects

Key steps in managing thrombophlebitis
- Activity limitation
- Antiembolism stockings
- Anticoagulants

Key nursing interventions for a patient with thrombophlebitis

- Assess for Homans' sign.
- Apply warm, moist compresses.
- Measure and record the circumference of thighs and calves.
- Keep patient in bed and elevate the affected extremity.

  - Avoid prolonged sitting or standing, constrictive clothing, or crossing the legs when seated
  - Don't take hormonal contraceptives
  - Have blood drawn periodically for prothrombin time if taking warfarin

Complications
- Pulmonary embolism
- Stroke

Possible surgical interventions
- Vena cava filter
- Vein ligation and stripping
- Thrombectomy

ENDOCARDITIS

Endocarditis

- Inflammation and infection of the endocardial lining
- Caused by formation of bacterial colonies on the endocardial lining, destroying heart valve leaflets

Definition
- Inflammation and infection of the endocardial lining

Causes
- Bacterial infection: Beta-hemolytic streptococcus, *Staphylococcus aureus*
- Rheumatic heart disease
- Dental procedures
- Invasive monitoring
- I.V. drug abuse

Pathophysiology
- Formation of bacterial colonies on the endocardial lining, destroying heart valve leaflets (see *Degenerative changes in endocarditis*)
- Disrupted blood flow, resulting in murmurs
- Vegetations that seed the bloodstream with bacteria

Assessment findings
- Elevated temperature
- Heart murmur
- Diaphoresis
- Malaise
- Anorexia
- Chills
- Dyspnea
- Tachypnea
- Crackles
- Tachycardia
- Arrhythmias
- S_3, S_4
- Peripheral edema
- Clubbing of fingers and toes
- Petechiae
- Night sweats

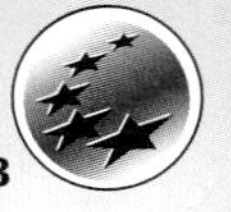

TOP 3

Assessment findings in endocarditis

1. Elevated temperature
2. Heart murmur
3. Malaise

Degenerative changes in endocarditis

This illustration shows typical vegetations on the endocardium produced by fibrin and platelet deposits on infection sites.

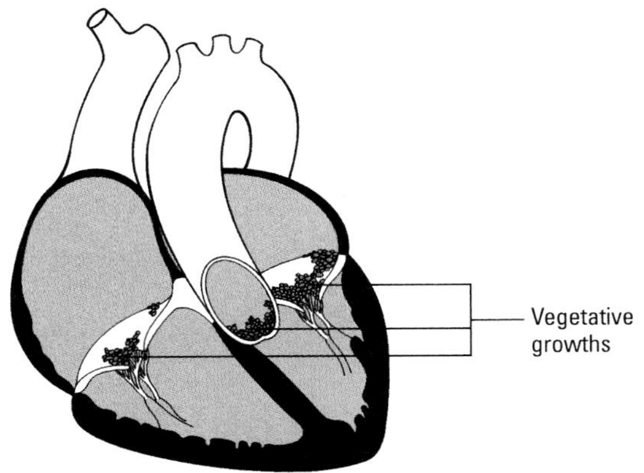

- Splinter hemorrhages in nail beds
- Hematuria
- Joint pain
- Headache

Diagnostic test findings

- Blood cultures: positive for specific organism
- Hematology: increased WBCs, ESR; decreased HCT
- Echocardiography: valvular damage, vegetations

Medical management

- I.V. therapy: hydration, saline lock
- Oxygen therapy
- Activity: bed rest
- Monitoring: vital signs, I/O, and neurovascular checks
- Laboratory studies: blood cultures, WBC, and HCT
- Antibiotics: penicillin G potassium (Pentids), vancomycin (Vancocin), cefazolin (Ancef), depending on organism
- Positive inotropic agents: digoxin (Lanoxin), dobutamine (Dobutrex)
- Fluids: increased intake
- Antipyretic: aspirin
- Anticoagulant: warfarin (Coumadin)

Nursing interventions

- Encourage fluids
- Administer I.V. fluids, oxygen, and medications, as prescribed
- Assess cardiovascular status
- Monitor and record vital signs, I/O, and laboratory studies

Key diagnostic findings in endocarditis

- Blood cultures: positive for specific organism
- Echocardiography: valvular damage, vegetations

Medications used to treat endocarditis

- Antibiotics
- Positive inotropic agents
- Antipyretics
- Anticoagulants

Key nursing interventions for a patient with endocarditis

- Administer medications, as prescribed.
- Assess cardiovascular status.
- Encourage rest periods.

Key home care instructions for a patient with endocarditis

- Avoid exposure to people with infections.
- Monitor for infection, particularly after a dental or gynecologic examination, and seek treatment if infection develops.
- Wear medical identification.

Abdominal aortic aneurysm highlights

- Dilation of or localized weakness in the medial layer of an abdominal artery
- Caused by degenerative changes from atherosclerosis and continued weakening from the force of blood flow

Common causes of abdominal aortic aneurysm

- Atherosclerosis
- Hypertension
- Smoking

- Encourage the patient to express his feelings such as a fear of dying
- Allay the patient's anxiety
- Encourage rest periods
- Individualize home care instructions
  - Recognize the signs and symptoms of endocarditis
  - Follow activity limitations; alternate rest periods with activity, and adhere to the prescribed exercise regimen
  - Avoid exposure to people with infections; monitor self for infection, particularly after a dental or gynecologic examination; and seek treatment if infection develops
  - Wear medical identification

Complications

- Embolism
- Heart failure
- Mycotic aneurysm

Possible surgical intervention

- Valve replacement

ABDOMINAL AORTIC ANEURYSM

Definition

- Dilation of or localized weakness in the medial layer of an abdominal artery

Causes

- Most common
  - Atherosclerosis
  - Hypertension
  - Smoking
- Less common
  - Congenital defect
  - Trauma
  - Syphilis
  - Infection
  - Marfan syndrome

Pathophysiology

- Degenerative changes from atherosclerosis, weakening the medial layer
- Continued weakening from the force of blood flow, resulting in outpouching of the artery
- Four types: saccular, fusiform, dissecting, false (see *Types of aortic aneurysms*)

Assessment findings

- Asymptomatic
- Lower abdominal pain, lower back pain
- Abdominal mass to the left of the midline
- Abdominal pulsations

Types of aortic aneurysms

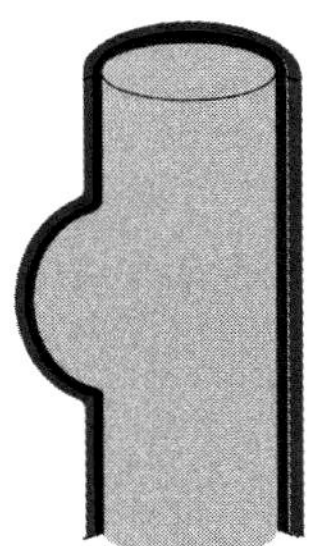

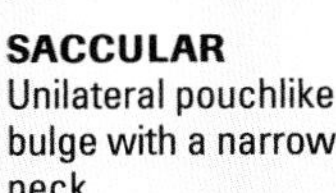

SACCULAR
Unilateral pouchlike bulge with a narrow neck

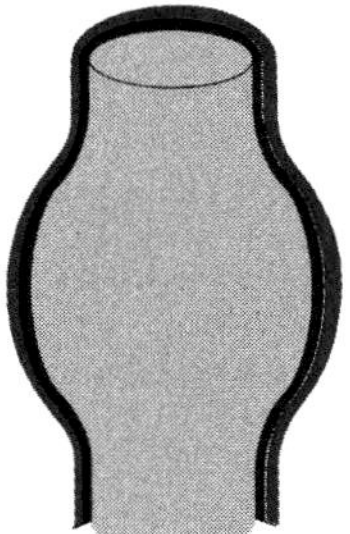

FUSIFORM
A spindle-shaped bulge encompassing the entire diameter of the vessel

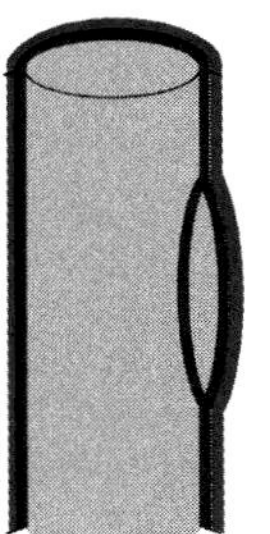

DISSECTING
A hemorrhagic separation of the medial layer of the vessel wall, which creates a false lumen

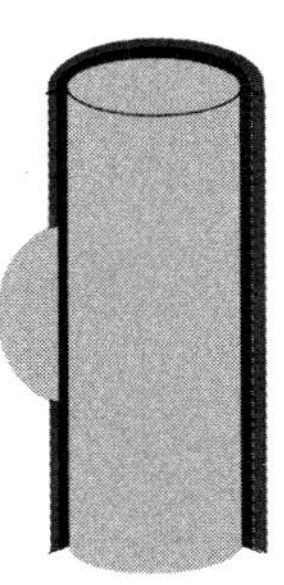

FALSE ANEURYSM
A pulsating hematoma resulting from trauma and often mistaken for an abdominal aneurysm

- Bruits
- Diminished femoral pulses
- Systolic blood pressure in the legs lower than that in the arms
- Deep, diffuse chest pain
- Hoarse voice
- Coughing
- Dyspnea
- Dysphagia
- Jugular vein distention
- Edema

Diagnostic test findings

- Chest X-ray: aneurysm
- ECG: differentiation of aneurysm from MI
- Abdominal ultrasound: aneurysm
- Aortography: aneurysm

Medical management

- Activity: bed rest
- Monitoring: vital signs, I/O, and neurovascular checks
- Analgesic: oxycodone (Tylox)
- Beta-adrenergic blocker: propranolol (Inderal)
- Antihypertensives: methyldopa (Aldomet), hydralazine (Apresoline), prazosin (Minipress)

Nursing interventions

- Assess cardiovascular status
- Monitor and record vital signs, I/O, neurovascular checks, and laboratory studies

4 types of abdominal aortic aneurysm

- Saccular: unilateral; pouchlike bulge
- Fusiform: spindle-shaped bulge; encompasses entire diameter of vessel
- Dissecting: hemorrhagic separation of medial layer of vessel wall; creates a false lumen
- False: pulsating hematoma; often mistaken for an abdominal aneurysm

Common assessment findings in aortic aneurysm

- Asymptomatic
- Lower abdominal pain, lower back pain
- Abdominal mass to the left of the midline
- Abdominal pulsations
- Bruits

Key diagnostic test finding

- Aneurysm apparent on chest X-ray, abdominal ultrasound, and aortography

Medications used to treat abdominal aortic aneurysm

- Analgesics
- Beta-adrenergic blockers
- Antihypertensives

- Administer medications, as prescribed
- Encourage the patient to express feelings such as a fear of dying
- Assess pain
- Check peripheral circulation: pulses, temperature, color, and complaints of abnormal sensations
- Allay the patient's anxiety
- Observe the patient for signs of shock, such as anxiety; restlessness; decreased pulse pressure; increased thready pulse; and pale, cool, moist, clammy skin
- Palpate the abdomen for distention
- Individualize home care instructions
  - Recognize the signs and symptoms of decreased peripheral circulation, such as change in skin color or temperature, complaints of numbness or tingling, and absent pulses
  - Adhere to activity limitations, alternate rest periods with activity, and adhere to prescribed exercise regimen
  - Maintain a quiet environment

Possible complication

- Rupture of aneurysm
- Hemorrhage
- Renal insufficiency

Possible surgical intervention

- Resection of aneurysm
- Endovascular graft repair

CARDIOMYOPATHY

Definition

- Disease of the muscle of the heart impacting the structure and function of the ventricle
- Types
  - Congestive (dilated)
  - Hypertrophic — two types
    - More common form is caused by pressure overload-hypertension or aortic valve stenosis
    - Hypertrophic obstructive cardiomyopathy is due to a genetic abnormality
  - Restrictive (obliterative)

Causes

- Infection
- Metabolic and immunologic disorders
- Pregnancy and postpartum disorders
- Congenital
- Ischemia
- Drug abuse
- Chronic alcoholism (congestive)

Key nursing interventions for a patient with aortic aneurysm

- Check peripheral circulation: pulses, temperature, color, and complaints of abnormal sensations.
- Observe the patient for signs of shock, such as anxiety; restlessness; decreased pulse pressure; increased thready pulse; and pale, cool, moist, clammy skin.
- Palpate the abdomen for distention.
- Teach the signs and symptoms of decreased peripheral circulation: change in skin color or temperature, complaints of numbness or tingling, and absent pulses.

Facts about cardiomyopathy

- Disease of the heart's muscle impacting the structure and function of the ventricle
- Heart failure develops in later stages
- Myocardium becomes flabby

Cardiomyopathy: types

- Congestive (dilated)
- Hypertrophic
- Hypertrophic obstructive
- Restrictive (obliterative)

- Idiopathic hypertrophic subaortic stenosis (hypertrophic)
- Amyloidosis (restrictive)
- Cancer and other infiltrative diseases (restrictive)

Pathophysiology

- Cardiac function is altered, resulting in decreased cardiac output
- Increased heart rate and increased muscle mass compensate in early stages
- Heart failure develops in later stages
- Myocardium becomes flabby

Assessment findings

- Major manifestations
  - Dyspnea
  - Dry cough
  - Fatigue
  - Palpitations
  - Weakness
- Other manifestations
  - Signs and symptoms of heart failure
  - Paroxysmal nocturnal dyspnea
  - Jugular vein distention
  - Dependent pitting edema
  - Enlarged liver
  - Murmur
  - Crackles
  - S_3, S_4

Diagnostic test findings

- ECG: left ventricular hypertrophy
- Echocardiogram: decreased myocardial function
- Cardiac catheterization: rule out CAD
- Chest X-ray: cardiomegaly

Medical management

- Diet: low-sodium, vitamin supplements
- I.V. therapy
- Oxygen therapy
- Bed rest
- Position: semi-Fowler's
- Monitoring: vital signs, ECG, hemodynamic variables, and I/O
- Laboratory studies: ABGs, sodium, potassium, CK and LD with isoenzymes
- Left ventricular assist device
- Intra-aortic balloon pump
- Arterial line for blood pressure monitoring
- Diuretics: furosemide (Lasix), bumetanide (Bumex), metolazone (Zaroxolyn)
- Beta-adrenergic blockers: propranolol (Inderal), nadolol (Corgard), metoprolol (Lopressor)

Major manifestations of cardiomyopathy

- Dyspnea
- Dry cough
- Fatigue
- Palpitations
- Weakness

Key cardiomyopathy test findings

- ECG: left ventricular hypertrophy
- Echocardiogram: decreased myocardial function
- Chest X-ray: cardiomegaly

Key steps in managing cardiomyopathy

- Low-sodium diet, vitamin supplements
- Left ventricular assist device
- Diuretics
- Beta-adrenergic blockers
- Calcium channel blockers
- ACE inhibitors
- Anticoagulants

Key nursing interventions for a patient with cardiomyopathy

- Keep the patient in semi-Fowler's position.
- Monitor ECG results.
- Administer oxygen and medications as prescribed.

Key home care instructions for cardiomyopathy

- Recognize signs and symptoms of heart failure.
- Weigh daily and report increases over 3 lb.
- Demonstrate exercises to increase cardiac output (raising arms).
- Refrain from smoking and drinking alcohol.

Cardiac arrhythmias defined

- Abnormal electrical conduction or automaticity
- Alter heart rate and rhythm
- Results from a disturbance in excitability, automaticity, or conductivity

- Calcium channel blockers: verapamil (Calan), diltiazem (Cardizem), nifedipine (Procardia), nicardipine (Cardene)
- ACE inhibitors: captopril (Capoten), enalapril (Vasotec), lisinopril (Prinivil)
- Anticoagulant: warfarin (Coumadin)

Nursing interventions

- Maintain the patient's prescribed diet
- Assess cardiovascular and respiratory status
- Monitor and record vital signs, I/O, hemodynamic variables, laboratory studies, and ECG results
- Maintain bed rest
- Administer oxygen and medications, as prescribed
- Allay the patient's anxiety
- Keep the patient in semi-Fowler's position
- Provide information about the American Heart Association
- Individualize home care instructions
  - Recognize signs and symptoms of heart failure
  - Avoid straining during bowel movements
  - Monitor pulses and blood pressure
  - Weigh daily and report increases over 3 lb (1.4 kg)
  - Demonstrate exercises to increase cardiac output (raising arms)
  - Refrain from smoking and drinking alcohol

Complications

- Heart failure
- Arterial emboli

Possible surgical interventions

- Ventricular myomectomy
- Heart transplant

CARDIAC ARRHYTHMIAS

Definition

- Abnormal electrical conduction or automaticity causing changes in heart rate and rhythm

Causes

- Congenital
- Myocardial ischemia
- MI
- Organic heart disease
- Drug effects and toxicity
- Conductive tissue degeneration
- Electrolyte imbalance
- Acid-base imbalances
- Cellular hypoxia

Pathophysiology

- Results from a disturbance in excitability, automaticity, or conductivity
- Heart rate and rhythm are altered, reducing cardiac output

Assessment findings

- Asymptomatic
- Palpitations
- Chest pain
- Dizziness
- Weakness, fatigue
- Feelings of impending doom
- Irregular heart rhythm
- Bradycardia or tachycardia
- Hypotension
- Syncope
- Altered level of consciousness
- Diaphoresis
- Pallor
- Nausea, vomiting
- Cold, clammy skin
- Life-threatening arrhythmias may result in pulselessness, absence of respirations, and no palpable blood pressure

Possible diagnostic findings

- ECG: changes in heart rate, rhythm (see *Types of cardiac arrhythmias,* pages 58 to 65)
- Blood chemistry: electrolyte imbalance

Medical management (see *Types of cardiac arrhythmias,* pages 58 to 65)

Nursing interventions

- Monitor pulse for irregular pattern or abnormally rapid or slow rate
- Observe for arrhythmias if the patient is receiving continuous cardiac monitoring
- Assess cardiovascular, respiratory, and neurovascular status
- If the patient has an arrhythmia, promptly assess airway, breathing, and circulation
- Initiate cardiopulmonary resuscitation (CPR), if indicated, until other advanced cardiac life support (ACLS) measures are available and successful
- Perform defibrillation early for ventricular tachycardia and ventricular fibrillation
- Administer medications, oxygen, and I.V. fluids, as needed
- Prepare for procedures, such as cardioversion or pacemaker insertion, if indicated
- Monitor for predisposing factors (such as fluid and electrolyte imbalance) and signs of drug toxicity, especially digoxin; correct the underlying cause — for example, if the patient has a toxic reaction to a drug, withhold the next dose
- Monitor and record vital signs, I/O, hemodynamic variables, laboratory studies, medication levels, and ECG readings
- Maintain prescribed diet
- Maintain bed rest, until patient is stable
- Provide support to the patient and family

(Text continues on page 65.)

Key assessment findings in the patient with a cardiac arrhythmia

- Chest pain
- Irregular heart rhythm
- Bradycardia or tachycardia
- Hypotension
- Syncope
- Altered level of consciousness
- Diaphoresis
- Pallor

Key nursing interventions for a patient with a cardiac arrhythmia

- Monitor pulse for irregular pattern or abnormally rapid or slow rate.
- Observe for arrhythmias if the patient is receiving continuous cardiac monitoring.
- If the patient has an arrhythmia, promptly assess airway, breathing, and circulation.
- Initiate CPR, if indicated, until other ACLS measures are available and successful.
- Perform defibrillation early for ventricular tachycardia and ventricular fibrillation.
- Prepare for procedures, such as cardioversion or pacemaker insertion, if indicated.
- Maintain bed rest, until patient is stable.

ECG characteristics: Sinus arrhythmia

- Irregular atrial and ventricular rhythms
- Normal P wave preceding each QRS complex

ECG characteristics: Sinus tachycardia

- Atrial and ventricular rhythms regular
- Rate > 100 beats/minute; rarely > 160 beats/minute
- Normal P wave preceding each QRS complex

ECG characteristics: Sinus bradycardia

- Atrial and ventricular rhythms regular
- Rate < 60 beats/minute
- Normal P waves preceding each QRS complex

Types of cardiac arrrhythmias

This chart reviews many common cardiac arrhythmias and outlines their features, causes, and treatments. Use a normal electrocardiogram strip, if available, to compare normal cardiac rhythm configurations with the rhythm strips below. Characteristics of normal rhythm include:

- ventricular and atrial rates of 60 to 100 beats/minute
- regular and uniform QRS complexes and P waves
- PR interval of 0.12 to 0.2 second
- QRS duration < 0.12 second
- identical atrial and ventricular rates, with constant PR interval.

ARRHYTHMIA AND FEATURES	CAUSES	TREATMENT
Sinus arrhythmia • Irregular atrial and ventricular rhythms • Normal P wave preceding each QRS complex	• A normal variation of normal sinus rhythm in athletes, children, and elderly people • Also seen in digoxin toxicity and inferior wall myocardial infarction (MI)	• Atropine if rate decreases below 40 beats/minute and the patient is symptomatic
Sinus tachycardia 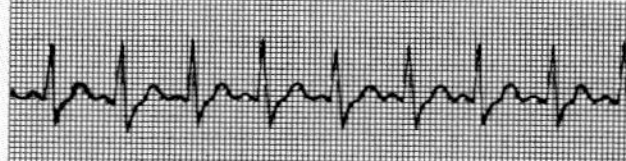 • Atrial and ventricular rhythms regular • Rate > 100 beats/minute; rarely, > 160 beats/minute • Normal P wave preceding each QRS complex	• Normal physiologic response to fever, exercise, anxiety, pain, dehydration; may also accompany shock, left ventricular failure, cardiac tamponade, hyperthyroidism, anemia, hypovolemia, pulmonary embolism, and anterior wall MI • May also occur with atropine, epinephrine, isoproterenol, quinidine, caffeine, alcohol, and nicotine use	• Correction of underlying cause • Beta-adrenergic blockers or calcium channel blockers for symptomatic patients
Sinus bradycardia 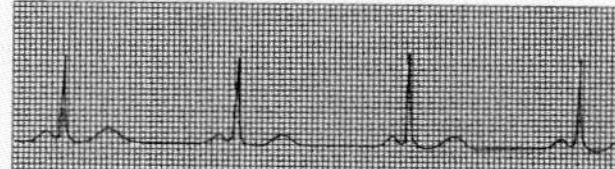 • Atrial and ventricular rhythms regular • Rate < 60 beats/minute • Normal P waves preceding each QRS complex	• Normal, in well-conditioned heart, as in an athlete • Increased intracranial pressure; increased vagal tone due to straining during defecation, vomiting, intubation, mechanical ventilation; sick sinus syndrome, hypothyroidism; inferior wall MI • May also occur with anticholinesterase, beta-adrenergic blocker, digoxin, and morphine use	• Correction of underlying cause • For low cardiac output, dizziness, weakness, altered level of consciousness, or low blood pressure; advanced cardiac life support (ACLS) protocol for administration of atropine • Temporary pacemaker or permanent pacemaker • Dopamine or epinephrine infusion

Types of cardiac arrhythmias *(continued)*

ARRHYTHMIA AND FEATURES	CAUSES	TREATMENT
Sinoatrial arrest or block (sinus arrest) 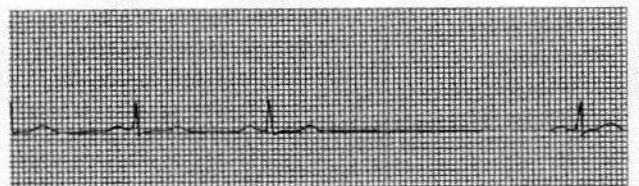 • Atrial and ventricular rhythms regular except for missing complex • Normal P waves preceding each QRS complex, missing during pause • Pause not equal to a multiple of the previous sinus rhythm	• Acute infection • Coronary artery disease, degenerative heart disease, acute inferior wall MI • Vagal stimulation, Valsalva's maneuver, carotid sinus massage • Digoxin, quinidine, or salicylate toxicity • Pesticide poisoning • Pharyngeal irritation caused by endotracheal (ET) intubation • Sick sinus syndrome	• Correction of underlying cause • Treat symptoms with atropine I.V. • Temporary or permanent pacemaker for repeated episodes
Wandering atrial pacemaker 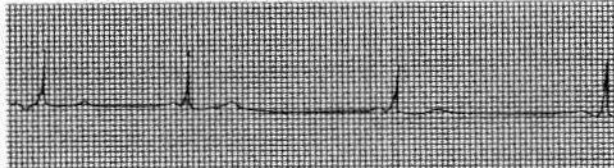 • Atrial and ventricular rhythms slightly irregular • PR interval varies • P waves irregular with changing configuration, indicating that they're not all from sinoatrial (SA) node or single atrial focus; may appear after the QRS complex • QRS complexes uniform in shape but irregular in rhythm	• Rheumatic carditis due to inflammation involving the SA node • Digoxin toxicity • Sick sinus syndrome	• No treatment if patient is asymptomatic • Treatment of underlying cause if patient is symptomatic
Premature atrial contraction (PAC) 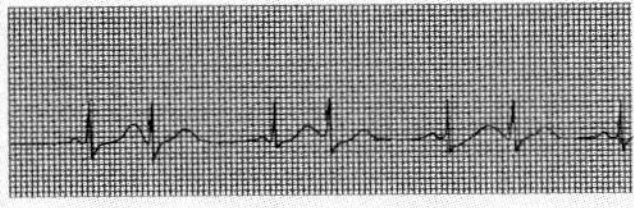 • Premature, abnormal-looking P waves that differ in configuration from normal P waves • QRS complexes after P waves, except in very early or blocked PACs • P wave often buried in the preceding T wave or identified in the preceding T wave	• Coronary or valvular heart disease, atrial ischemia, coronary atherosclerosis, heart failure, acute respiratory failure, chronic obstructive pulmonary disease (COPD), electrolyte imbalance, and hypoxia • Digoxin toxicity; use of aminophylline, adrenergics, or caffeine • Anxiety	• Usually no treatment needed • Treatment of underlying cause

(continued)

ECG characteristics: Sinoatrial arrest or block

- Atrial and ventricular rhythms regular except for missing complex
- Normal P waves preceding each QRS complex, missing during pause
- Pause not equal to a multiple of the previous sinus rhythm

ECG characteristics: Wandering atrial pacemaker

- Atrial and ventricular rhythms slightly irregular
- PR interval varies
- P waves irregular with changing configuration, indicating that they aren't all from sinoatrial node or single atrial focus; may appear after the QRS complex
- QRS complexes uniform in shape but irregular in rhythm

ECG characteristics: Premature atrial contraction

- Premature, abnormal-looking P waves that differ in configuration from normal P waves
- QRS complexes after P waves, except in very early or blocked PACs
- P wave often buried in the preceding T wave or identified in the preceding T wave

ECG characteristics: Paroxysmal supraventricular tachycardia

- Atrial and ventricular rhythms regular
- Heart rate > 160 beats/minute; rarely exceeds 250 beats/minute
- P waves regular but aberrant; difficult to differentiate from preceding T wave
- P wave preceding each QRS complex
- Sudden onset and termination of arrhythmia

ECG characteristics: Atrial flutter

- Atrial rhythm regular, rate 250 to 400 beats/minute
- Ventricular rate variable, depending on degree of AV block (usually 60 to 100 beats/minute)
- Sawtooth P-wave configuration possible (F waves)
- QRS complexes uniform in shape but often irregular in rate

ECG characteristics: Atrial fibrillation

- Atrial rhythm grossly irregular; rate > 400 beats/minute
- Ventricular rate grossly irregular
- QRS complexes of uniform configuration and duration
- PR interval indiscernible
- No P waves, or P waves that appear as erratic, irregular, baseline fibrillatory waves

Types of cardiac arrhythmias *(continued)*

ARRHYTHMIA AND FEATURES	CAUSES	TREATMENT
Paroxysmal supraventricular tachycardia 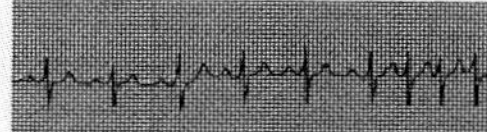 • Atrial and ventricular rhythms regular • Heart rate > 160 beats/minute; rarely exceeds 250 beats/minute • P waves regular but aberrant; difficult to differentiate from preceding T wave • P wave preceding each QRS complex • Sudden onset and termination of arrhythmia	• Intrinsic abnormality of atrioventricular (AV) conduction system • Physical or psychological stress, hypoxia, hypokalemia, cardiomyopathy, congenital heart disease, MI, valvular disease, Wolff-Parkinson-White syndrome, cor pulmonale, hyperthyroidism, and systemic hypertension • Digoxin toxicity; use of caffeine, marijuana, or central nervous system stimulants	• If patient is unstable: immediate cardioversion • If patient is stable: vagal stimulation, Valsalva's manuever, and carotid sinus massage • If cardiac function is preserved, treatment priority: calcium channel blocker, beta-adrenergic blocker, digoxin, and cardioversion; then consider procainamide, amiodarone, or sotalol if each preceding treatment is ineffective in rhythm conversion • If the ejection fraction is less than 40% or if the patient is in heart failure, treatment order: digoxin, amiodarone, then diltiazem.
Atrial flutter 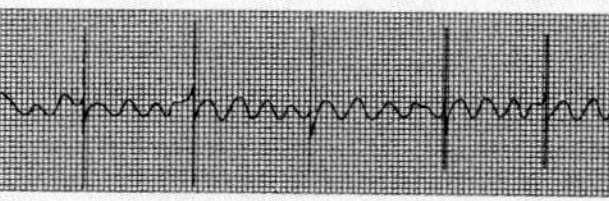 • Atrial rhythm regular, rate 250 to 400 beats/minute • Ventricular rate variable, depending on degree of AV block (usually 60 to 100 beats/minute) • Sawtooth P-wave configuration possible (F waves) • QRS complexes uniform in shape but often irregular in rate	• Heart failure, tricuspid or mitral valve disease, pulmonary embolism, cor pulmonale, inferior wall MI, and carditis • Digoxin toxicity	• If patient is unstable with a ventricular rate > 150 beats/minute, immediate cardioversion. • If patient is stable, drug therapy may include calcium channel blockers, diltiazem, beta-adrenergic blockers, or antiarrhythmics. • Anticoagulation therapy (heparin, enoxparin [Lovenox], or warfarin) may also be necessary • Radiofrequency ablation to control rhythm
Atrial fibrillation 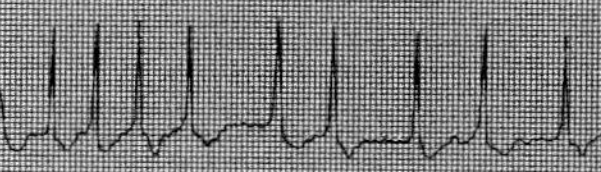 • Atrial rhythm grossly irregular; rate > 400 beats/minute • Ventricular rate grossly irregular • QRS complexes of uniform configuration and duration • PR interval indiscernible • No P waves, or P waves that appear as erratic, irregular, baseline fibrillatory waves	• Heart failure, COPD, thyrotoxicosis, constrictive pericarditis, ischemic heart disease, sepsis, pulmonary embolus, rheumatic heart disease, hypertension, mitral stenosis, atrial irritation, complication of coronary bypass or valve replacement surgery • Nifedipine and digoxin use	• If patient is unstable with a ventricular rate > 150 beats/minute, immediate cardioversion. • If patient is stable, follow ACLS protocol for cardioversion and drug therapy which may include calcium channel blockers, beta-adrenergic blockers, or antiarrhythmics • Anticoagulants, such as heparin, enoxaparin, or warfarin

Types of cardiac arrhythmias *(continued)*

ARRHYTHMIA AND FEATURES	CAUSES	TREATMENT
Atrial fibrillation *(continued)*		• Class III antiarrhythmic, dofetilide (Tikosyn) for conversion of atrial fibrillation and atrial flutter to normal sinus rhythm • Radiofrequency catheter ablation to the His bundle to interrupt all conduction between atria and the ventricles (in resistant patients with recurring symptomatic atrial fibrillation) • Maze procedure in which sutures are placed in stragetic places in the atrial myocardium to prevent electrical circuits from developing perpetuating atrial fibrillation
Premature junctional contractions (junctional premature beats) 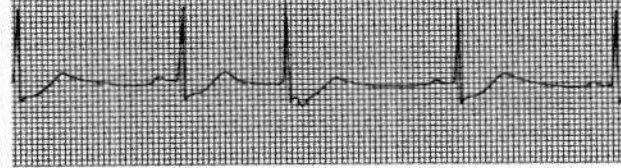 • Atrial and ventricular rhythms irregular • P waves inverted; may precede, be hidden within, or follow QRS complex • PR interval < 0.12 second if P wave precedes QRS complex • QRS complex configuration and duration normal	• MI or ischemia • Digoxin toxicity and excessive caffeine or amphetamine use	• Correction of underlying cause • Discontinuation of digoxin if appropriate
Junctional rhythm 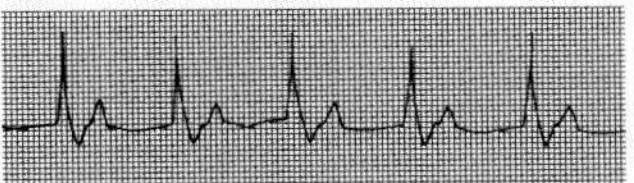 • Atrial and ventricular rhythms regular; atrial rate 40 to 60 beats/minute; ventricular rate usually 40 to 60 beats/minute (60 to 100 beats/minute is accelerated junctional rhythm) • P waves preceding, hidden within (absent), or after QRS complex; inverted if visible • PR interval (when present) < 0.12 second • QRS complex configuration and duration normal, except in aberrant conduction	• Inferior wall MI or ischemia, hypoxia, vagal stimulation, sick sinus syndrome • Acute rheumatic fever • Valve surgery • Digoxin toxicity	• Correction of underlying cause • Atropine for symptomatic slow rate • Pacemaker insertion if patient doesn't respond to drugs • Discontinuation of digoxin if appropriate

(continued)

ECG characteristics: Premature junctional contractions

- Atrial and ventricular rhythms irregular
- P waves inverted; may precede, be hidden within, or follow QRS complex
- PR Interval < 0.12 second if P wave precedes QRS complex
- QRS complex configuration and duration normal

ECG characteristics: Junctional rhythm

- Atrial and ventricular rhythms regular; atrial rate 40 to 60 beats/minute; ventricular rate usually 40 to 60 beats/minute (60 to 100 beats/minute is accelerated junctional rhythm)
- P waves preceding, hidden within (absent), or after QRS complex; inverted if visible
- PR interval (when present) < 0.12 second
- QRS complex configuration and duration normal, except in aberrant conduction

ECG characteristics: Junctional tachycardia

- Atrial and ventricular rhythms regular
- Atrial rate > 100 beats/minute
- Ventricular rate > 100 beats/minute
- P wave inverted; may occur before or after QRS complex, may be hidden in QRS complex, or may be absent
- QRS complex configuration and duration normal

ECG characteristics: First-degree AV block

- Atrial and ventricular rhythms regular
- PR interval > 0.20 second
- P wave precedes QRS complex
- QRS complex normal

ECG characteristics: Second-degree AV block (Mobitz I)

- Atrial rhythm regular
- Ventricular rhythm irregular
- Atrial rate exceeds ventricular rate
- PR interval progressively longer with each cycle until QRS complex disappears; PR interval shorter after dropped beat

ECG characteristics: Second-degree AV block (Mobitz II)

- Atrial rhythm regular
- Ventricular rhythm regular or irregular; varying degree of block
- PR interval constant except with dropped beat
- QRS complexes periodically absent

Types of cardiac arrhythmias *(continued)*

ARRHYTHMIA AND FEATURES	CAUSES	TREATMENT
Junctional tachycardia 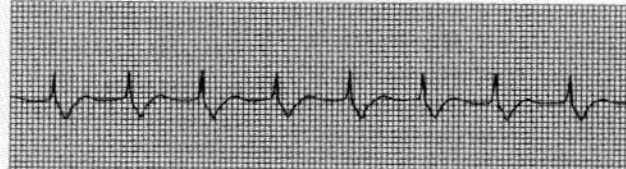 • Atrial and ventricular rhythms regular • Atrial rate > 100 beats/minute; however, P waves may be absent, hidden in QRS complex, or preceding T wave • Ventricular rate > 100 beats/minute • P wave inverted; may occur before or after QRS complex, may be hidden in QRS complex, or may be absent • QRS complex configuration and duration normal	• Myocarditis, cardiomyopathy, inferior wall MI or ischemia, acute rheumatic fever, complication of valve replacement surgery • Digoxin toxicity	• Correction of underlying cause • Beta-adrenergic blockers, calcium channel blockers, or amiodarone • Discontinuation of digoxin if appropriate
First-degree AV block 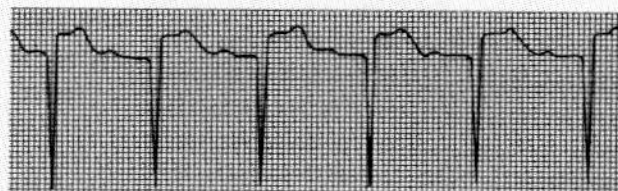 • Atrial and ventricular rhythms regular • PR interval > 0.20 second • P wave precedes QRS complex • QRS complex normal	• May be seen in a healthy person • Inferior wall MI or ischemia, hypothyroidism, hypokalemia, hyperkalemia • Digoxin toxicity; use of quinidine, procainamide, or beta-adrenergic or calcium channel blockers, or amiodarone	• Correction of underlying cause • Possibly atropine if severe bradycardia develops, and the patient is symptomatic • Cautious use of digoxin, calcium channel blockers, and beta-adrenergic blockers
Second-degree AV block Mobitz I (Wenckebach) 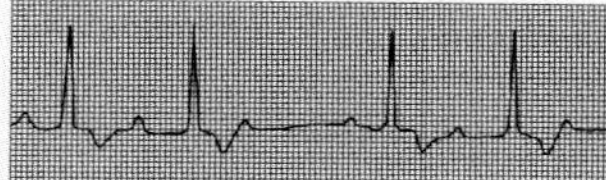 • Atrial rhythm regular • Ventricular rhythm irregular • Atrial rate exceeds ventricular rate • PR interval progressively longer, but only slightly, with each cycle until QRS complex disappears (dropped beat); PR interval shorter after dropped beat	• Inferior wall MI, cardiac surgery, acute rheumatic fever, and vagal stimulation • Digoxin toxicity; use of propranolol, quinidine, or procainamide	• Treatment of underlying cause • Atropine or temporary pacemaker for symptomatic bradycardia • Discontinuation of digoxin if appropriate
Second-degree AV block Mobitz II 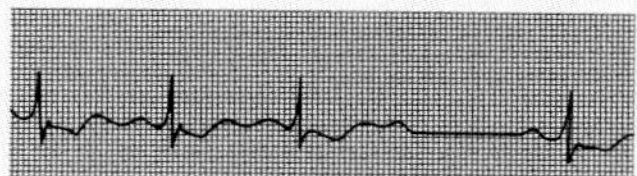 • Atrial rhythm regular • Ventricular rhythm regular or irregular, with varying degree of block • PR interval constant, except with dropped beat • QRS complexes periodically absent	• Severe coronary artery disease, anterior wall MI, acute myocarditis • Digoxin toxicity	• Temporary or permanent pacemaker • Atropine, dopamine, or epinephrine for symptomatic bradycardia • Discontinuation of digoxin if appropriate

Types of cardiac arrhythmias *(continued)*

ARRHYTHMIA AND FEATURES	CAUSES	TREATMENT
Third-degree AV block (complete heart block) 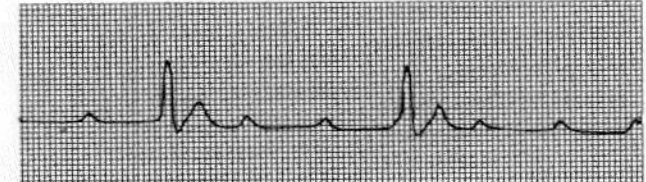 • Atrial rhythm regular • Ventricular rate slow and rhythm regular • No relation between P waves and QRS complexes • No constant PR interval • QRS interval normal (nodal pacemaker) or wide and bizarre (ventricular pacemaker) rates regular • PR interval varies • P wave may be buried in QRS complexes or T wave • QRS complex normal	• Inferior or anterior wall MI, congenital abnormality, rheumatic fever, hypoxia, postoperative complication of mitral valve replacement, Lev's disease (fibrosis and calcification that spreads from cardiac structures to the conductive tissue), Lenegre's disease (conductive tissue fibrosis) • Digoxin toxicity	• Atropine, dopamine, or epinephrine for symptomatic bradycardia • Temporary or permanent pacemaker
Premature ventricular contraction (PVC) 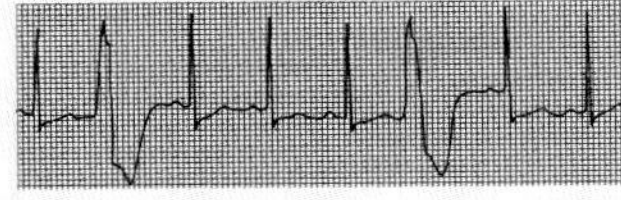 • Atrial rhythm regular • Ventricular rhythm irregular • QRS complex premature, usually followed by a complete compensatory pause • QRS complex wide and distorted, usually > 0.14 second • Premature QRS complexes occurring singly, in pairs, or in threes, alternating with normal beats; focus from one or more sites • Ominous when clustered, multifocal, with R wave on T pattern	• Heart failure; old or acute MI, ischemia, or contusion; myocardial irritation by ventricular catheter or a pacemaker; hypercapnia; hypokalemia; hypocalcemia • Drug toxicity (cardiac glycosides, aminophylline, tricyclic antidepressants, beta-adrenergic blockers [isoproterenol or dopamine]) • Caffeine, tobacco, or alcohol use • Psychological stress, anxiety, pain, exercise	• If warranted, procainamide, lidocaine, or amiodarone I.V. • Treatment of underlying cause • Discontinuation of drug causing toxicity • Potassium chloride I.V. if PVC induced by hypokalemia • Magnesium sulfate I.V. if PVC induced by hypomagnesemia

(continued)

ECG characteristics: Third-degree AV block

- Atrial rhythm regular
- Ventricular rate slow and rhythm regular
- No relation between P waves and QRS complexes
- No constant PR interval
- QRS interval normal (nodal pacemaker) or wide and bizarre (ventricular pacemaker) rates regular
- PR interval varies
- P wave may be buried in QRS complexes or T wave
- QRS complex normal

ECG characteristics: PVC

- Atrial rhythm regular
- Ventricular rhythm irregular
- QRS complex premature, usually followed by a complete compensatory pause
- QRS complex wide and distorted, usually > 0.14 second
- Premature QRS complexes occurring singly, in pairs, or in threes, alternating with normal beats; focus from one or more sites
- Ominous when clustered, multifocal, with R wave on T pattern

ECG characteristics: Ventricular tachycardia

- Ventricular rate 140 to 220 beats/minute, rhythm regular or irregular
- QRS complexes wide, bizarre, and independent of P waves
- P waves not discernible
- May start and stop suddenly

ECG characteristics: Ventricular fibrillation

- Ventricular rhythm chaotic; rate rapid
- QRS complexes wide and irregular; no visible P waves

Types of cardiac arrhythmias *(continued)*

ARRHYTHMIA AND FEATURES	CAUSES	TREATMENT
Ventricular tachycardia 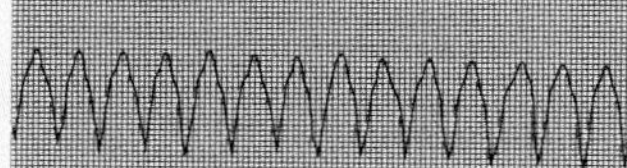 • Ventricular rate 140 to 220 beats/minute, rhythm regular or irregular • QRS complexes wide, bizarre, and independent of P waves • P waves not discernible • May start and stop suddenly	• Myocardial ischemia, infarction, or aneurysm; coronary artery disease; rheumatic heart disease; mitral valve prolapse; heart failure; cardiomyopathy; ventricular catheters; hypokalemia; hypercalcemia; pulmonary embolism • Digoxin, procainamide, epinephrine, or quinidine toxicity • Anxiety	• Pulseless: Initiate cardiopulmonary resuscitation (CPR); follow ACLS protocol for defibrillation, ET intubation, and administration of epinephrine or vasopressin, followed by amiodarone or lidocaine; if ineffective, magnesium sulfate or procainamide. • With pulse: If hemodynamically stable monomorphic VT follow ACLS protocol for administration of procainamide, sotalol, amiodarone, or lidocaine; if drugs are ineffective, initiate synchronized cardioversion. • If polymorphic VT, follow ACLS protocol for administration of beta-adrenergic blockers, lidocaine, amiodarone, procainamide, or sotalol. If drugs are ineffective, initiate synchronized cardioversion. • If torsades: administer magnesium, then overdose pacing if rythm perisists; isoproterenol, phenytoin, or lidocaine may also be given. • Implanted cardioverter defibrillator if recurrent VT
Ventricular fibrillation 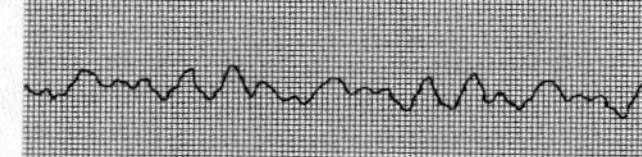 • Ventricular rhythm chaotic; rate rapid • QRS complexes wide and irregular; no visible P waves	• Myocardial ischemia or infarction, untreated ventricular tachycardia, R-on-T phenomenon, hypokalemia, hyperkalemia, hypercalcemia, alkalosis, electric shock, hypothermia • Digoxin, epinephrine, or quinidine toxicity	• Pulseless: Initiate CPR; follow ACLS protocol for defibrillation, ET intubation, and administration of epinephrine or vasopressin, followed by lidocaine or amiodarone; if ineffective, magnesium sulfate or procainamide. • Implantable cardioverter defibrillator if risk for recurrent ventricular fibrillation

Types of cardiac arrhythmias *(continued)*

ARRHYTHMIA AND FEATURES	CAUSES	TREATMENT
Asystole • No atrial or ventricular rate or rhythm • No discernible P waves, QRS complexes, or T waves	• Myocardial ischemia or infarction, aortic valve disease, heart failure, hypoxia, hypokalemia, severe acidosis, electric shock, ventricular arrhythmia, AV block, pulmonary embolism, heart rupture, cardiac tamponade, hyperkalemia, electromechanical dissociation • Cocaine overdose	• Continue CPR, follow ACLS protocol for ET intubation, transcutaneous pacing, administration of epinephrine and atropine

- Individualize home care instructions
  - Know the signs and symptoms of an arrhythmia to report
  - Take pulse regularly and report abnormal values
  - Understand all procedures, such as pacemaker insertion

Complications
- Death
- Stroke
- MI
- Hypotension
- Heart failure
- Shock

Possible surgical interventions
- Pacemaker insertion
- Catheter ablation therapy
- Endocardial resection

PERICARDITIS

Definition
- Inflammation of the pericardium, the fibrous sac that envelops, supports, and protects the heart

Causes
- Bacterial, fungal, or viral infection
- Neoplasms (primary or metastases from lungs, breasts, or other organs)
- High dose radiation to the chest
- Hypersensitivity or autoimmune disease, such as acute rheumatic fever (most common cause of pericarditis in children)
- Medications, such as hydralazine or procainamide

ECG characteristics: Asystole
- No atrial or ventricular rate or rhythm
- No discernible P waves, QRS complexes, or T waves

Key facts about pericarditis
- Inflammation of the pericardium
- May be fibrinous or effusive
- Caused by an attack by a pathogen or other substance that starts the inflammatory response

Common causes of pericarditis
- Bacterial, fungal, or viral infection
- Neoplasms (primary or metastases from lungs, breasts, or other organs)
- Postcardiac injury such as MI

- Postcardiac injury, such as MI (which later causes an autoimmune reaction in the pericardium), trauma, and surgery that leaves the pericardium intact but allows blood to leak into the pericardial cavity
- Aortic aneurysm with pericardial leakage (less common)
- Myxedema with cholesterol deposits in the pericardium (less common)

Pathophysiology

- A pathogen or other substance attacks the pericardium starting the inflammatory response
- Acute pericarditis may be fibrinous or effusive, with serous, purulent, or hemorrhagic exudate
- Chronic pericarditis (also called constrictive pericarditis) is characterized by dense, fibrous pericardial thickening

Assessment findings

- Acute pericarditis
  - Sharp, usually sudden pain over the sternum, radiating to the neck, shoulders, back, and arms
  - Pain increases with deep inspiration or when lying down and decreases when sitting up and leaning forward
  - Pericardial friction rub
  - Distant heart sounds
  - Increased cardiac dullness
  - Diminished or absent apical impulse
- Chronic pericarditis
  - Increased systemic venous pressure
  - Signs similar to chronic right-sided heart failure, including fluid retention, ascites, and hepatomegaly

Diagnostic test findings

- Hematologic studies: WBC may normal or elevated, especially in infectious pericarditis; ESR is elevated
- Blood chemistries: Serum CK-MB levels are slightly elevated with associated myocarditis; BUN levels detect uremia
- Serologic testing: antistreptolysin-O titers detect rheumatic fever
- Skin testing: purified protein derivative skin test detects tuberculosis
- Cultures: pericardial fluid culture may identify causative organism in bacterial or fungal pericarditis
- ECG: elevated ST segments; QRS segments may be diminished with pericardial effusion; rhythm changes may occur, including atrial ectopic rhythms, such as atrial fibrillation and sinus arrhythmia
- Echocardiography: detects pericarditis and pericardial effusion

Medical management

- Bed rest as long as fever and pain persist
- Nonsteroidal anti-inflammatory drugs: aspirin, indomethacin (Indocin)
- Corticosteroids, if the cause isn't tuberculosis
- Antibiotics: depending on causative organism
- Surgical drainage

Pain associated with acute pericarditis

- Sharp, usually sudden pain over the sternum
- Radiates to the neck, shoulders, back, and arms
- Increases with deep inspiration or when lying down
- Decreases when sitting up and leaning forward

Key pericarditis diagnostic test findings

- ECG
  - Elevated ST segments
  - QRS segments may be diminished with pericardial effusion
  - Rhythm changes may occur, including atrial ectopic rhythms, such as atrial fibrillation and sinus arrhythmia
- Echocardiography
  - Detects pericarditis and pericardial effusion

Key ways to manage pericarditis medically

- Bed rest as long as fever and pain persist
- Nonsteroidal anti-inflammatory drugs
- Corticosteroids
- Antibiotics

- Pericardiocentesis
- Oxygen therapy
- Pericardectomy

Nursing interventions
- Maintain complete bed rest
- Assess pain and provide analgesics if necessary
- Assess cardiovascular and respiratory status
- Administer I.V. fluids, oxygen, and medications, as prescribed
- Place the patient in an upright position
- Monitor and record vital signs, I/O, and hemodynamic variables
- Provide reassurance and explain all test, procedures, and treatments
- Monitor for signs of cardiac compression and cardiac tamponade, such as decreased blood pressure, increased CVP, and pulsus paradoxus
- Individualize home care instructions
  - Take medications, as ordered
  - Follow activity restrictions
  - Report signs and symptoms of pericarditis, pericardial effusion, and cardiac tamponade to physician immediately

Complications
- Pericardial effusion
- Heart failure
- Chronic right-sided heart failure
- Cardiac tamponade

Possible surgical intervention
- Pericardectomy

ARTERIAL OCCLUSIVE DISEASE

Definition
- Obstruction or narrowing of the aorta's lumen and its major branches, causing an interruption of blood flow, usually to the legs and feet

Causes and risk factors
- Causes
  - Atherosclerosis
  - Emboli
  - Thrombosis
  - Trauma or fracture
- Risk factors
  - Age
  - Diabetes
  - Family history of vascular disorders, MI, or stroke
  - Hyperlipidemia
  - Hypertension
  - Smoking

Key nursing interventions for a patient with pericarditis

- Maintain complete bed rest.
- Place the patient in an upright position.
- Monitor and record vital signs, I/O, and hemodynamic variables.
- Assess pain and provide analgesics, if necessary.

Key facts about arterial occlusive disease

- Obstruction or narrowing of the aorta's lumen and it's major branches that causes an interruption of blood flow
- Reduced perfusion results in tissue ischemia, skin ulceration, and gangrene
- Obstruction may be endogenous or exogenous

Causes of arterial occlusive disease

- Atherosclerosis
- Emboli
- Thrombosis
- Trauma or fracture

Key assessment findings in arterial occlusive disease

- Femoral, popliteal, or innominate arteries
  - Decreased pulses distal to the occlusion
  - Mottling and pallor of the extremity
  - Paralysis and paresthesia in the affected extremity
  - Sudden and localized pain in the affected extremity (most common symptom)
- Internal and external carotid arteries
  - Stroke
  - TIA
- Subclavian artery
  - Subclavian steal syndrome
- Vertebral and basilar arteries
  - TIA

Arteriography findings in a patient with arterial occlusive disease

- The type (thrombus or embolus), location, and degree of obstruction
- Collateral circulation

Pathophysiology

- Occlusive mechanism may be endogenous, due to emboli formation or thrombosis, or exogenous, due to trauma or fracture
- Arteries unable to respond to increased needs related to physical activity or sympathetic nervous system responses
- Reduced perfusion results in tissue ischemia, skin ulceration, and gangrene
- May affect carotid, vertebral, innominate, subclavian, mesenteric, celiac, femoral, and popliteal arteries

Assessment findings

- Femoral, popliteal, or innominate arteries
  - Decreased pulses distal to the occlusion
  - Mottling of the extremity
  - Pallor
  - Paralysis and paresthesia in the affected arm or leg
  - Sudden and localized pain in the affected arm or leg (most common symptom)
  - Temperature change that occurs distal to the occlusion
- Internal and external carotid arteries
  - Absent or decreased pulsation with an auscultatory bruit over affected arteries
  - Stroke
  - Transient ischemic attacks (TIAs)
- Subclavian artery
  - Subclavian steal syndrome (characterized by the backflow of blood from the brain through the vertebral artery on the same side as the occlusion, into the subclavian artery distal to the occlusion; clinical effects of vertebrobasilar occlusion and exercise-induced arm claudication)
- Vertebral and basilar arteries
  - TIAs

Diagnostic test findings

- Arteriography: demonstrates the type (thrombus or embolus), location, and degree of obstruction, and the collateral circulation
- Doppler ultrasonography and plethysmography: show decreased blood flow distal to the occlusion in acute disease
- EEG and computed tomography scan: to rule out brain lesions
- Ophthalmodynamometry: Determines the degree of obstruction in the internal carotid artery by comparing ophthalmic artery pressure to brachial artery pressure on the affected side

Medical management

- Diet: low-cholesterol
- Antilipemics: lovastatin (Mevacor), pravastatin (Pravachol), simvastatin (Zocor)
- Antiplatelets: aspirin, ticlopidine (Ticlid), clopidogrel (Plavix)
- Pentoxifylline (Trental)

- Anticoagulants: heparin, warfarin (Coumadin)
- Thrombolytics: alteplase (Activase), streptokinase (Streptase), urokinase (Abbokinase)
- Surgery: atherectomy, balloon angioplasty, bypass grafting, embolectomy, laser angioplasty, patch grafting, stent placement, thromboendarterectomy, or amputation
- Smoking cessation
- Activity: walking

Nursing interventions

- Assess distal pulses, skin color, and temperature
- Assess pain and provide pain relief as needed
- Assist the patient to gradually increase activity as tolerated
- Maintain prescribed diet
- Administer I.V. fluids, oxygen, and medications, as prescribed
- Monitor and record vital signs, I/O, laboratory values, and hemodynamic variables
- Monitor the patient with carotid, innominate, vertebral, or subclavian artery occlusion for signs of stroke

Key medications used to manage a patient with arterial occlusive disease

- Antilipemics
- Antiplatelets
- Pentoxifylline
- Anticoagulants
- Thrombolytics

Key nursing interventions for a patient with arterial occlusive disease

- Assess distal pulses, skin color, and temperature.
- Assess pain and provide pain relief as needed.
- Administer I.V. fluids, oxygen, and medications, as prescribed.
- Monitor the patient with carotid, innominate, vertebral, or subclavian artery occlusion for signs of stroke.

NCLEX CHECKS

It's never too soon to begin your NCLEX preparation. Now that you've reviewed this chapter, carefully read each of the following questions and choose the best answer. Then compare your responses to the correct answers.

1. While auscultating the heart sounds of a patient with mitral insufficiency, the nurse hears an extra heart sound immediately after the second heart sound (S_2). The nurse should document this extra heart sound as a:

☐ **A.** first heart sound (S_1).
☐ **B.** third heart sound (S_3).
☐ **C.** fourth heart sound (S_4).
☐ **D.** mitral murmur.

2. The nurse administers warfarin (Coumadin) to a patient with deep vein thrombophlebitis. Which laboratory value should the nurse monitor to determine the effectiveness of warfarin?

☐ **A.** Partial thromboplastin time (PTT)
☐ **B.** Hematocrit (HCT)
☐ **C.** Complete blood count (CBC)
☐ **D.** Prothrombin time (PT)

3. A patient has just returned from cardiac catheterization. Which nursing intervention would be most appropriate?

☐ **A.** Assist the patient to ambulate to the bathroom.
☐ **B.** Restrict fluids.
☐ **C.** Monitor peripheral pulses.
☐ **D.** Insert an indwelling urinary catheter.

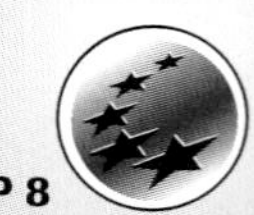

TOP 8

Items to study for your next test on the cardiovascular system

1. Myocardial blood supply
2. Cardiac conduction system
3. Significance of assessment findings, such as chest pain, edema, and blood pressure changes
4. Patient preparation and postoperative care for diagnostic procedures such as cardiac catheterization
5. Modifiable and nonmodifiable risk factors for developing cardiovascular disorders
6. Patient preparation and postoperative care for surgical procedures, such as coronary artery bypass grafting, aneurysm repair, and pacemaker insertion
7. Medical management and nursing interventions for key disorders, such as CAD, hypertension, heart failure, and MI
8. Patient teaching points

4. A patient is in the first postoperative day following left femoropopliteal revascularization. Which position would be most appropriate for this patient?

☐ **A.** On his left side
☐ **B.** In high Fowler's position
☐ **C.** On his right side
☐ **D.** In a left lateral decubitus position

5. The nurse is admitting a patient with left-sided heart failure. Which finding would the nurse expect to assess?

☐ **A.** Ascites
☐ **B.** Dyspnea
☐ **C.** Hepatomegaly
☐ **D.** Jugular vein distention

6. A patient has developed acute pulmonary edema. Which test result should the nurse expect?

☐ **A.** Interstitial edema by chest X-ray
☐ **B.** Metabolic alkalosis by arterial blood gas (ABG) analysis
☐ **C.** Bradycardia by electrocardiogram (ECG)
☐ **D.** Decreased pulmonary artery wedge pressure (PAWP) by hemodynamic monitoring

7. The nurse is performing discharge teaching for a patient with peripheral vascular disease. The nurse should teach the patient to:

☐ **A.** inspect his feet weekly.
☐ **B.** begin a daily walking program.
☐ **C.** wear constrictive clothing.
☐ **D.** stand when possible, rather than sit.

8. If the nurse knows the patient's heart rate, what other value does she need to know to determine cardiac output? ______________________

ANSWERS AND RATIONALES

1. CORRECT ANSWER: B

An S_3 is heard following an S_2. This indicates that the patient is experiencing heart failure and results from increased filling pressures. An S_1 is a normal heart sound made by the closing of the mitral and tricuspid valves. An S_4 is heard before S_1 and is caused by resistance to ventricular filling. A murmur of mitral insufficiency occurs during systole and is heard when there's turbulent blood flow across the valve.

2. CORRECT ANSWER: D

The therapeutic effectiveness of warfarin is determined by monitoring the patient's PT. PTT, HCT, and CBC don't monitor the therapeutic effectiveness of warfarin. Monitoring the PTT determines heparin's effectiveness.

3. CORRECT ANSWER: C

After cardiac catheterization, monitor the peripheral pulses to assess peripheral perfusion. Assisting the patient to ambulate to the bathroom is incorrect because the patient should be on bed rest for 4 to 8 hours after the procedure to reduce the risk of bleeding at the insertion site. Restricting fluids is incorrect because the patient should be encouraged to drink fluids after the procedure, unless contraindicated. Adequate hydration reduces the risk of nephrotoxicity that can occur with the use of contrast dye. Although urine output is monitored following cardiac catheterization, the insertion of a urinary catheter isn't necessary.

4. CORRECT ANSWER: C

Following revascularization, avoid positioning the patient on the surgical side. Because this patient had left femoropopliteal revascularization, he may be positioned on the right side. Placing the patient on the left side is incorrect because this would position the patient on the operative side. Positioning the patient in high Fowler's position is incorrect because the patient should avoid flexion at the surgical site. Placing the patient in a left lateral decubitus position is incorrect because this would place the patient on the surgical side and cause flexion at the site.

5. CORRECT ANSWER: B

Dyspnea may occur in a patient with left-sided heart failure. Ascites, hepatomegaly, and jugular vein distention are assessment findings in right-sided heart failure.

6. CORRECT ANSWER: A

The chest X-ray of a patient with acute pulmonary edema shows interstitial edema as a result of the heart's failure to pump adequately. Metabolic alkalosis is incorrect because the ABG analysis of a patient in acute pulmonary edema shows respiratory alkalosis or acidosis. Bradycardia is incorrect because the ECG would most likely indicate tachycardia. Decreased PAWP is incorrect because PAWP rises in the patient in acute pulmonary edema.

7. CORRECT ANSWER: B

The nurse should encourage the patient with peripheral vascular disease to follow a program of walking and other leg exercises. Inspecting the feet weekly is incorrect because the nurse should teach the patient to inspect his feet daily. Wearing constrictive clothing is incorrect because the patient should wear loose clothing that doesn't restrict circulation. Standing when possible — rather than sitting — is incorrect because the patient should avoid standing for long periods of time.

8. CORRECT ANSWER: STROKE VOLUME

Cardiac output equals stroke volume (the amount of blood ejected with each beat) times heart rate.

2

Respiratory system

LEARNING OBJECTIVES

After studying this chapter, you should be able to:

- Describe the psychosocial impact of respiratory disorders.
- Differentiate between modifiable and nonmodifiable risk factors in the development of a respiratory disorder.
- List three probable and three possible nursing diagnoses for a patient with any respiratory disorder.
- Identify the nursing interventions for a patient with a respiratory disorder.
- Write three goals for teaching a patient with a respiratory disorder.

CHAPTER OVERVIEW

Caring for the patient with a respiratory disorder requires a sound understanding of respiratory anatomy and physiology as well as the diffusion of oxygen. A thorough assessment is essential to planning and implementing appropriate care. The assessment should include a complete history, a physical examination, diagnostic testing, identification of modifiable and nonmodifiable risk factors, and information related to the psychosocial impact of respiratory dysfunction on the patient.

Nursing diagnoses focus primarily on ineffective breathing patterns and impaired gas exchange. Patient teaching — a crucial nursing activity — involves giving the patient information about medical follow-up, medication regimens, signs and symptoms of possible complications, and reducing modifiable risk factors (avoiding people with infections, activity and diet restrictions, stress management, and smoking cessation).

ANATOMY AND PHYSIOLOGY REVIEW

- **Nares**
  - Filter out particles
  - Humidify inspired air
  - Contain olfactory receptor sites
- **Paranasal sinuses**
  - Air-filled, cilia-lined cavities
  - Function: to trap particles
- **Pharynx**
  - Serves as a passageway to digestive and respiratory tracts
  - Maintains air pressure in the middle ear
  - Contains a mucosal lining that humidifies and warms inspired air and traps particles
- **Larynx**
  - Known as the "voice box"
  - Connects the upper and lower airways
  - Contains vocal cords that produce sounds and initiate the cough reflex
- **Trachea**
  - Consists of smooth muscle
  - Contains C-shaped cartilaginous rings
  - Connects the larynx to the bronchi
- **Bronchi and bronchioles**
  - Formed by branching of the trachea
  - Right main bronchus is slightly larger and more vertical than the left
  - Bronchioles branch into terminal bronchioles, which end in alveoli
- **Alveoli**
  - Clustered microscopic sacs enveloped by capillaries
  - Gases exchange in the alveoli
  - Coating of surfactant reduces surface tension to keep alveoli from collapsing
  - Diffusion of gases occurs across the alveolar-capillary membrane
- **Lungs**
  - Composed of three lobes on the right side and two lobes on the left side
  - Covered by pleura
  - Regulate air exchange by concentration gradient
- **Pleura**
  - Visceral pleura covers the lungs
  - Parietal pleura lines the thoracic cavity
  - Pleural fluid lubricates the pleura to reduce friction during respiration

Nares

- Filter out particles
- Humidify inspired air
- Contain olfactory receptor sites

Bronchi

- Formed by trachea branching
- Right main bronchus is slightly larger and more vertical than the left
- Bronchioles branch into terminal bronchioles

Alveoli

- Site of gas exchange
- Occurs across the alveolar-capilillary exchange

Lungs

- Three lobes on the right side
- Two lobes on the left side
- Covered by pleura
- Regulate air exchange

ASSESSMENT FINDINGS

History

- Difficulty breathing, shortness of breath, dyspnea
- Chest pain
- Voice change
- Dysphagia
- Fatigue
- Weight change
- Cough

Physical examination

- Respiratory system changes
  - Nasal flaring
  - Decreased respiratory excursion
  - Decreased diaphragmatic excursion
  - Accessory muscle use
  - Retractions
  - Heaving
- Sputum characteristics
- Clubbing of fingers
- Adventitious sounds: crackles, rhonchi, wheezing, and pleural friction rub (see *Abnormal breath sounds*)
- Fremitus
- Crepitus
- Pattern and character of respirations
- Shape of thoracic anatomy (such as barrel chest)
- Change in mentation
- Skin color and temperature

Key assessment findings indicating a respiratory disorder

- Dyspnea
- Fatigue
- Cough
- Accessory muscle use
- Retractions
- Heaving
- Adventitious sounds: crackles, rhonchi, wheezing, and pleural friction rub
- Pattern and character of respirations
- Change in mentation
- Skin color and temperature

DIAGNOSTIC TESTS AND PROCEDURES

Bronchoscopy

- Definition and purpose
  - Procedure using a bronchoscope for direct visualization of the trachea and bronchial tree
  - Allows physicians to take biopsies and perform deep tracheal suctioning
- Nursing interventions before the procedure
  - Withhold food and fluids
  - Allay the patient's anxiety
  - Explain the procedure and what to expect following the procedure
  - Place obtained written informed consent in the patient's chart
- Nursing interventions after the procedure
  - Check cough and gag reflexes — this minimizes the risk of aspiration
  - Assess sputum
  - Assess respiratory status
  - Withhold food and fluids until gag reflex returns
  - Check vasovagal response

Bronchoscopy

- Invasive test
- Allows for visualization of the trachea and bronchial tree
- Allows the physician to take biopsies
- Allows for deep tracheal suctioning
- Intervention: check cough and gag reflexes after procedure

Abnormal breath sounds

Characteristics of abnormal breath sounds are described here.

- *Crackles* – intermittent, nonmusical, crackling sounds heard during inspiration; classified as fine or coarse
- *Wheezes* – high-pitched sounds heard on exhalation that are caused by blocked airflow
- *Rhonchi* – low-pitched snoring or rattling sound heard primarily on exhalation
- *Stridor* – loud, high-pitched sound heard during inspiration
- *Pleural friction rub* – low-pitched, grating sound heard during inspiration and expiration; accompanied by pain

Chest X-ray

- Definition and purpose
  - Noninvasive examination
  - Radiographic picture of lung tissue
- Nursing interventions
  - Determine the patient's ability to inhale and hold breath
  - Ensure that the patient removes jewelry
  - Determine pregnancy status, for the female patient

Pulmonary angiography

- Definition and purpose
  - Procedure using an injection of a radiopaque dye through a catheter
  - Radiographic examination of the pulmonary circulation
- Nursing interventions before the procedure
  - **Note the patient's allergies to iodine, seafood, and radiopaque dyes**
  - Instruct the patient about possible flushing of the face or burning in the throat after the dye is injected
  - Place obtained written informed consent in the patient's chart
- Nursing interventions after the procedure
  - Assess neurovascular status
  - Check the insertion site for bleeding
  - Monitor for delayed allergic response

Sputum studies

- Definition and purpose
  - Laboratory test
  - Microscopic evaluation of sputum that includes culture and sensitivity, Gram stain, and acid-fast bacillus
- Nursing interventions
  - Obtain early-morning sterile specimen from suctioning or expectoration

Thoracentesis

- Definition and purpose
  - Procedure using needle aspiration of intrapleural fluid under local anesthesia
  - Specimen examination or removal of pleural fluid

Abnormal breath sounds found in respiratory disorders

- Crackles
- Wheezes
- Rhonchi
- Stridor
- Pleural friction rub

Chest X-ray

- Noninvasive test
- Provides radiographic picture of lung tissue
- Intervention: determine pregnancy status for the female patient

Pulmonary angiography

- Invasive test involving injection of radiopaque dye
- Allows for radiographic examination of pulmonary circulation
- Intervention: note allergies to iodine, seafood, and radiopaque dyes before test

Sputum studies

- Noninvasive laboratory test
- Microscopic evaluation of sputum: culture and sensitivity, Gram stain, and acid-fast bacillus
- Intervention: obtain early-morning sterile specimen

Thoracentesis

- Invasive procedure using needle aspiration
- Allows for removal of pleural fluid and specimen examination
- Intervention: place the patient in the proper position

PFTs

- Noninvasive test
- Measure lung volume, ventilation, and diffusing capacity
- Intervention: document bronchodilators or narcotics used before testing

ABG analysis

- Blood test
- Arterial blood measurements of tissue oxygenation, ventilation, acid-base status
- Intervention: apply pressure to puncture site for 5 minutes after procedure

Lung scan

- Invasive test involving inhalation or injection of radioisotopes
- Provides imaging of distribution and blood flow in lungs
- Interventions:
  - Assess for allergies to isotopes
  - Check catheter insertion site for bleeding after lung scan

Mantoux test

- Invasive test to detect TB antibodies
- Follow-up reading should be obtained 48 to 72 hours after injection
- Intervention: circle and record the test site

- Nursing interventions during the procedure
  - Reassure the patient
  - Place the patient in the proper position (either sitting on the edge of the bed or lying partially on the side, partially on the back)
- Nursing interventions after the procedure
  - Assess the patient's respiratory status
  - Monitor vital signs frequently
  - Position the patient on the affected side, as ordered, for at least 1 hour to seal the puncture site
  - Check the puncture site for fluid leakage
  - **Auscultate lungs to assess for pneumothorax**
  - Monitor oxygen saturation ($Sa{O_2}$) levels

Pulmonary function tests (PFTs)

- Definition and purpose
  - Noninvasive test
  - Measurement of lung volume, ventilation, and diffusing capacity
- Nursing interventions
  - Document bronchodilators or narcotics used before testing
  - Allay the patient's anxiety during testing

Arterial blood gas (ABG) analysis

- Definition and purpose
  - Laboratory test
  - Assessment of arterial blood for tissue oxygenation, ventilation, and acid-base status
- Nursing interventions before the procedure
  - Note temperature
  - Document oxygen and assisted mechanical ventilation used
- Nursing interventions after the procedure
  - **Apply pressure to the site for 5 minutes**
  - Apply a pressure dressing

Lung scan

- Definition and purpose
  - Procedure using inhalation or I.V. injection of radioisotopes
  - Imaging of distribution and blood flow in the lungs
- Nursing interventions before the procedure
  - Allay the patient's anxiety
  - Determine the patient's ability to lie still during the procedure
- Nursing interventions after the procedure
  - Check the catheter insertion site for bleeding
  - Assess for allergies to injected radioisotopes
  - Increase fluid intake, unless contraindicated

Mantoux intradermal skin test

- Definition and purpose
  - Procedure involving the administration of tuberculin
  - Detection of tuberculosis (TB) antibodies

- Nursing interventions
  - Document current dermatitis or rashes
  - Document history of positive results in past skin testing
  - Note history of receiving the bacille Calmette-Guèrin vaccine as a child (may be contraindication for Mantoux skin test)
  - Circle and record the test site
  - Note date for follow-up reading (48 to 72 hours after injection)

Laryngoscopy

- Definition and purpose
  - Procedure using a laryngoscope
  - Direct visualization of the larynx
- Nursing interventions before the procedure
  - Withhold food and fluids for 6 to 8 hours before the test
  - Explain to the patient that he'll receive a sedative to promote relaxation
  - Place obtained written informed consent in the patient's chart
- Nursing interventions after the procedure
  - Assess the patient's respiratory status
  - Allay the patient's anxiety
  - Withhold food and fluids until gag reflex returns
  - Assess for trauma to oropharynx
  - Assess for hemoptysis

Lung biopsy

- Definition and purpose
  - Procedure involving the percutaneous removal of a small amount of lung tissue
  - Histologic evaluation
- Nursing interventions before the procedure
  - Withhold food and fluids
  - Place obtained written informed consent in the patient's chart
- Nursing interventions after the procedure
  - Observe the patient for signs of pneumothorax and air embolism
  - Check the patient for hemoptysis and hemorrhage
  - Monitor and record vital signs
  - Check the insertion site for bleeding
  - Monitor for signs of respiratory distress

Hematologic studies

- Definition and purpose
  - Laboratory test of a blood sample
  - Analysis for red blood cells (RBCs), white blood cells (WBCs), prothrombin time (PT), partial thromboplastin time (PTT), erythrocyte sedimentation rate (ESR), platelets, hemoglobin (Hb), and hematocrit (HCT)
- Nursing interventions
  - Note current drug therapy before the procedure
  - Check the site for bleeding after the procedure

Laryngoscopy

- Invasive test
- Allows for direct visualization of larynx
- Interventions:
  - Withhold food and fluids for 6 to 8 hours before test
  - Withhold flood and fluids after test until gag reflex returns

Lung biopsy

- Invasive test
- Removal of a small amount of lung tissue for histologic evaluation
- Intervention: observe the patient for signs of pneumothorax and air embolism after procedure

Hematologic studies

- Blood test
- Analysis of:
  - RBCs
  - WBCs
  - PT and PTT
  - ESR
  - Platelets
  - Hb and HCT
- Intervention: check the site for bleeding after the procedure

Blood chemistry

- Blood test
- Analysis of:
- – Potassium, sodium, calcium, phosphorus
- – Glucose
- – Bicarbonate
- – Blood urea nitrogen and creatinine
- – Protein and albumin
- – Osmolality
- – $Alpha_1$-antitrypsin
- Intervention: withhold food and fluids before the procedure

Respiratory disease's impact on patient life

- Fear of dying
- Restrictions in work activity
- Changes in leisure activities, sexual function, and role performance
- Social isolation

Key risk factors for a respiratory disorder

- Modifiable: cigarette or pipe smoking; morbid obesity
- Nonmodifiable: aging; history of allergies; previous respiratory illness

Blood chemistry
- Definition and purpose
  - Laboratory test of a blood sample
  - Analysis for potassium, sodium, calcium, phosphorus, glucose, bicarbonate (HCO_3^-), blood urea nitrogen, creatinine, protein, albumin, osmolality, and $alpha_1$-antitrypsin
- Nursing interventions
  - Withhold food and fluids before the procedure, as directed
  - Check the site for bleeding after the procedure

PSYCHOSOCIAL IMPACT OF RESPIRATORY DISORDERS

Developmental impact
- Decreased self-esteem
- Fear of dying

Economic impact
- Disruption or loss of employment
- Cost of hospitalizations and home health care

Occupational and recreational impact
- Restrictions in work activity
- Changes in leisure activities

Social impact
- Changes in sexual function
- Social isolation
- Changes in role performance

RISK FACTORS

Modifiable risk factors
- Crowded living conditions
- Inadequate knowledge of risk factors
- Exposure to chemical and environmental pollutants
- Cigarette or pipe smoking
- Use of chewing tobacco
- Alcohol abuse
- Morbid obesity

Nonmodifiable risk factors
- Aging
- History of allergies
- Previous respiratory illness
- Family history of respiratory illness
- Family history of allergies

NURSING DIAGNOSES

Probable nursing diagnoses
- Impaired physical mobility
- Ineffective breathing pattern
- Impaired gas exchange
- Ineffective airway clearance
- Disturbed sleep pattern
- Activity intolerance
- Ineffective tissue perfusion (cardiopulmonary)

Possible nursing diagnoses
- Impaired spontaneous ventilation
- Dysfunctional ventilatory weaning response
- Anxiety
- Fear
- Imbalanced nutrition: Less than body requirements
- Impaired verbal communication
- Noncompliance
- Risk for aspiration

Key probable nursing diagnoses for a respiratory disorder
- Impaired physical mobility
- Ineffective breathing pattern
- Impaired gas exchange
- Ineffective airway clearance

LARYNGECTOMY

Description
- Partial laryngectomy: surgical excision of a lesion on one vocal cord
- Total laryngectomy: surgical removal of the larynx, hyoid bone, and tracheal rings, with closure of the pharynx and formation of a permanent tracheostomy

Laryngectomy defined
- Partial: excision of a lesion on one vocal cord
- Total: removal of larynx, hyoid bone, and tracheal rings; closure of pharynx; formation of permanent tracheostomy

Preoperative nursing interventions
- Complete patient and family preoperative teaching
  - Determine the patient's understanding of the procedure
  - Describe the operating room, postanesthesia care unit (PACU), and preoperative and postoperative routines
  - Demonstrate postoperative turning, coughing, deep breathing, splinting, and range-of-motion (ROM) exercises
  - Explain the postoperative need for drainage tubes, surgical dressings, oxygen therapy, I.V. therapy, and pain control
- Complete a preoperative checklist
- Administer preoperative medications, as prescribed
- Allay the patient's and his family's anxiety about surgery
- Document the patient's history and physical assessment database
- Establish methods of communication: writing, call bell, "magic slate," picture board
- Encourage the patient to express his feelings about changes in his body image and loss of his voice

Key interventions before laryngectomy
- Demonstrate postoperative turning, coughing, deep breathing, splinting, and ROM exercises.
- Explain the postoperative need for drainage tubes, surgical dressings, oxygen therapy, I.V. therapy, and pain control.
- Establish methods of communication: writing, call bell, "magic slate," picture board.
- Encourage the patient to express feelings about changes in body image and loss of voice.

Postoperative nursing interventions
- Assess respiratory status

Key nursing interventions after laryngectomy

- Assess respiratory status.
- Keep the patient in semi-Fowler's position.
- Provide tracheal suction.
- Administer high-humidity oxygen.
- Monitor and maintain position and patency of drainage tubes.
- Assess the color, amount, and consistency of sputum.
- Encourage the patient to express feelings about changes in body image and loss of voice.
- Provide oral hygiene.
- Reinforce method of communication established preoperatively.
- Reinforce speech therapy.
- Assess gag and cough reflex and ability to swallow.
- Provide stoma and laryngectomy care.
- Observe for hemorrhage and edema in the neck.

Radical neck dissection

- Excision of:
  - Sternocleidomastoid and omohyoid muscles
  - Muscles of the floor of the mouth
  - Submaxillary gland
  - Internal jugular vein
  - External carotid artery
  - Cervical chain of lymph nodes
- Laryngectomy

- Assess pain and administer postoperative analgesics, as prescribed
- Assess for return of peristalsis; provide solid foods and liquids, as tolerated; increase calories and protein
- Administer I.V. fluids and nasogastric (NG) tube feedings
- Allay the patient's anxiety
- Inspect the surgical dressing and change, as directed
- Reinforce turning, coughing, and deep breathing
- Keep the patient in semi-Fowler's position
- Provide tracheal suction
- Increase activity, as tolerated
- Administer oxygen via high-humidity tracheostomy mask
- Monitor and record vital signs, intake and output (I/O), laboratory studies, and pulse oximetry
- Monitor and maintain position and patency of drainage tubes: wound drainage
- Assess the color, amount, and consistency of sputum
- Encourage the patient to express his feelings about changes in his body image and loss of his voice
- Provide oral hygiene
- Reinforce method of communication established preoperatively
- Reinforce speech therapy
- Assess gag and cough reflexes and ability to swallow
- Provide stoma and laryngectomy care
- Reinforce increased intake of fluids
- Observe for hemorrhage and edema in the neck
- Arrange referrals to community agencies
- Individualize home care instructions
  - Communicate using esophageal speech or artificial larynx
  - Avoid swimming, showering, and using aerosol sprays
  - Complete stoma and laryngectomy care daily
  - Suction laryngectomy using clean technique
  - Protect the neck from injury
  - Demonstrate ways to prevent debris from entering the stoma

Possible surgical complications

- Hemorrhage
- Atelectasis
- Pneumonia
- Aspiration

RADICAL NECK DISSECTION

Description

- Surgical excision of the sternocleidomastoid and omohyoid muscles, muscles of the floor of the mouth, submaxillary gland, internal jugular vein, external carotid artery, and cervical chain of lymph nodes, in addition to laryngectomy

Preoperative nursing interventions

- Complete patient and family preoperative teaching
  - Determine the patient's understanding of the procedure
  - Describe the operating room, PACU, and preoperative and postoperative routines
  - Demonstrate postoperative turning, coughing, deep breathing, splinting, and ROM exercises
  - Explain the postoperative need for drainage tubes, surgical dressings, oxygen therapy, I.V. therapy, and pain control
- Complete a preoperative checklist
- Administer preoperative medications, as prescribed
- Allay the patient's and his family's anxiety about surgery
- Document the patient's history and physical assessment database
- Establish methods of communication: writing, call bell, "magic slate," picture board
- Discuss alteration in body image

Postoperative nursing interventions

- Assess cardiac, respiratory, and neurologic status
- Assess pain and administer postoperative analgesics, as prescribed
- Assess for the return of peristalsis; provide nutrition and liquids, as indicated
- Administer I.V. fluids, NG tube feedings, and transfusion therapy, as prescribed
- Allay the patient's anxiety
- Inspect the surgical dressing and change it, as directed
- Reinforce turning, coughing, and deep breathing
- Keep the patient in high Fowler's position
- Provide tracheal suction
- Maintain activity: active and passive ROM and isometric exercises, as tolerated
- Administer oxygen via high-humidity tracheostomy mask
- Monitor and record vital signs, I/O, laboratory studies, and pulse oximetry
- Monitor and maintain position and patency of drainage tubes: NG, indwelling urinary catheter, and wound drainage
- **Assess gag and cough reflexes and ability to swallow**
- Encourage the patient to express his feelings about changes in his body image and loss of his voice
- Provide stoma and laryngectomy care; arrange for referrals to community agencies for follow-up care
- Reinforce increased intake of fluids
- Observe the patient for hemorrhage and edema in the neck
- Provide suture line care
- Reinforce method of communication established preoperatively
- Reinforce speech therapy
- Individualize home care instructions
  - Communicate using esophageal speech or artificial larynx
  - Recognize the signs and symptoms of tracheostomy stenosis

Key steps before radical neck dissection

- Demonstrate turning, coughing, deep breathing, splinting and ROM exercises.
- Establish methods of communication.

Key care steps after radical neck dissection

- Assess cardiac, respiratory, and neurologic status.
- Reinforce turning, coughing, and deep breathing.
- Keep the patient in high Fowler's position.
- Provide tracheal suction.
- Administer high-humidity oxygen.
- Monitor and maintain position and patency of drainage tubes.
- Assess gag and cough reflexes and ability to swallow.
- Encourage the patient to express his feelings about changes in his body image and loss of his voice.
- Provide stoma and laryngectomy care.
- Observe the patient for hemorrhage and edema in the neck.

Key home care instructions after radical neck dissection

- Communicate using esophageal speech or artificial larynx.
- Recognize the signs and symptoms of tracheostomy stenosis.
- Suction laryngectomy using clean technique.
- Complete incision, stoma, and laryngectomy care daily.

- Avoid swimming, showers, and using aerosol sprays
- Protect the neck from injury
- Suction laryngectomy using clean technique
- Complete incision, stoma, and laryngectomy care daily
- Demonstrate ways to prevent debris from entering the stoma
- Complete ROM exercises for arms, shoulders, and neck daily

3 types of pulmonary resection

- Lobectomy
- Wedge resection
- Pneumonectomy

Possible surgical complications

- Tracheostomy stenosis
- Aspiration
- Pneumonia
- Hemorrhage

PULMONARY RESECTION

Description

- Lobectomy: surgical removal of one lobe of the lung
- Wedge resection: surgical removal of a wedge-shaped section of a lobe
- Pneumonectomy: surgical removal of a lung

Key nursing steps before pulmonary resection

- Demonstrate postoperative turning, coughing, deep breathing, splinting, and ROM exercises, and the use of incentive spirometry.
- Explain the postoperative need for drainage tubes, chest tubes, surgical dressings, oxygen therapy, I.V. therapy, and pain control.

Preoperative nursing interventions

- Complete patient and family preoperative teaching
  - Determine the patient's understanding of the procedure
  - Describe the operating room, PACU, and preoperative and postoperative routines
  - Demonstrate postoperative turning, coughing, deep breathing, splinting, and ROM exercises, and the use of incentive spirometry
  - Explain the postoperative need for drainage tubes, chest tubes, surgical dressings, oxygen therapy, I.V. therapy, and pain control (see *Checking in on chest tubes*)
- Complete a preoperative checklist and obtain informed consent
- Administer preoperative medications, as prescribed
- Allay the patient's and his family's anxiety about surgery
- Document the patient's history and physical assessment database

Key nursing steps after pulmonary resection

- Assess cardiac and respiratory status.
- Reinforce turning, coughing, and deep breathing, and splinting of incision.

Postoperative nursing interventions

- Assess cardiac and respiratory status
- Assess pain and administer postoperative analgesics, as prescribed
- Assess for return of peristalsis; provide solid foods and liquids, as tolerated
- Administer I.V. fluids
- Allay the patient's anxiety
- Inspect the surgical dressing and change it, as directed
- Reinforce turning, coughing, and deep breathing, and splinting of incision
- **Maintain the patient's position: for pneumonectomy patient, keep him on his back or on the side of the surgery; for lobectomy or wedge resection patient, keep him on his back or on the side opposite the surgery**
- Provide incentive spirometry, suction, chest physiotherapy, and postural drainage

Checking in on chest tubes

Caring for a patient with a chest tube requires taking actions to ensure the patient's health. Here are typical nursing steps regarding chest tubes, beginning when the chest tube is first placed:

- First, have the patient take several deep breaths to fully inflate the lungs and help push pleural air out through the tube.
- Next, palpate his chest around the tube for subcutaneous emphysema and notify the physician of any increase.
- Routinely assess the function of the chest tube. Describe and record the amount of drainage on the intake and output sheet.

If there's a leak:

- Bubbling in the water-seal chamber or air leak meter indicates that there's an air leak. If there's no air leak, the water level in this chamber will rise and fall with the patient's respirations, reflecting normal pressure changes in the pleural cavity.
- If the water fluctuates with respirations (for example, fluctuation occurs on exhalation in the patient breathing spontaneously), the lung is most likely the source of the air leak.
- If the lung isn't the source of the air leak, check and tighten the connections. If the leak is in the tubing, replace the unit.

If the tube becomes dislodged:

- Cover the opening immediately with petroleum gauze and apply pressure to prevent negative inspiratory pressure from sucking air into the patient's chest. Call the physician and continue to keep the opening closed. Then get ready to start the chest tube process over.
- If the chest tube becomes cracked, place the distal end of the tube in sterile water and call the physician.

- Maintain activity: active and passive ROM and isometric exercises, as tolerated
- Administer oxygen and maintain endotracheal tube to ventilator
- Monitor and record vital signs, I/O, laboratory studies, electrocardiogram (ECG), hemodynamic variables, and pulse oximetry
- Monitor and maintain position and patency of drainage tubes: NG tube, indwelling urinary catheter, and chest tube
- **Assess chest tube insertion site for subcutaneous air and drainage (except pneumonectomy)**
- Encourage the patient to express his feelings about a fear of dying
- Administer antibiotics, as prescribed
- Individualize home care instructions
  - Recognize the signs and symptoms of respiratory distress
  - Complete incision care daily
  - Maintain active ROM exercises to operative shoulder

Possible surgical complications

- Hemorrhage
- Pneumonia

Chest tube care

- If there's an air leak:
  - Lung may be the source.
  - Check and tighten connections.
  - Replace the unit if the leak is in the tubing.
- If the tube becomes dislodged:
  - Cover chest opening with petroleum gauze and apply pressure.
  - Notify the physician.
- If the chest tube is cracked:
  - Place distal end of tube in sterile water.
  - Notify the physician.

Mandatory monitoring after pulmonary resection

- Maintain the patient's position: for pneumonectomy patient, keep him on his back or on the side of the surgery; for lobectomy or wedge resection patient, keep him on his back or on the side opposite the surgery.
- Monitor and maintain position and patency of drainage tubes: NG tube, indwelling urinary catheter, and chest tube.
- Assess chest tube insertion site for subcutaneous air and drainage (except pneumonectomy).

EMBOLECTOMY

Description

- Removal of an embolus from an artery using a balloon-tipped catheter

Preoperative nursing interventions

- Complete patient and family preoperative teaching
  - Determine the patient's understanding of the procedure
  - Describe the operating room, PACU, and preoperative and postoperative routines
  - Demonstrate postoperative turning, coughing, deep breathing, splinting, and ROM exercises
  - Explain the postoperative need for drainage tubes, surgical dressings, oxygen therapy, I.V. therapy, and pain control
- Complete a preoperative checklist
- Administer preoperative medications, as prescribed
- Allay the patient's and his family's anxiety about surgery
- Document the patient's history and physical assessment database
- Obtain a baseline vascular assessment
- Administer anticoagulants, as prescribed
- Maintain the extremity in slightly dependent position
- Administer thrombolytics, as prescribed
- Provide a bed cradle

Postoperative nursing interventions

- Assess cardiac, respiratory, and neurologic status
- Assess pain and administer postoperative analgesics, as prescribed
- Assess for return of peristalsis; provide solid foods and liquids, as tolerated
- Administer I.V. fluids
- Allay the patient's anxiety
- Inspect the surgical dressing and change it, as directed
- Reinforce turning, coughing, and deep breathing
- Keep the patient in semi-Fowler's position
- Provide incentive spirometry
- Maintain activity: active and passive ROM and isometric exercises, as tolerated
- Administer oxygen
- Monitor and record vital signs, I/O, laboratory studies, neurovascular checks, and pulse oximetry
- Administer anticoagulants, as prescribed
- Provide bed cradle
- Check site for bleeding
- Maintain pressure dressing
- Individualize home care instructions
  - Recognize the signs and symptoms of bleeding
  - Avoid prolonged sitting
  - State precautions of long-term anticoagulant therapy
  - Complete incision care daily

Embolectomy

- Removal of an embolus from an artery
- Involves use of a balloon-tipped catheter

Key interventions before embolectomy

- Administer thrombolytics, as prescribed.
- Demonstrate postoperative turning, coughing, and deep breathing, splinting, and leg and ROM exercises.

Key interventions after embolectomy

- Assess cardiac, respiratory, and neurologic status.
- Inspect the surgical dressing and change it, as directed.
- Reinforce turning, coughing, and deep breathing.
- Keep the patient in semi-Fowler's position.
- Monitor and record vital signs, I/O, laboratory studies, neurovascular checks, and pulse oximetry.
- Administer anticoagulants, as prescribed.

- **Possible surgical complications**
  - Hemorrhage
  - Embolism
  - Thrombosis
  - Respiratory distress

VENA CAVAL FILTER INSERTION AND PLICATION OF INFERIOR VENA CAVA

- **Description**
  - Vena caval filter (for example, Greenfield filter) insertion: surgical placement of an intracaval filter (umbrella) to partially occlude the inferior vena cava and prevent pulmonary emboli
  - Plication: surgical suturing and placement of Teflon clips to partially occlude the inferior vena cava and prevent pulmonary emboli
- **Preoperative nursing interventions**
  - Complete patient and family preoperative teaching
    - Determine the patient's understanding of the procedure
    - Describe the operating room, PACU, and preoperative and postoperative routines
    - Demonstrate postoperative turning, coughing, deep breathing, splinting, and ROM exercises
    - Explain the postoperative need for drainage tubes, surgical dressings, oxygen therapy, I.V. therapy, and pain control
  - Complete a preoperative checklist
  - Administer preoperative medications, as prescribed
  - Allay the patient's and his family's anxiety about surgery
  - Document the patient's history and physical assessment database
- **Postoperative nursing interventions**
  - Assess cardiac and respiratory status
  - Assess pain and administer postoperative analgesics, as prescribed
  - Assess for return of peristalsis; provide solid foods and liquids, as tolerated
  - Administer I.V. fluids
  - Allay the patient's anxiety
  - Inspect the surgical dressing and change it, as directed
  - Reinforce turning, coughing, and deep breathing
  - Keep the patient in semi-Fowler's position, with the foot of the bed elevated
  - Provide incentive spirometry
  - Maintain activity: active and passive ROM and isometric exercises, as tolerated
  - Administer oxygen
  - Monitor and record vital signs, I/O, laboratory studies, neurovascular checks, and pulse oximetry
  - Check the insertion site for bleeding and hematoma
  - Assess peripheral edema

Vena caval filter insertion and plication of inferior vena cava

- Vena caval filter insertion: surgical placement of an intracaval filter (umbrella) to partially occlude inferior vena cava
- Plication of inferior vena cava: surgical suturing and placement of Teflon clips to partially occlude inferior vena cava

Key preoperative steps for vena caval filter insertion and plication of inferior vena cava

- Demonstrate turning, coughing, deep breathing, splinting, and ROM exercises.
- Provide emotional support to the patient and his family.

Key postoperative steps for vena caval filter insertion and plication of inferior vena cava

- Check the insertion site for bleeding and hematoma.
- Assess peripheral edema.
- Apply antiembolism stockings.

- Apply antiembolism stockings
- Avoid hip flexion
- Individualize home care instructions
  - Recognize the signs and symptoms of infection and edema
  - Avoid prolonged sitting or crossing legs when sitting
  - Complete incision care daily
  - Walk daily
  - Elevate legs when sitting
  - Wear antiembolism stockings
  - Adhere to long-term anticoagulant therapy

Possible surgical complications

- Embolism
- Infection

Key orders for home care after vena caval filter insertion and plication of inferior vena cava

- Elevate legs when sitting.
- Avoid prolonged sitting or crossing legs when sitting.
- Wear antiembolism stockings.
- Adhere to long-term anticoagulant therapy.

PNEUMONIA

Definition

- Bacterial, viral, parasitic, or fungal infection that causes inflammation of the alveolar spaces

Causes

- Organisms: *Escherichia coli, Haemophilus influenzae, Staphylococcus aureus, Pneumocystis carinii, Pneumococcus,* and *Pseudomonas* (see Pneumocystis carinii *pneumonia*)
- Aspiration of food
- Aspiration of fluid
- Chemical irritants

Pathophysiology

- Microorganisms enter the alveolar spaces by droplet inhalation
- Inflammation occurs and alveolar fluid increases
- Ventilation decreases as secretions thicken

Assessment findings

- Cough
- Malaise
- Chills
- Shortness of breath
- Dyspnea
- Elevated temperature
- Crackles
- Rhonchi
- Pleural friction rub
- Pleuritic pain
- Sputum production
  - Rusty, green, or bloody (pneumococcal pneumonia)
  - Yellow-green (bronchopneumonia)

Pneumonia defined

- Inflammation of alveolar spaces
- Causes:
- – Bacteria
- – Viruses
- – Parasites
- – Fungi

Key assessment findings in pneumonia

- Cough
- Chills
- Dyspnea
- Elevated temperature
- Crackles
- Rhonchi
- Pleural friction rub
- Sputum production

Significance of sputum color in a patient with pneumonia

- Rusty, green, or bloody: indicates pneumococcal pneumonia
- Yellow-green: indicates bronchopneumonia

Pneumocystis carinii pneumonia

Pneumocystis carinii pneumonia (PCP) is a communicable, opportunistic infection frequently associated with human immunodeficiency virus (HIV) infection as well as other immunocompromising conditions, such as organ transplantation, leukemia, lymphoma, and steroid use.

It has an insidious onset, with increasing shortness of breath and a nonproductive cough. Other signs and symptoms include low-grade, intermittent fever; tachypnea and dyspnea; cyanosis (with acute illness); dullness on percussion (with consolidation); crackles; and decreased breath sounds.

Diagnostic tests may include chest X-ray, arterial blood gas analysis to check for hypoxemia, and fiber-optic bronchoscopy to obtain lung tissue specimens for culture. PCP may respond to drug therapy with co-trimoxazole or pentamidine (which may be administered I.V. or in aerosol form). Prophylactic therapy with co-trimoxazole in the patient with HIV with low immune function has prevented PCP from high mortality rates.

Care for a patient with PCP resembles that of a patient with other types of pneumonia. Key nursing interventions include administering oxygen and an analgesic, as needed; assessing the patient's respiratory status frequently; practicing good handwashing techniques throughout care; limiting activity and encouraging rest periods; and teaching techniques to reduce the spread of infection and reduce stress.

Diagnostic test findings

- Sputum studies: identification of organism
- Chest X-ray: pulmonary infiltrates
- Hematology: increased WBCs, ESR
- ABG analysis: hypoxemia, respiratory alkalosis

Medical management

- Diet: high-calorie, high-protein
- Dietary recommendation: encourage fluids
- I.V. therapy: hydration, saline lock
- Oxygen therapy
- Intubation and mechanical ventilation
- Position: semi-Fowler's
- Activity: bed rest, active and passive ROM and isometric exercises
- Monitoring: vital signs, ABG values, and I/O
- Laboratory studies: WBCs, sputum culture, blood culture, and throat culture
- Nutritional support: total parental nutrition (TPN)
- Treatments: indwelling urinary catheter, chest physiotherapy, postural drainage, incentive spirometry, and high-flow nebulizer treatments
- Antibiotics: penicillin G potassium (Pentids), ampicillin (Omnipen), pentamidine (NebuPent), amoxicillin with clavulanic acid (Augmentin)
- Antipyretics: aspirin, acetaminophen (Tylenol)
- Bronchodilators: metaproterenol (Alupent), isoetharine (Bronkosol), albuterol (Proventil)

Pneumocystis carinii pneumonia

- Opportunistic infection
- Frequently associated with HIV infection and other immunocompromising conditions
- Key signs and symptoms: increasing shortness of breath, nonproductive cough, and low-grade fever
- Treatment: co-trimoxazole, pentamidine

Key test findings in pneumonia

- Sputum studies: positive for specific organism
- Chest X-ray: pulmonary infiltrates
- ABG analysis: respiratory alkalosis

Main treatments for pneumonia

- Oxygen therapy
- Antibiotics
- Antipyretics
- Bronchodilators

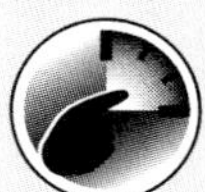

TIME-OUT FOR TEACHING

Patients with respiratory disorders

Be sure to include these topics in your teaching plan for the patient with a respiratory disorder.

- Follow-up appointments
- Smoking cessation; avoidance of irritants
- Self-monitoring for infection, including avoiding exposure to people with infections
- Signs of infection and respiratory distress
- Optimal weight maintenance
- Medication therapy, including action, adverse effects, and scheduling
- Dietary recommendations and restrictions
- Rest and activity patterns
- Community agencies and resources

Key teaching topics for a patient with a respiratory disorder

- Self-monitoring for infection
- Signs of infection and respiratory distress
- Medication therapy
- Dietary recommendations

Important nursing interventions for a patient with pneumonia

- Encourage fluids to 3 to 4 L/day.
- Administer oxygen.
- Assess respiratory status.
- Monitor and record vital signs, I/O, laboratory studies, and pulse oximetry.
- Monitor and record color, consistency, and amount of sputum.

Home care checklist for a patient with pneumonia

- Recognize the signs and symptoms of respiratory infections.
- Avoid exposure to people with infections.
- Increase fluid intake to 3 L/day.

- Specialized bed: rotation (Rotorest)
- Pulse oximetry

Nursing interventions

- Maintain the patient's diet
- Encourage fluids to 3 to 4 L/day
- Administer I.V. fluids
- Administer oxygen
- Provide suction and turn the patient; encourage coughing and deep breathing
- Assess respiratory status
- Keep the patient in semi-Fowler's position
- Monitor and record vital signs, I/O, laboratory studies, and pulse oximetry
- Administer medications, as prescribed
- Encourage the patient to express his feelings about a fear of suffocation
- Monitor and record color, consistency, and amount of sputum
- Allay the patient's anxiety
- Prevent spread of infection
- Provide oral hygiene
- Provide information about the American Lung Association
- Individualize home care instructions (for more information about teaching, see *Patients with respiratory disorders*)
  - Recognize the signs and symptoms of respiratory infections
  - Avoid exposure to people with infections
  - Increase fluid intake to 3 L/day

Complications

- Heart failure
- Pulmonary edema
- Respiratory failure

Possible surgical interventions

- None

CHRONIC OBSTRUCTIVE PULMONARY DISEASE (COPD)

Definition
- COPD is group of diseases that results in persistent obstruction of bronchial airflow
- Diseases include emphysema, asthma, bronchiectasis, and chronic bronchitis
- **In emphysema, the stimulus to breathe is low partial pressure of arterial oxygen (PaO_2) instead of increased partial pressure of arterial carbon dioxide ($PaCO_2$)**

Causes
- Congenital weakness
- Respiratory irritants: smoke, polluted air, chemical irritants
- Respiratory tract infections
- Genetic predisposition

Pathophysiology
- Bronchiectasis: infection destroys the bronchial mucosa, which is replaced by fibrous scar tissue; loss of resilience and dilation of airways causes pooling of secretions, obstruction of air flow, and decreased perfusion
- Asthma: irritants to bronchial tree cause bronchoconstriction, resulting in narrowed inflamed airways, dyspnea, and mucus production — all of which are reversible
- Bronchitis: excessive bronchial mucus production causes chronic or recurrent productive cough
- Emphysema: destruction of elastin alters alveolar walls and narrows airways, resulting in enlargement of air spaces distal to terminal bronchioles, trapped air, and coalesced alveoli

Assessment findings
- Cough
- Dyspnea
- Sputum production
- Weight loss
- Barrel chest (emphysema)
- Hemoptysis
- Exertional dyspnea
- Clubbing of fingers
- Malaise
- Wheezes
- Crackles
- Anemia
- Anxiety
- Diaphoresis
- Use of accessory muscles
- Orthopnea

COPD
- Group of diseases
- Results in persistent obstruction of bronchial airflow
- In emphysema, the stimulus to breathe is low PaO_2 instead of increased $PaCO_2$

4 forms of COPD
- Bronchiectasis
- Asthma
- Bronchitis
- Emphysema

Common COPD assessment findings
- Cough
- Dyspnea
- Sputum production
- Clubbing of fingers
- Use of accessory muscles

Key test findings in COPD

- Chest X-ray: congestion, hyperinflation
- ABG analysis: respiratory acidosis
- PFTs: increased residual volume and functional residual capacity; decreased vital capacity

Key ways to manage COPD

- High-protein, high-vitamin C, high-calorie, and high-nitrogen diet
- Encourage fluids to 3 L/day
- Antibiotics
- Bronchodilators
- Corticosteroids
- Beta-adrenergic medication
- Mast cell stabilizers

Key interventions for a patient with COPD

- Administer small, frequent feedings.
- Encourage fluids.
- Administer low-flow oxygen.
- Provide chest physiotherapy, intermittent positive pressure breathing, turning, postural drainage, and suction; encourage coughing, deep breathing, and use of incentive spirometer.
- Assess respiratory status.
- Reinforce pursed-lip breathing to prolong exhalation and to increase airway pressure.
- Keep the patient in high Fowler's position.

Diagnostic test findings

- Chest X-ray: congestion, hyperinflation
- ABG analysis: respiratory acidosis, hypoxemia
- Sputum studies: positive identification of organism
- PFTs: increased residual volume, increased functional residual capacity, decreased vital capacity

Medical management

- Diet: high in protein, vitamin C, calories, and nitrogen
- Dietary recommendations: encourage fluids to 3 L/day, as tolerated
- I.V. therapy: saline lock
- Oxygen therapy: 2 to 3 L/minute
- Intubation and mechanical ventilation
- Position: high Fowler's
- Activity: as tolerated
- Monitoring: vital signs and I/O
- Laboratory studies: ABG values, WBCs, and sputum studies
- Treatments: chest physiotherapy, postural drainage, intermittent positive pressure breathing, high-flow nebulizer treatments, and incentive spirometry
- Antibiotics: ampicillin (Omnipen), tetracycline (Achromycin), cefixime (Suprax)
- Antacid: aluminum hydroxide gel (AlternaGEL)
- Bronchodilators: terbutaline (Brethine), aminophylline (Truphylline), isoproterenol (Isuprel), theophylline (Theo-Dur); via nebulizer: albuterol (Proventil), ipratropium (Atrovent), metaproterenol (Alupent)
- Corticosteroids: hydrocortisone (Solu-Cortef), methylprednisolone sodium succinate (Solu-Medrol)
- Expectorant: guaifenesin (Robitussin)
- Beta-adrenergic medication: epinephrine (Adrenalin)
- Mast cell stabilizer: cromolyn (Intal)

Nursing interventions

- Maintain the patient's diet
- Administer small, frequent feedings
- Encourage fluids
- Administer low-flow oxygen
- Provide chest physiotherapy, intermittent positive pressure breathing, turning, postural drainage, and suction; encourage coughing, deep breathing, and use of incentive spirometer
- Assess respiratory status
- **Reinforce pursed-lip breathing to prolong exhalation and to increase airway pressure**
- Keep the patient in high Fowler's position
- Monitor and record vital signs, I/O, and laboratory studies
- Administer medications, as prescribed
- Encourage the patient to express his feelings about fear of suffocation
- Allow activity, as tolerated

- Monitor and record the color, amount, and consistency of sputum
- Allay the patient's anxiety
- Weigh the patient daily
- Provide information about the American Lung Association
- Individualize home care instructions
  - Identify ways to reduce stress
  - Recognize the signs and symptoms of respiratory infection and hypoxia
  - Adhere to activity limitations
  - Know proper use of home oxygen
  - Demonstrate pursed-lip and diaphragmatic breathing
  - Avoid exposure to chemical irritants and pollutants
  - Demonstrate deep-breathing and coughing exercises
  - Avoid eating gas-producing foods, spicy foods, and extremely hot or cold foods

Complications

- From emphysema
  - Pulmonary hypertension
  - Right-sided heart failure
  - Spontaneous pneumothorax
- Carbon dioxide narcosis
- Acute respiratory failure
- Pneumonia

Possible surgical interventions

- None

ACUTE RESPIRATORY DISTRESS SYNDROME (ARDS, SHOCK LUNG)

Definition

- Clinical syndrome of respiratory insufficiency

Causes

- Viral pneumonia
- Fat emboli
- Sepsis
- Decreased surfactant production
- Fluid overload
- Shock
- Trauma
- Neurologic injuries
- Oxygen toxicity

Pathophysiology

- Damaged capillary membranes cause interstitial edema and intra-alveolar hemorrhage (see *What happens in ARDS,* page 92)
- Decreased gas exchange results

Key home care steps for a patient with COPD

- Recognize the signs and symptoms of respiratory infection and hypoxia.
- Know proper use of home oxygen.
- Demonstrate pursed-lip and diaphragmatic breathing.
- Avoid exposure to chemical irritants and pollutants.
- Demonstrate deep-breathing and coughing exercises.

ARDS defined

- Clinical syndrome of respiratory insufficiency
- Damaged capillary membranes cause interstitial edema and intra-alveolar hemorrhage
- Hypoxemia results

Common causes of ARDS

- Viral pneumonia
- Fat emboli
- Sepsis
- Decreased surfactant production

Pathophysiology of ARDS

- Lung injury causes platelets to aggregate.
- Platelets release substances that inflame and damage the alveolar membrane, increasing capillary permeability.
- Fluids shift into the interstitial space.
- As capillary permeability increases, pulmonary edema results.
- Alveoli collapse, impairing gas exchange.
- Oxygen and carbon dioxide levels in the blood decrease.
- Pulmonary edema worsens, inflammation leads to fibrosis, and gas exchange is further impeded.
- Metabolic acidosis results.

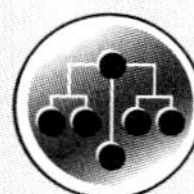

GO WITH THE FLOW

What happens in ARDS

This flow chart shows the process and progress of acute respiratory distress syndrome (ARDS).

Injury reduces blood flow to the lungs, allowing platelets to aggregate.

↓

These platelets release substances, such as serotonin, bradykinin and, especially, histamine. These substances inflame and damage the alveolar membrane and later increase capillary permeability. At this early stage, signs and symptoms of ARDS are undetectable.

↓

Histamines and other inflammatory substances increase capillary permeability, allowing fluid to shift into the interstitial space. As a result, the patient may experience tachypnea, dyspnea, and tachycardia.

↓

As capillary permeability increases, proteins and more fluid leak out, increasing interstitial osmotic pressure and causing pulmonary edema. At this stage, the patient may experience increased tachypnea, dyspnea, and cyanosis. Hypoxia (usually unresponsive to increased fraction of inspired oxygen), decreased pulmonary compliance, and crackles and rhonchi also may develop.

↓

Fluid in the alveoli and decreased blood flow damage surfactant in the alveoli, reducing the cells' ability to produce more. Without surfactant, alveoli collapse, impairing gas exchange. Look for thick, frothy sputum and marked hypoxemia with increased respiratory distress.

↓

The patient breathes faster, but sufficient oxygen can't cross the alveolocapillary membrane. Carbon dioxide, however, crosses more easily and is lost with every exhalation. Oxygen and carbon dioxide levels in the blood decrease. Look for increased tachypnea, hypoxemia, and hypocapnia.

↓

Pulmonary edema worsens. Meanwhile, inflammation leads to fibrosis, which further impedes gas exchange. The resulting hypoxemia leads to metabolic acidosis. At this stage, look for increased partial pressure of arterial carbon dioxide, decreased pH, partial pressure of arterial oxygen, and bicarbonate levels, and mental confusion.

- Cellular damage causes decreased surfactant production, resulting in hypoxemia

Assessment findings

- Dyspnea
- Tachypnea
- Cyanosis
- Cough
- Crackles
- Rhonchi
- Anxiety
- Restlessness
- Decreased breath sounds

Diagnostic test findings

- ABG analysis: respiratory acidosis, hypoxemia that doesn't respond to increased percentage of oxygen
- Chest X-ray: interstitial edema
- Sputum studies: may identify offending organism
- Blood cultures: may identify offending organism

Medical management

- Diet: restrict fluid intake
- I.V. therapy: saline lock
- Oxygen therapy
- Intubation and mechanical ventilation using positive end expiratory pressure (PEEP)
- Position: high-Fowler's
- Activity: bed rest; active ROM and isometric exercises
- Monitoring: vital signs, I/O, central venous pressure (CVP), ECG, and hemodynamic variables
- Laboratory studies: ABG values, sputum studies, blood cultures, Hb, and HCT
- Nutritional support: TPN
- Treatments: indwelling urinary catheter, chest physiotherapy, postural drainage, and suction
- Transfusion therapy: platelets, packed RBCs
- Antibiotics: amoxicillin (Amoxil), ampicillin (Omnipen)
- Analgesic: morphine
- Diuretics: furosemide (Lasix), ethacrynic acid (Edecrin)
- Anticoagulant: heparin
- Steroids: hydrocortisone (Solu-Cortef), methylprednisolone sodium succinate (Solu-Medrol)
- Antacid: aluminum hydroxide gel (AlternaGEL)
- Neuromuscular blocking agents: pancuronium (Pavulon), vecuronium bromide (Norcuron)
- Mucosal barrier fortifier: sucralfate (Carafate)
- Pulse oximetry

Key assessment findings in ARDS

- Dyspnea
- Tachypnea
- Crackles
- Rhonchi
- Anxiety
- Decreased breath sounds

ABG and X-ray findings in ARDS

- ABG analysis: respiratory acidosis, hypoxemia that doesn't respond to increased percentage of oxygen
- Chest X-ray: interstitial edema

Key steps in managing ARDS

- Intubation and mechanical ventilation using PEEP
- Antibiotics
- Analgesics
- Steroids
- Neuromuscular blocking agents

Important nursing interventions for a patient with ARDS

- Monitor mechanical ventilation.
- Monitor and record vital signs, hemodynamic variables, I/O, specific gravity, laboratory studies, and pulse oximetry.

- **Nursing interventions**
  - Maintain fluid restrictions
  - Administer I.V. fluids
  - Monitor mechanical ventilation
  - Provide suction, turning, and postural drainage; encourage coughing and deep breathing
  - Assess respiratory status
  - Keep the patient in high Fowler's position
  - Monitor and record vital signs, hemodynamic variables, I/O, specific gravity, laboratory studies, and pulse oximetry
  - Administer TPN
  - Administer medications, as prescribed
  - Encourage the patient to express his feelings about fear of suffocation
  - Organize nursing care to allow rest periods
  - Weigh the patient daily
  - Allay the patient's anxiety
  - Maintain bed rest
  - Individualize home care instructions
    - Recognize the signs and symptoms of respiratory distress
    - Demonstrate deep breathing and coughing exercises
    - Avoid exposure to chemical irritants and pollutants
- **Complications**
  - Pulmonary edema
  - Atelectasis
- **Possible surgical interventions**
  - None

Pulmonary TB defined

- Airborne, infectious, communicable disease
- Can occur acutely or chronically
- Caused by *M. tuberculosis*

TUBERCULOSIS (TB), PULMONARY

- **Definition**
  - Airborne, infectious, communicable disease that can occur acutely or chronically
- **Causes**
  - *Mycobacterium tuberculosis*
- **Pathophysiology**
  - Alveoli become the focus of infection from inhaled droplets containing bacteria
  - Tubercle bacilli multiply, spread through the lymphatics, and drain into the systemic circulation
  - In the lung tissue, macrophages surround the bacilli and form tubercles
  - Tubercles go through the process of caseation, liquefaction, and cavitation
- **Assessment findings**
  - Fatigue
  - Malaise
  - Irritability

Pathophysiology of TB

- Tubercle bacilli multiply, spread through the lymphatics and drain into the systemic circulation
- Macrophages surround bacilli and form tubercles
- Tubercles caseate, liquify, and cavitate

- Night sweats
- Tachycardia
- Weight loss
- Anorexia
- Cough
- Yellow and mucoid sputum
- Dyspnea
- Hemoptysis
- Crackles
- Elevated temperature

Diagnostic test findings

- Chest X-ray: active or calcified lesions
- Sputum cultures: positive acid-fast bacillus; positive *M. tuberculosis*
- Hematology: increased WBCs, ESR
- Mantoux skin test: positive

Medical management

- Diet: high-carbohydrate, high-protein, high-vitamin B_6 and C, high-calorie
- I.V. therapy: saline lock
- Activity: bed rest, active ROM and isometric exercises
- Monitoring: vital signs and I/O
- Laboratory studies: ABG values, hepatic studies (due to medications), and sputum studies (to guide treatment and determine effectiveness of antibiotics and antituberculosis agents)
- Treatments: chest physiotherapy, postural drainage, and incentive spirometry
- Precautions: standard
- Antibiotic: streptomycin
- Antituberculosis: isoniazid (INH), ethambutol (Myambutol), rifampin (Rifadin), pyrazinamide (pms-Pyrazinamide)

Nursing interventions

- Maintain the patient's diet
- Provide small, frequent meals
- Provide suctioning, turning, chest physiotherapy, and postural drainage; encourage coughing and deep breathing
- Assess respiratory status
- Monitor and record vital signs, I/O, and laboratory studies
- Administer medications, as prescribed
- Allay the patient's anxiety
- Maintain infection control precautions
- Encourage fluids
- Maintain bed rest
- Instruct the patient to cover nose and mouth when sneezing
- Provide frequent oral hygiene
- Provide ultraviolet light, negative pressure, or well-ventilated room
- Provide information about the American Lung Association

Hallmarks of TB

- Night sweats
- Elevated temperature

TOP 3

TB test findings

1. Chest X-ray: active or calcified lesions
2. Sputum cultures: positive acid-fast bacillus; positive *M. tuberculosis*
3. Mantoux skin test: positive

Key antituberculosis medications

- Isoniazid
- Ethambutol
- Rifampin
- Pyrazinamide

Key nursing interventions for a patient with TB

- Maintain the patient's diet.
- Provide suctioning, turning, chest physiotherapy, and postural drainage; encourage coughing and deep breathing.
- Assess respiratory status.
- Monitor and record vital signs, I/O, and laboratory studies.
- Maintain infection control precautions.
- Encourage fluids.
- Instruct the patient to cover his nose and mouth when sneezing.
- Provide frequent oral hygiene.
- Provide ultraviolet light, negative pressure, or well-ventilated room.

Pneumothorax

- Loss of negative intrapleural pressure
- Results in collapse of the lung
- Three types: spontaneous, open, and tension

Main causes of pneumothorax

- Blunt chest trauma
- Rupture of a bleb
- CVP line insertion

- Individualize home care instructions
  - Demonstrate methods to prevent spread of sputum droplets
  - Provide adequate air ventilation in rooms
  - Reinforce need to finish entire course of medication (6 to 18 months)

Complications
- Atelectasis
- Spontaneous pneumothorax

Possible surgical intervention
- Lobectomy

PNEUMOTHORAX

Definition
- Loss of negative intrapleural pressure results in collapse of the lung
- Types include spontaneous, open, tension

Causes
- Blunt chest trauma
- Rupture of a bleb
- CVP line insertion
- Thoracentesis
- Penetrating chest injuries
- Thoracic surgery

Pathophysiology
- The loss of negative intrapleural pressure causes lung collapse
- Surface area for gas exchange is reduced, resulting in hypoxia and hypercarbia
- Spontaneous pneumothorax occurs with bleb rupture
- Open pneumothorax occurs when an opening through the chest wall allows positive atmospheric pressure to enter the pleural space
- Tension pneumothorax occurs when positive pressure builds up in the pleural space

Assessment findings
- Sharp pain that increases with exertion
- Diminished or absent breath sounds unilaterally
- Dyspnea
- Tracheal shift
- Anxiety
- Diaphoresis
- Tachycardia
- Tachypnea
- Decreased chest expansion unilaterally
- Subcutaneous emphysema
- Pallor
- Cough

Diagnostic test findings

- Chest X-ray: pneumothorax
- ABG analysis: respiratory acidosis, hypoxemia
- Ventilation-perfusion ($\dot{V}/\dot{Q}$) scintigraphy: decreased
- $\dot{V}/\dot{Q}$ defects: $\dot{V}/\dot{Q}$ mismatches

Medical management

- Oxygen therapy
- Position: high Fowler's
- Activity: out of bed to chair, active ROM exercises to affected arm
- Monitoring: vital signs and I/O
- Laboratory studies: ABG values
- Treatments: incentive spirometry
- Insertion: chest tube to water-seal drainage
- Thoracentesis
- Analgesic: oxycodone (Tylox)

Nursing interventions

- Administer oxygen
- Turn the patient and encourage coughing,deep breathing, and the use of incentive spirometer
- Assess respiratory status
- Maintain chest tube to water-seal drainage
- Keep the patient in high Fowler's position
- Monitor and record vital signs, chest tube drainage, air leak or subcutaneous emphysema, and laboratory studies
- Administer medications, as prescribed
- Allay the patient's anxiety
- Assess the patient's pain
- Individualize home care instructions
  - Recognize the signs and symptoms of pneumothorax and respiratory infection
  - Avoid heavy lifting

Complications

- Mediastinal shift
- Respiratory insufficiency
- Infection

Possible surgical interventions

- None

PULMONARY EMBOLISM

Definition

- Undissolved substance in the pulmonary vasculature that obstructs blood flow
- Three types
  - Fat

Common pneumothorax symptoms

- Sharp pain that increases with exertion
- Diminished or absent breath sounds unilaterally
- Dyspnea
- Tachypnea

Key therapies for pneumothorax

- Oxygen therapy
- Insertion: chest tube to water-seal drainage
- Thoracentesis

Key nursing steps for a patient with pneumothorax

- Assess respiratory status.
- Monitor vital signs and chest tube drainage.
- Administer medications, as ordered.

Pulmonary embolism

- Undissolved substance in pulmonary vasculature obstructs blood flow
- Three types: fat, air, and thrombus

- Air
- Thrombus

Causes
- Flat or long bone fractures
- Thrombophlebitis
- Venous stasis
- Hypercoagulability
- Abdominal surgery
- Malignant tumors
- Prolonged bed rest
- Obesity
- CVP line insertion
- Trauma

Pathophysiology
- Air, fat, or the tail of a thrombus that breaks off travels from the venous circulation to the right side of the heart and pulmonary artery
- The embolism obstructs blood flow, resulting in pulmonary hypertension and possible infarction

Assessment findings
- Dyspnea
- Tachycardia
- Elevated temperature
- Cough
- Hemoptysis
- Chest pain
- Tachypnea
- Anxiety
- Crackles
- Hypotension
- Arrhythmias
- Frothy, pink-tinged sputum

Diagnostic test findings
- Chest X-ray: dilated pulmonary arteries
- ABG analysis: respiratory alkalosis, hypoxemia
- Lung scan: decreased pulmonary circulation, blood flow obstruction
- Angiography: location of embolism, filling defect of pulmonary artery
- Blood chemistry: increased lactate dehydrogenase
- ECG: tachycardia, nonspecific ST changes

Medical management
- I.V. therapy: hydration, saline lock
- Oxygen therapy
- Intubation and mechanical ventilation
- Position: high Fowler's
- Activity: bed rest; active and passive ROM and isometric exercises
- Monitoring: vital signs, CVP, ECG, I/O, and neurovascular checks

Key causes of pulmonary embolism
- Flat or long bone fractures
- Thrombophlebitis
- Venous stasis

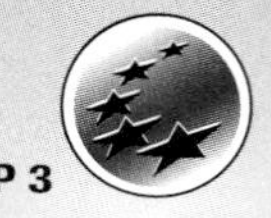

TOP 3

Assessment findings in pulmonary embolism
1. Dyspnea
2. Tachypnea
3. Crackles

Key pulmonary embolism test results
- ABG analysis: respiratory alkalosis, hypoxemia
- Lung scan: decreased pulmonary circulation, blood flow obstruction
- Angiography: location of embolism, filling defect of pulmonary artery

- Laboratory studies: ABG analysis, PT, and PTT
- Treatments: indwelling urinary catheter, incentive spirometry
- Analgesics: meperidine (Demerol), oxycodone (Percocet, Tylox)
- Diuretics: furosemide (Lasix), ethacrynic acid (Edecrin)
- Anticoagulants: heparin (Lipo-Hepin), warfarin (Coumadin)
- Thrombolytics: streptokinase, urokinase
- Pulse oximetry

Nursing interventions

- Administer I.V. fluids
- Administer oxygen
- Provide suction and turning; encourage coughing, and deep breathing
- Assess respiratory status
- Keep the patient in high Fowler's position
- Monitor and record vital signs, CVP, I/O, urine for blood, laboratory studies, and pulse oximetry
- Administer medications, as prescribed
- Allay the patient's anxiety
- Monitor and record color, consistency, and amount of sputum
- **Assess for positive Homans' sign**
- **Monitor PT and PTT to maintain therapeutic anticoagulation levels**
- Individualize home care instructions
  - Recognize the signs and symptoms of respiratory distress
  - Avoid activities that promote venous stasis
    - **Prolonged sitting and standing**
    - **Wearing constrictive clothing**
    - **Crossing legs when seated**
    - Using hormonal contraceptives
  - Recognize signs and symptoms of excessive anticoagulation

Complications

- Pulmonary infarction

Possible surgical interventions

- Vein ligation
- Plication of inferior vena cava
- Embolectomy
- Vena cava filter insertion

LUNG CANCER

Definition

- Malignant tumor of the lung that may be primary or metastatic

Causes

- Cigarette smoking
- Exposure to environmental pollutants
- Exposure to occupational pollutants

Main medical approaches to pulmonary embolism

- Intubation and mechanical ventilation
- Anticoagulants
- Thrombolytics

Key nursing interventions for a patient with pulmonary embolism

- Assess for positive Homans' sign.
- Monitor PT and PTT to maintain therapeutic anticoagulation levels.
- Teach the patient to recognize signs and symptoms of excessive anticoagulation.

Key facts about lung cancer

- Malignant tumor of the lung
- May be primary or metastatic
- Caused by cigarette smoking and exposure to pollutants
- Four types: epidermoid, adenocarcinoma, large cell anaplastic, and small cell anaplastic

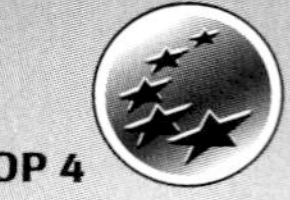

TOP 4

Assessment findings in lung cancer

1. Cough
2. Hemoptysis
3. Weight loss
4. Anorexia

Diagnostic test results in lung cancer

- Bronchoscopy: positive biopsy
- Chest X-ray and lung scan: mass
- Pulmonary angiography: involvement of pulmonary artery or veins
- Sputum studies: positive cytology for cancer cells

Key therapies for lung cancer

- Radiation therapy
- Antineoplastics

Pathophysiology

- Unregulated cell growth and uncontrolled cell division result in the development of a neoplasm
- Four histologic types include epidermoid (squamous), adenocarcinoma, large cell anaplastic, and small cell anaplastic
- The lungs are a common target site for metastasis from other organs

Assessment findings

- Cough
- Dyspnea
- Hemoptysis
- Chest pain
- Chills
- Fever
- Weight loss
- Weakness
- Anorexia
- Wheezing
- Fatigue

Diagnostic test findings

- Chest X-ray: lesion or mass
- Bronchoscopy: positive biopsy
- Pulmonary angiography: involvement of pulmonary artery or pulmonary veins
- Sputum studies: positive cytology for cancer cells
- Lung scan: mass

Medical management

- Diet: high-protein, high-calorie
- I.V. therapy: saline lock
- Oxygen therapy
- Intubation and mechanical ventilation
- Position: semi-Fowler's
- Activity: active and passive ROM exercises, as tolerated
- Monitoring: vital signs and I/O
- Laboratory studies: ABG analysis
- Nutritional support: TPN
- Radiation therapy
- Antineoplastics: cisplatin (Platinol), cyclophosphamide (Cytoxan), doxorubicin (Adriamycin), vinblastine (Velban)
- Treatment: incentive spirometry
- Isotope implant
- Laser photocoagulation
- Diuretics: furosemide (Lasix), ethacrynic acid (Edecrin)
- Analgesics: meperidine (Demerol), morphine (Roxanol)
- Antiemetic: prochlorperazine (Compazine), ondansetron (Zofran)
- Pulse oximetry

Nursing interventions
- Maintain the patient's diet
- Encourage fluids
- Administer I.V. fluids
- Administer oxygen
- Provide suction and turning; encourage coughing and deep breathing
- Assess respiratory status
- Keep the patient in semi-Fowler's position
- Monitor and record vital signs, I/O, laboratory studies, and pulse oximetry
- Administer TPN
- Administer medications, as prescribed
- Encourage the patient to express his feelings about changes in his body image and a fear of dying
- Assess the patient's pain and administer analgesics, as prescribed
- Provide postchemotherapeutic and postradiation nursing care
  - Provide skin and mouth care
  - Monitor dietary intake
  - Administer antiemetics and antidiarrheals, as prescribed
  - Monitor for bleeding, infection, and electrolyte imbalance
  - Provide rest periods
- Provide information about the American Cancer Society
- Individualize home care instructions
  - Demonstrate deep breathing and coughing exercises
  - Alternate rest periods with activity
  - Follow dietary recommendations and restrictions

Key nursing interventions for a patient with lung cancer
- Assess respiratory status.
- Administer oxygen.
- Provide emotional support.
- Administer medications, as ordered.
- Provide postchemotherapeutic and postradiation nursing care.

Complications
- Respiratory insufficiency
- Pneumonia
- Death

Possible surgical interventions
- Lung resection
- Lobectomy
- Wedge resection
- Pneumonectomy

LARYNGEAL CANCER

Laryngeal cancer
- Benign or malignant tumor of the larynx
- Main cause is cigarette smoking
- Most are squamous cell carcinomas
- Either intrinsic or extrinsic

Definition
- Benign or malignant tumor of the larynx

Causes
- Cigarette smoking
- Alcohol abuse
- Exposure to environmental pollutants
- Exposure to radiation
- Voice strain

Pathophysiology

- Unregulated cell growth and uncontrolled cell division result in the development of a neoplasm through the growth of abnormal cells
- Most laryngeal cancers are squamous cell carcinomas
- Intrinsic cancer is cancer within the larynx
- Extrinsic cancer is cancer outside the larynx

Common assessment findings in laryngeal cancer

- Throat pain
- Palpable lump in neck
- Dysphagia
- Progressive hoarseness
- Sore throat

Assessment findings

- Throat pain
- Burning sensation
- Palpable lump in neck
- Dysphagia
- Dyspnea
- Cough
- Hemoptysis
- Progressive hoarseness
- Sore throat
- Weakness
- Weight loss
- Foul breath

Key diagnostic test findings in laryngeal cancer

- Laryngoscopy: lesions, ulcerations, positive biopsy
- Biopsy: cytology positive for cancer cells

Diagnostic test findings

- Laryngoscopy: lesions, ulcerations, positive biopsy
- Biopsy: cytology positive for cancer cells
- Computed tomography scan: laryngeal tumor
- Magnetic resonance imaging: laryngeal tumor

Main medical therapies for laryngeal cancer

- Speech therapy
- Radiation therapy
- Antineoplastics

Medical management

- Diet: high-calorie, high-vitamin, high-protein
- I.V. therapy: saline lock
- Oxygen therapy
- Position: semi-Fowler's
- Activity: as tolerated
- Monitoring: vital signs and I/O
- Laboratory studies: Hb, HCT, and ABG analysis
- Nutritional support: TPN, NG tube feedings, and gastrostomy feedings
- Speech therapy
- Radiation therapy
- Treatment: incentive spirometry
- Analgesic: oxycodone (Tylox)
- Antineoplastics: methotrexate (Mexate), vincristine (Oncovin), bleomycin (Blenoxane), cisplatin (Platinol)
- Antiemetic: prochlorperazine (Compazine)

Nursing interventions

- Maintain high-calorie, high-vitamin, high-protein diet
- Administer I.V. fluids
- Administer oxygen
- Turn the patient and encourage coughing, deep breathing, and use of incentive spirometer

- Assess respiratory status
- Maintain activity, as tolerated
- Keep the patient in semi-Fowler's position
- Monitor and record vital signs, I/O, and laboratory studies
- Administer TPN, NG tube feedings, and gastrostomy feedings
- Administer medications, as prescribed
- Encourage the patient to express his feelings about the potential loss of his voice and changes in his body image
- Monitor and record the color, amount, and consistency of sputum
- Provide postchemotherapeutic and postradiation nursing care
  - Provide prophylactic skin and mouth care
  - Monitor dietary intake
  - Administer antiemetics and antidiarrheals, as prescribed
  - Monitor for bleeding, infection, and electrolyte imbalance
  - Provide rest periods
- Provide information about the Lost Chord Club, New Voice Club, and International Association of Laryngectomies
- Individualize home care instructions
  - Recognize the signs and symptoms of respiratory distress
  - Limit using voice
  - Demonstrate tracheostomy care, suctioning, alternative communication

Complications

- Laryngeal obstruction
- Respiratory distress

Possible surgical interventions

- Partial laryngectomy
- Total laryngectomy
- Radical neck dissection

OCCUPATIONAL LUNG DISEASE

Definition

- A variety of obstructive or restrictive respiratory disorders that occur with exposure to occupational fumes, dust, vapors, or gases
- Four main categories of occupational lung disease: occupational asthma, pneumoconiosis, diffuse interstitial fibrosis, and extrinsic allergic alveolitis

Causes

- Exposure to occupational fumes, dust, vapors, or gases
- Smoking worsens the disease

Pathophysiology

- Occupational asthma is associated with variable airway narrowing related to an exposure in the workplace
- Pneumoconiosis is due to lodging of inhaled dust in the lungs
  - Silicosis is caused by long-term inhalation of free crystalline silica dust

Key steps in caring for a patient with laryngeal cancer

- Maintain high-calorie, high-vitamin, high-protein diet.
- Encourage the patient to express his feelings about the potential loss of his voice and changes in his body image.
- Provide postchemotherapeutic and postradiation nursing care.

Key home care instructions for a patient with laryngeal cancer

- Tracheostomy care
- Suctioning
- Alternative communication

Occupational lung disease

- Obstructive or restrictive respiratory disorders
- Occurs with exposure to occupational fumes, dust, vapors, or gases
- Four main categories:
  - Occupational asthma
  - Pneumoconiosis
  - Diffuse interstitial fibrosis
  - Extrinsic allergic alveolitis

Pathophysiology of occupational lung disease

- Occupational asthma: exposure in the workplace causes variable airway narrowing
- Pneumoconiosis: inhaled dust becomes lodged in the lungs
- Diffuse interstitial fibrosis: caused by occupational exposure to irritants
- Extrinsic allergic alveolitis: immunological response causes a hypersensitivity pneumonitis

Key assessment findings in occupational lung disease

- Exertional dyspnea
- Blood-streaked sputum
- Cough
- Tachypnea

Medical treatment options for occupational lung disease

- Oxygen therapy: 1 to 2 L/minute; mechanical ventilation in advanced cases
- Chest physiotherapy, turning, coughing, deep breathing, postural drainage, intermittent positive pressure breathing
- Antibiotics
- Fluid restriction for cor pulmonale
- Laboratory studies: ABG values, WBCs, and sputum studies

  - Coal miner's pneumoconiosis (black lung disease) is due to deposits of coal dust in the lungs
- Diffuse interstitial fibrosis is caused by occupational exposure to irritants
  - Asbestosis: common among asbestos miners, millers, and those employed in building trades and shipping yards (see *A close look at asbestosis*)
  - Talcosis occurs after years of exposure to high concentrations of talc dust
  - Berylliosis, a chronic granulomatous disorder, caused by inhalation of beryllium
- Extrinsic allergic alveolitis is a hypersensitivity pneumonitis caused by an immunologic response to inhaled organic dust or chemicals containing bacteria or fungal antigens
  - Includes farmer's lung, bird fancier's lung, and machine operator's lung

Assessment findings

- Exertional dyspnea
- Anxiety
- Frequent respiratory infections
- Blood-streaked sputum
- Cough
- Tachypnea

Diagnostic test findings

- Chest X-ray: nodular lesions, enlarged hilar nodes
- Lung biopsy: to establish diagnosis
- PFTs: reveal decreased volume and forced vital capacity
- ABG analysis: may reveal decreased $Pa{O_2}$ and $Sa{O_2}$ levels; increased $Pa{CO_2}$

Medical management

- Oxygen therapy: 1 to 2 L/minute; mechanical ventilation in advanced cases
- Treatments: chest physiotherapy, turning, coughing, deep breathing, postural drainage, and intermittent positive pressure breathing
- Dietary recommendations: increase fluids, unless contraindicated
- Aerosol therapy
- Bronchodilators: aminophylline (Phyllocontin), theophylline (Theo-Dur), metaproterenol (Alupent), cromolyn (Intal)
- Corticosteroids: oral prednisone or aerosol corticosteroid
- Inhaled mucolytic therapy: acetylcysteine (Mucomyst)
- Antibiotics: according to susceptibility of infecting organism
- Diuretic: furosemide (Lasix)
- Cardiac glycoside: digoxin (Lanoxin)
- Fluid restriction for cor pulmonale
- Activity: as tolerated
- Monitoring: vital signs and I/O

A close look at asbestosis

After years of exposure to asbestos, healthy lung tissue progresses to massive pulmonary fibrosis, as shown here.

HEALTHY LUNG TISSUE

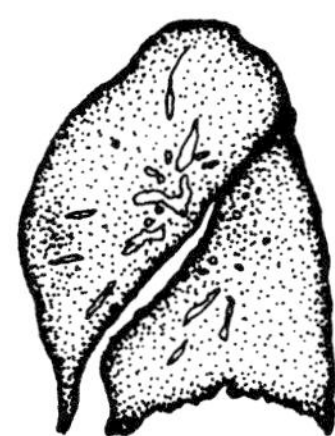

SIMPLE ASBESTOSIS

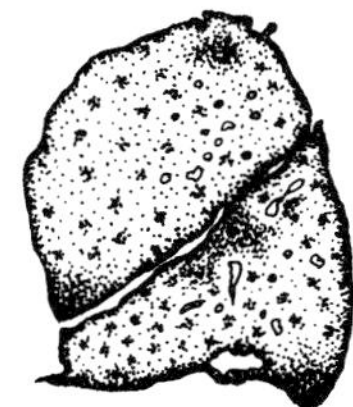

PROGRESSIVE MASSIVE FIBROSIS

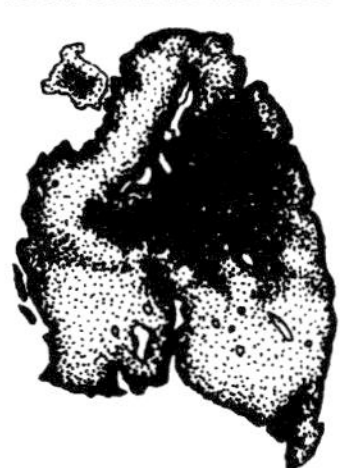

- Laboratory studies: ABG analysis, WBCs, and sputum studies
- I.V. therapy: saline lock

Nursing interventions

- Maintain patient's diet
- Administer small, frequent feedings
- **Encourage fluids, unless the patient has cor pulmonale**
- Administer oxygen
- Provide chest physiotherapy, intermittent positive pressure breathing, turning and postural drainage; encourage coughing and deep breathing
- Assess cardiovascular and respiratory status
- Monitor and record vital signs, I/O, and laboratory studies
- Administer medications, as prescribed
- Encourage activity, as tolerated
- Monitor sputum for amount, color, and consistency
- Individualize home care instructions
  - Prevent infection by avoiding crowds and persons with respiratory infections
  - Receive influenza and pneumococcal vaccines
  - Pace activities and provide rest periods
  - Know proper use of home oxygen
  - Take measures to stop smoking

Complications

- Cor pulmonale
- Right-sided heart failure
- Respiratory infection
- TB
- Respiratory insufficiency

Possible surgical interventions

- None

Key nursing interventions for a patient with occupational lung disease

- Encourage fluids, unless the patient has cor pulmonale.
- Administer oxygen.
- Provide chest physiotherapy, intermittent positive pressure breathing, turning, coughing, deep breathing, and postural drainage.
- Assess cardiovascular and respiratory status.
- Monitor and record vital signs, I/O, and laboratory studies.
- Monitor sputum for amount, color, and consistency.

ARF highlights

- Acute deterioration in ABG values with corresponding clinical deterioration
- In normal lung tissue, ARF usually means $Paco_2$ above 50 mm Hg and Pao_2 below 50 mm Hg
- COPD patient usually has consistently high $Paco_2$ and low Pao_2

Chief causes of ARF

- Respiratory infection
- Bronchospasm
- CNS depression
- Cardiovascular disorders

What happens in ARF

- Causative condition increases work of breathing and decreases respiratory drive.
- Increased $\dot{V}/\dot{Q}$ mismatch and reduced alveolar ventilation result in hypoxemia and acidemia.

Key assessment findings in ARF

- Tachypnea
- Crackles
- Restlessness
- Confusion
- Tachycardia
- Arrhythmias

ACUTE RESPIRATORY FAILURE (ARF) IN COPD

Definition

- Acute deterioration in ABG values with corresponding clinical deterioration

Causes

- Respiratory infection, such as bronchitis or pneumonia (most common)
- Bronchospasm
- Accumulating secretions secondary to cough suppression
- Central nervous system (CNS) depression
  - Head trauma
  - Injudicious use of sedatives, narcotics, tranquilizers, or oxygen
- Cardiovascular disorders
  - Myocardial infarction
  - Heart failure, or pulmonary emboli
- Airway irritants
- Endocrine and metabolic disorders
  - Myxedema
  - Metabolic alkalosis
- Thoracic abnormalities
  - Chest trauma
  - Pneumothorax
  - Thoracic or abdominal surgery

Pathophysiology

- In the patient with normal lung tissue, ARF usually means $Paco_2$ above 50 mm Hg and Pao_2 below 50 mm Hg
- These limits don't apply to the patient with COPD, who commonly has a consistently high $Paco_2$ and low Pao_2
- ARF may develop in the patient with COPD as a result of any condition that increases the work of breathing and decreases the respiratory drive
- Increased $\dot{V}/\dot{Q}$ mismatch and reduced alveolar ventilation decrease Pao_2 (hypoxemia) and increase $Paco_2$ (hypercapnia)
- The resulting hypoxemia and acidemia affect all body organs, especially the CNS and respiratory and cardiovascular systems

Assessment findings

- Respiratory
  - Increased or normal respiratory rate, depending on cause
  - Shallow or deep respirations, or alternating between the two
  - Air hunger
  - Cyanosis
  - Crackles, rhonchi, wheezes, or diminished breath sounds
- CNS
  - Restlessness
  - Confusion
  - Loss of concentration

  - Irritability
  - Tremulousness
  - Diminished tendon reflexes
  - Papilledema
  - Coma
- Cardiovascular
  - Tachycardia
  - Arrhythmias
  - Jugular vein distention
  - Hepatomegaly
  - Peripheral edema

Diagnostic test findings

- ABG analysis: progressive deterioration in ABG levels and pH
- Blood chemistry: increased HCO_3^-, indicating metabolic alkalosis or metabolic compensation for chronic respiratory acidosis; hypokalemia and hypochloremia from diuretic and corticosteroid therapies that treat ARF
- Hematology: elevated WBCs due to bacterial infection
- Chest X-ray: identifies pathologic conditions, such as emphysema, atelectasis, lesions, pneumothorax, infiltrates, or effusions
- ECG: arrhythmias suggest cor pulmonale or myocardial hypoxia

Medical management

- **Oxygen therapy: use minimum fraction of inspired air (FIO_2) required, by nasal prongs or Venturi mask, to maintain ventilation or oxygen saturation greater than 85%**
- Intubation and mechanical ventilation
- Position: high Fowler's
- Activity: as tolerated
- Treatments: chest physiotherapy, postural drainage, intermittent positive pressure breathing, and incentive spirometry
- Monitoring: vital signs and I/O
- Laboratory studies: ABG analysis, WBCs, and sputum studies
- Antibiotics: ampicillin (Omnipen), tetracycline (Achromycin), cefixime (Suprax)
- Bronchodilators: terbutaline (Brethine), aminophylline (Phyllocontin), isoproterenol (Isuprel), theophylline (Theo-Dur); via nebulizer: albuterol (Proventil), ipratropium (Atrovent), metaproterenol (Alupent)
- Corticosteroids: hydrocortisone (Solu-Cortef), methylprednisolone sodium succinate (Solu-Medrol)
- Antacid: aluminum hydroxide gel (AlternaGel)
- I.V. therapy: saline lock

Nursing interventions

- Maintain the patient's diet
- Administer small, frequent feedings
- Encourage fluids, unless contraindicated
- Administer low-flow oxygen

Key diagnostic findings in ARF

- ABG analysis: progressive deterioration
- Chest X-ray: identifies pathologic conditions
- ECG: arrhythmias

Main treatment options for ARF

- Oxygen therapy: use minimum FIO_2 required, by nasal prongs or Venturi mask, to maintain ventilation or SaO_2 greater than 85%
- Intubation and mechanical ventilation
- Position: high Fowler's
- Chest physiotherapy, postural drainage, intermittent positive pressure breathing, and incentive spirometry
- Antibiotics
- Bronchodilators
- Corticosteroids

Key steps in providing care to patients with ARF

- Administer low-flow oxygen.
- Provide chest physiotherapy, intermittent positive pressure breathing, turning, postural drainage, and suctioning; encourage coughing, deep breathing, and use of incentive spirometer.
- Assess cardiovascular and respiratory status.
- Reinforce pursed-lip breathing.
- Keep the patient in high Fowler's position.
- Weigh the patient daily.

Asthma defined

- Form of COPD
- Heightened response to various stimuli causes widespread airway constriction

2 forms of asthma

- Extrinsic (atopic) asthma is caused by sensitivity to specific external allergens
- Intrinsic (nonatopic) asthma is caused by a reaction to internal, nonallergic factors

- Provide chest physiotherapy, intermittent positive pressure breathing, turning, postural drainage, and suctioning; encourage coughing, deep breathing, and use of incentive spirometer
- Assess cardiovascular and respiratory status
- Reinforce pursed-lip breathing
- Keep the patient in high Fowler's position
- Monitor and record vital signs, I/O, and laboratory studies
- Administer medications, as prescribed
- Encourage the patient to express concerns, and allay his anxieties
- Allow activity, as tolerated
- Monitor and record the color, amount, and consistency of sputum
- Weigh the patient daily
- Individualize home care instructions
  - Recognize the signs and symptoms of respiratory infection and hypoxia
  - Adhere to activity limitations
  - Know proper use of home oxygen
  - Demonstrate pursed-lip breathing and coughing exercises
  - Receive influenza and pneumococcal vaccines

Complications
- Severe respiratory failure
- Death

Surgical interventions
- None

ASTHMA

Definition
- A form of COPD in which a heightened response to various stimuli causes widespread airway constriction
- Two forms
  - Extrinsic (atopic) asthma is caused by sensitivity to specific external allergens
  - Intrinsic (nonatopic) asthma is caused by a reaction to internal, nonallergic factors

Causes
- Extrinsic asthma
  - Allergens (pollen, dust, dander, sulfite food additives)
- Intrinsic asthma
  - Endocrine changes
  - Noxious fumes
  - Respiratory infection
  - Stress
  - Temperature and humidity

Pathophysiology

- Bronchial linings overreact to various stimuli, causing episodic spasms and inflammation that severely restrict the airways
- Narrowed airways trap the air; as the airways becomes occluded by thick secretions, the lungs hyperinflate

Assessment findings

- Absent or diminished breath sounds during severe obstruction
- Chest tightness
- Dyspnea
- Productive cough with thick mucus
- Prolonged expiration
- Tachypnea
- Tachycardia
- Use of accessory muscles
- Usually asymptomatic between attacks
- Wheezing, primarily on expiration, but also sometimes on inspiration

Diagnostic test findings

- ABG analysis: in severe acute asthma, decreased PaO_2 and decreased, normal, or increased $PaCO_2$
- Laboratory values: serum immunoglobulin E may increase from an allergic reaction; WBC count may reveal increased eosinophil count
- Chest X-ray: hyperinflated lungs with air trapping during an attack
- PFTs: during attacks show decreased forced expiratory volumes that improve with therapy, and increased residual volume and total lung capacity
- Skin tests: may identify allergens

Medical management

- Dietary recommendations: encourage fluids to 3 L/day as tolerated
- Oxygen therapy: 2 L/minute
- Intubation and mechanical ventilation, if respiratory status worsens
- Position: high Fowler's
- Activity: as tolerated
- Monitoring: vital signs, I/O, ABG values, laboratory values, and PFTs
- Treatments: turning, coughing, deep breathing, and breathing retraining
- Desensitization to allergens
- Antacid: aluminum hydroxide gel (AlternaGEL)
- Antibiotics: according to sensitivity of infective organism
- Antasthmatics: zileuton (Zyflo), zafirlukast (Accolate)
- Bronchodilators: terbutaline (Brethine), aminophylline (Phyllocontin), theophylline (Theo-Dur); via nebulizer: albuterol (Proventil), ipratropium (Atrovent), metaproterenol (Alupent)
- Mast cell stabilizer: cromolyn (Intal)
- Corticosteroids: hydrocortisone (Solu-Cortef), methylprednisolone sodium succinate (Solu-Medrol); via nebulizer: beclomethasone (Vanceril), triamcinolone (Azmacort)
- Beta-adrenergics: epinephrine (Adrenalin), salmeterol (Serevent)
- I.V. therapy: saline lock

Key assessment findings in asthma

- Absent or diminished breath sounds during severe obstruction
- Usually asymptomatic between attacks
- Wheezing, primarily on expiration, but also sometimes on inspiration

PFT findings during attacks

- Decreased forced expiratory volumes that improve with therapy,
- Increased residual volume and total lung capacity

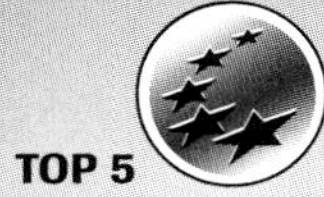

TOP 5

Most common asthma medications

1. Antasthmatics
2. Bronchodilators
3. Corticosteroids
4. Beta-adrenergics
5. Mast cell stabilizers

Key nursing interventions for a patient with asthma

- Encourage fluids.
- Administer low-flow oxygen.
- Keep the patient in high Fowler's position.

Key home care instructions for a patient with asthma

- Identify triggers to asthma attacks.
- Demonstrate use of a metered-dose inhaler and peak flow meter.
- Recognize early signs and symptoms of respiratory infection and hypoxia.

Blunt chest trauma

- Trauma to the chest
- Caused by sudden compression or positive pressure to chest wall
- With cardiac tamponade, intrapericardial pressure increases, compressing the heart; cardiac output decreases; and cardiogenic shock occurs

Nursing interventions

- Maintain the patient's diet, as tolerated
- Administer small, frequent feedings
- Encourage fluids
- Administer low-flow oxygen
- Provide turning; teach pursed-lip and diaphragmatic breathing; and encourage coughing and deep breathing
- Assess respiratory status
- Keep the patient in high Fowler's position
- Monitor and record vital signs, I/O, and laboratory studies
- Administer medications, as prescribed
- Encourage patient to express his feelings about his fear of suffocation
- Allow activity, as tolerated
- Monitor and record the color, amount, and consistency of sputum
- Individualize home care instructions
  - Identify triggers to asthma attacks
  - Demonstrate use of a metered-dose inhaler and peak flow meter
  - Demonstrate pursed-lip and diaphragmatic breathing
  - Recognize early signs and symptoms of respiratory infection and hypoxia

Complications

- Status asthmaticus

Possible surgical interventions

- None

BLUNT CHEST TRAUMA

Definition

- Trauma to the chest caused by sudden compression or positive pressure to the chest wall

Causes

- Motor vehicle accidents
- Falls
- Bicycle handlebar injuries
- Sports injuries
- Blast injuries

Pathophysiology

- Blunt trauma may result in rib fracture, flail chest, pneumothorax, tension pneumothorax, and cardiac tamponade
- Rib fracture causes pain with resultant hypoventilation, leading to atelectasis (see *A close look at atelectatic alveoli*)
- Flail chest results in paradoxical breathing and inadequate ventilation
- Pneumothorax impairs lung expansion, compromising gas exchange
- With cardiac tamponade, intrapericardial pressure increases, compressing the heart; cardiac output decreases, and cardiogenic shock occurs

A close look at atelectatic alveoli

Normally, air-filled alveoli exchange oxygen and carbon dioxide with capillary blood. However, in atelectasis, airless, shrunken alveoli can't accomplish gas exchange.

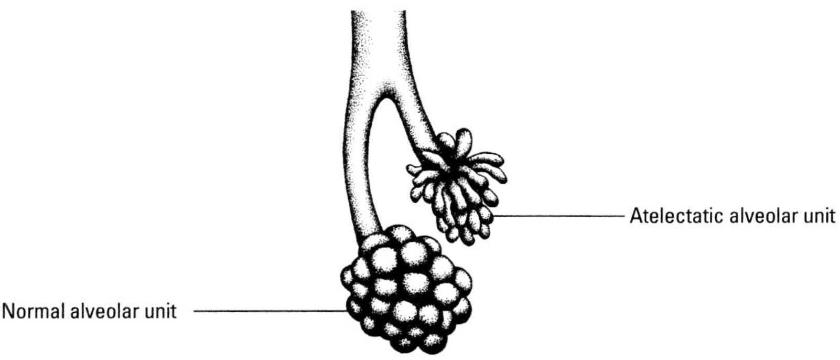

Assessment findings

- Cardiac tamponade
  - Chest pain
  - Hypotension
  - Muffled heart sounds
  - Tachycardia
  - Cyanosis
  - Diaphoresis
  - Restlessness
  - Jugular vein distention
  - Narrowed pulse pressure and paradoxical pulse
- Flail chest
  - Cyanosis
  - Dyspnea
  - Increased respiratory effort
  - Pain on inspiration and on palpation of the injured area
  - Paradoxical movement of the flail segment
- Pneumothorax
  - Asymmetrical lung expansion
  - Chest pain
  - Crepitus
  - Dyspnea
  - Decreased or absent breath sounds on the affected side
  - Restlessness
  - Signs of mediastinal shift and tension pneumothorax
- Rib fractures
  - Pain on inspiration
  - Pain and tenderness of injured area upon palpation
  - Hypoventilation

Chief assessment findings in cardiac tamponade

- Muffled heart sounds
- Restlessness
- Jugular vein distention
- Narrowed pulse pressure and paradoxical pulse

Chief assessment findings in flail chest pain

- Pain on inspiration and on palpation of the injured area
- Paradoxical movement of the flail segment

Chief assessment findings in pneumothorax

- Asymmetrical lung expansion
- Dyspnea
- Decreased or absent breath sounds on the affected side
- Restlessness
- Signs of mediastinal shift and tension pneumothorax

Chief assessment findings in rib fracture pain

- Pain on inspiration
- Pain and tenderness of injured area upon palpation

Chief assessment findings in tension pneumothorax

- Asymmetrical lung expansion and tracheal deviation to the affected side
- Hypotension
- Decreased or absent breath sounds on the affected side
- Jugular vein distention
- Severe chest pain and respiratory distress
- Subcutaneous emphysema

Key management options for blunt chest trauma

- Food and oral fluids restriction
- I.V. therapy: rapid I.V. fluids with lactated Ringer's or normal saline solution, if hypovolemic
- Oxygen therapy: high flow rates
- Intubation and mechanical ventilation using positive pressure
- Position: semi-Fowler's (unless patient requires shock position)
- Monitoring: vital signs, I/O, hemodynamic parameters, ECG, and pulse oximetry
- Transfusion therapy: RBCs, whole blood, plasma, autotransfusion
- Supportive medications to control heart failure and arrhythmias
- Thoracotomy
- Pericardiocentesis

- Tension pneumothorax
  - Asymmetrical lung expansion and tracheal deviation to the affected side
  - Cyanosis
  - Hypotension
  - Decreased or absent breath sounds on the affected side
  - Jugular vein distention
  - Severe chest pain and respiratory distress
  - Subcutaneous emphysema

Diagnostic test findings

- Chest X-rays: may confirm rib and sternal fractures, pneumothorax, flail chest, pulmonary contusions, lacerated or ruptured aorta, tension pneumothorax, diaphragmatic rupture, lung compression, or atelectasis with hemothorax
- ECG: with cardiac damage, may show abnormalities, including tachycardia, atrial fibrillation, bundle-branch block, ST-segment changes, and ventricular arrhythmias
- Laboratory tests: serial aspartate aminotransferase, alanine aminotransferase, lactate dehydrogenase, creatine kinase (CK), CK-MB, troponin I, and troponin T levels are elevated
- Retrograde aortography and transesophageal echocardiography: reveal aortic laceration or rupture
- Contrast studies and liver and spleen scans: detect diaphragmatic rupture
- Echocardiography, CT scans, and cardiac and lung scans: show the injury's extent

Medical management

- Diet: food and oral fluids restriction
- I.V. therapy: rapid I.V. fluids with lactated Ringer's or normal saline solution, if hypovolemic
- Oxygen therapy: high flow rates
- Intubation and mechanical ventilation using positive pressure
- Activity: bed rest
- Position: semi-Fowler's (unless patient requires shock position)
- Monitoring: vital signs, I/O, hemodynamic parameters, ECG, and pulse oximetry
- Laboratory studies: ABG analysis, CBC, cardiac enzymes, type, and crossmatch
- Treatments: indwelling urinary catheter, chest tube, turning, coughing, deep breathing, incentive spirometry, and suction
- Transfusion therapy: RBCs, whole blood, plasma, autotransfusion
- Analgesic: morphine
- Supportive medications to control heart failure and arrhythmias
- Corticosteroids
- Thoracotomy
- Pericardiocentesis
- I.V. therapy: saline lock

- **Nursing interventions**
  - Maintain food and oral fluid restrictions
  - Administer I.V. fluids
  - Monitor mechanical ventilation
  - Maintain bed rest or shock position
  - Assess cardiovascular and respiratory status
  - Monitor and record vital signs, hemodynamic variables, I/O, laboratory studies, ABG values, and pulse oximetry
  - Assess for pain and provide analgesics, as indicated
  - Administer medications, as ordered
  - Maintain and monitor chest tubes; monitor chest tube drainage
  - Administer oxygen therapy
  - Provide suctioning and turning; encourage coughing, deep breathing, and the use of incentive spirometer
  - Support the patient during this potentially life-threatening event
  - Teach the patient to splint the chest to minimize pain and maximize lung expansion in flail chest
  - **Monitor for complications, such as tension pneumothorax, hemorrhagic shock, and cardiac tamponade**
  - Individualize home care instructions
    - Demonstrate coughing and deep-breathing exercises
    - Recognize signs and symptoms of respiratory distress
    - Take analgesics for pain, as needed
    - Splint chest to relieve pain
- **Complications**
  - Hemothorax
  - Pneumothorax
  - Hemorrhagic shock
  - Diaphragmatic rupture
  - Tension pneumothorax
- **Possible surgical interventions**
  - Surgical repair of injured area, such as flail rib segments, myocardial rupture, septal perforation, and aortic rupture

NCLEX CHECKS

It's never too soon to begin your NCLEX preparation. Now that you've reviewed this chapter, carefully read each of the following questions and choose the best answer. Then compare your responses to the correct answers.

1. In a patient with emphysema, the initiative to breathe is triggered by:

☐ **A.** high $PaCO_2$ levels.
☐ **B.** low $PaCO_2$ levels.
☐ **C.** high PaO_2 levels.
☐ **D.** low PaO_2 levels.

Key nursing interventions for a patient with blunt chest trauma

- Maintain food and oral fluid restrictions.
- Monitor mechanical ventilation.
- Assess cardiovascular and respiratory status.
- Monitor and record vital signs, hemodynamic variables, I/O, laboratory studies, ABG values, and pulse oximetry.
- Assess for pain and provide analgesics, as indicated.
- Maintain and monitor chest tubes and chest tube drainage
- Administer oxygen therapy.
- Provide suctioning and turning; encourage coughing, deep breathing, and use of incentive spirometer.
- Teach the patient to splint the chest to minimize pain and maximize lung expansion in flail chest.

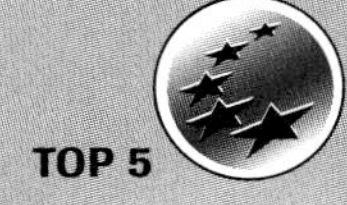

TOP 5 Items to study for your next test on the respiratory system

1. Role of alveoli in gas exchange
2. Signs of respiratory changes
3. Abnormal breath sounds
4. Care of the patient with a chest tube
5. Common disorders of the respiratory system, such as COPD, ARDS, TB, and asthma

2. Extrinsic asthma is caused by:

- ☐ **A.** temperature changes.
- ☐ **B.** sensitivity to specific allergens.
- ☐ **C.** respiratory tract infection.
- ☐ **D.** emotional stress.

3. The nurse is assessing a patient with suspected pneumothorax. Which key signs and symptoms should she expect? (Select all that apply.)

- ☐ **A.** Barrel chest
- ☐ **B.** Night sweats
- ☐ **C.** Diminished or absent breath sounds unilaterally
- ☐ **D.** Dysphagia
- ☐ **E.** Dyspnea

4. The nurse is teaching the patient about the respiratory system. She explains that which of the following is the basic unit of gas exchange?

- ☐ **A.** Alveoli
- ☐ **B.** Larynx
- ☐ **C.** Bronchioles
- ☐ **D.** Surfactant

5. The nurse is assessing a patient with fractured ribs from a motor vehicle accident. Which of the following findings indicates the patient has flail chest?

- ☐ **A.** Mediastinal shift
- ☐ **B.** Paradoxical chest movement
- ☐ **C.** Muffled heart sounds
- ☐ **D.** Subcutaneous emphysema

6. In which of the following positions should the nurse place a patient who has just had a pneumonectomy?

- ☐ **A.** On his back or on the side of surgery
- ☐ **B.** On his abdomen or on the side opposite the surgery
- ☐ **C.** Prone
- ☐ **D.** Any position is acceptable

7. When planning the care of a patient suspected of having tuberculosis (TB), the nurse understands that which of the following mechanisms transmits TB?

- ☐ **A.** Airborne
- ☐ **B.** Fomites
- ☐ **C.** Hand to mouth
- ☐ **D.** Blood

8. The nurse is teaching a patient with chronic bronchitis how to do pursed-lip breathing. What is the rationale for this type of exercise?

- ☐ **A.** Provides more time for gas exchange
- ☐ **B.** Increases airway pressure
- ☐ **C.** Increases the oxygen concentration
- ☐ **D.** Stimulates coughing

ANSWERS AND RATIONALES

1. CORRECT ANSWER: D
Because of long-standing hypercapnia, low PaO_2 levels trigger breathing in a patient with emphysema. In a patient with a normal respiratory drive, increased $PaCO_2$ levels trigger the initiative to breathe.

2. CORRECT ANSWER: B
Extrinsic, or atopic, asthma is caused by sensitivity to specific external allergens, such as pollen, dust, and dander. Temperature changes, respiratory tract infection, and emotional stress cause intrinsic (nonatopic) asthma.

3. CORRECT ANSWER: C, E
Diminished or absent breath sounds unilaterally and dyspnea are key signs and symptoms of a pneumothorax. A barrel chest typically develops with emphysema. Night sweats may occur with tuberculosis, and dysphagia may occur with laryngeal cancer.

4. CORRECT ANSWER: A
The alveoli are the basic unit of gas exchange in the lungs. The larynx contains the vocal cords that produce sounds and initiate the cough reflex. The bronchioles are formed by the branching of the trachea, and aren't involved in gas exchange. Surfactant reduces surface tension to keep alveoli from collapsing.

5. CORRECT ANSWER: B
Multiple rib fractures may cause flail chest, in which a portion of the chest wall moves in during inspiration, creating a paradoxical chest movement. Mediastinal shift may occur with pneumothorax. Muffled heart sounds may occur in cardiac tamponade. Subcutaneous emphysema is found in the patient with tension pneumothorax.

7. CORRECT ANSWER: A
Immediately following a pneumonectomy, place the patient on his back or on the side of surgery. Positioning the patient on the unaffected side or in another position may increase the stress on the bronchial stump and risk disruption of the suture line.

7. CORRECT ANSWER: A
TB is transmitted by droplet nuclei produced when the infected person coughs or sneezes. It isn't spread by fomites, hand to mouth, or through blood.

8. CORRECT ANSWER: B
Pursed-lip breathing is a technique that uses the mild resistance of partially opposed lips to prolong exhalation and to increase airway pressure, causing a delay of the airway's dynamic compression and minimizing the effects of airway trapping. Pursed-lip breathing doesn't provide more time for air exchange, increase the oxygen concentration, or stimulate coughing.

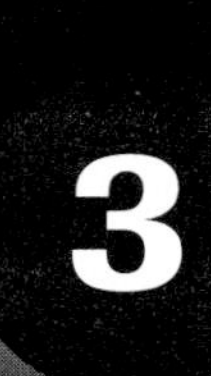

3 Nervous system

LEARNING OBJECTIVES

After studying this chapter, you should be able to:

- Describe the psychosocial impact of nervous system disorders.
- Differentiate between modifiable and nonmodifiable risk factors in the development of a nervous system disorder.
- List three probable and three possible nursing diagnoses for a patient with a nervous system disorder.
- Identify the nursing interventions for a patient with a nervous system disorder.
- Write three goals for teaching a patient with a nervous system disorder.

CHAPTER OVERVIEW

Caring for the patient with a neurologic disorder requires a sound understanding of the anatomy and physiology of the nervous system. A thorough assessment is essential in planning and implementing appropriate patient care. The assessment includes a complete history, a physical examination, diagnostic testing, identification of modifiable and nonmodifiable risk factors, and information related to the psychosocial impact of the disorder on the patient.

Nursing diagnoses focus primarily on self-care deficits, ineffective cerebral tissue perfusion, and decreased intracranial adaptive capacity. Nursing interventions are designed to increase the transmission of nerve impulses, which improves muscular function. Patient teaching — a crucial nursing activity — involves information about medical follow-up, medication regimens, providing a safe environment, signs and symptoms of possible complications, and reducing modifiable risk factors through weight control, activity and diet restrictions, stress management, and smoking cessation. With self-care deficits, consider the impact of neurologic dysfunction on self-esteem.

ANATOMY AND PHYSIOLOGY REVIEW

Neuron

- The nerve cell, or neuron, is the basic functional unit of the nervous system
- The neuron consists of a cell body, dendrites, and an axon; some axons are surrounded by a myelin sheath (myelinated neuron)
- The neuron conducts impulses across a synapse to muscles, glands, and organs
- Neurotransmitters (acetylcholine, serotonin, dopamine, endorphins, gamma-aminobutyric acid, and norepinephrine) excite the next neuron in the chain
  - Produce an action potential
  - Some neurotransmitters inhibit; others excite

Central nervous system (CNS)

- The CNS includes the brain and the spinal cord
  - Brain
    - The *cerebrum* is divided into two hemispheres, separated by a fissure and joined by the corpus callosum, that contain four lobes each (see *A close look at the cerebrum and its functions,* page 118)
      - The frontal lobe is the site of personality, intellectual functioning, and motor speech
      - The parietal lobe is the site of sensation, integration of sensory information, and spatial relationships
      - The temporal lobe is the site of hearing, taste, smell, and speech
      - The occipital lobe is the site of vision
    - The *corpus callosum* consists of nerve fibers that transmit nerve impulses from one hemisphere of the brain to the other
    - The *basal ganglia,* located deep in the cerebral hemispheres, is responsible for body movements
    - The *diencephalon* consists of the thalamus and hypothalamus
      - The thalamus relays sensory impulses of pain, temperature, and touch to the cortex
      - The hypothalamus controls temperature regulation, emotional states, appetite, sleep-wake cycle, thirst, autonomic nervous system (ANS), and endocrine functions
    - The *brain stem* comprises the midbrain, pons, and medulla oblongata
      - The midbrain consists of the tectum and the cerebral peduncles; it serves as the nerve pathway between the cerebral hemispheres
      - The pons consists of the pons dorsalis and pons ventralis; portions of the pons control the respiratory system
      - The medulla oblongata contains the vomiting, vasomotor, respiratory, and cardiac centers

Neuron

- Basic functional unit of the nervous system
- Components: cell body, dendrites, and axon

Parts of the CNS

- Spinal cord
- Brain
  - Cerebrum
  - Corpus callosum
  - Basal ganglia
  - Diencephalon
  - Brain stem
  - Cerebellum

Thalamus and hypothalamus

- Components of the diencephalon
- The thalamus relays sensory impulses of pain, temperature, and touch to the cortex
- The hypothalamus controls temperature regulation, emotional states, appetite, sleep-wake cycle, thirst, ANS, and endocrine functions

Components of the brain stem

- Midbrain: serves as the nerve pathway between the cerebral hemispheres
- Pons: portions control the respiratory system
- Medulla oblongata: contains the vomiting, vasometer, respiratory, and cardiac centers

4 lobes of the cerebrum

- Frontal lobe: the site of personality, intellectual functioning, and motor speech
- Parietal lobe: the site of sensation, integration of sensory information, and spatial relationships
- Temporal lobe: the site of hearing, taste, smell, and speech
- Occipital lobe: the site of vision

Cerebellum's coordination functions

- Muscle tone
- Movement
- Balance
- Posture

The blood-brain barrier

- The endothelial cells within the capillaries of the brain
- Prevents substances in plasma from reaching the brain and CSF

A close look at the cerebrum and its functions

The cerebrum is divided into four lobes, based on anatomic landmarks and functional differences. The lobes – parietal, occipital, temporal, and frontal – are named for the cranial bones that lie over them.

The illustration shows the locations of the cerebral lobes and explains their functions. It also shows the location of the cerebellum.

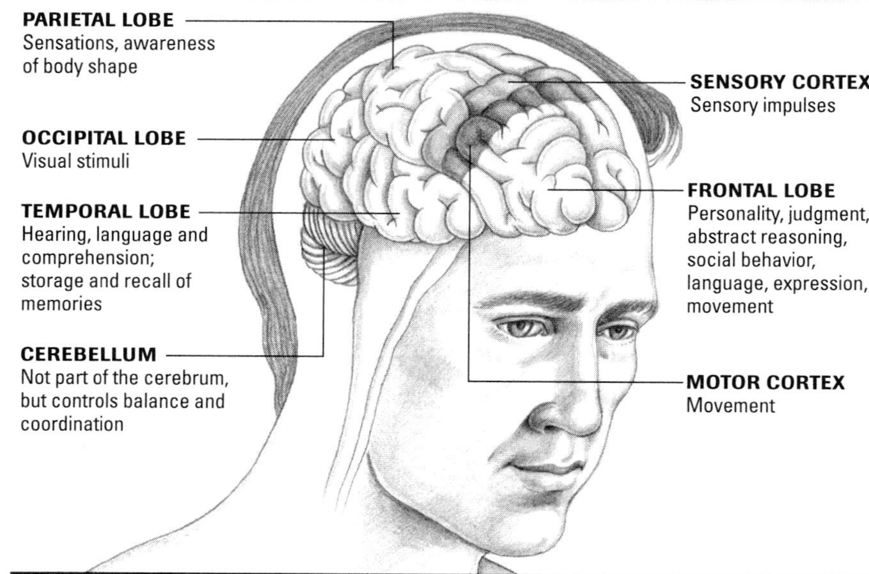

- Pyramidal tracts decussate at the medulla oblongata
- The *cerebellum* coordinates muscle tone, movement, balance, and posture
- Blood is supplied to the brain via the internal carotid arteries, vertebral arteries, and circle of Willis; these interconnecting arteries allow for collateral circulation
- The *reticular activating system* coordinates sensory input and regulates level of arousal, attention, sleep-wake cycles, consciousness, and response to stimuli
- The *blood-brain barrier* is a term for the endothelial cells within the capillaries of the brain that prevent substances in plasma from reaching the brain and cerebrospinal fluid (CSF)
- The *limbic system* stores recent memories and is involved in basic emotional drives, such as fear, hunger, and sexual drives, as well as the visceral response that accompanies them

– Spinal cord
- The *spinal cord* consists of gray matter and white matter
  - Gray matter forms an H-shaped core in the spinal cord
  - White matter includes the spinal cord's ascending (sensory) and descending (motor) tracts
- The spinal cord's reflex arc is an involuntary response to a stimulus

Identifying cranial nerves

The cranial nerves have either sensory or motor function or both. They're assigned Roman numerals and are written this way: CN I, CN II, CN III, and so forth. This illustration lists the function of each cranial nerve.

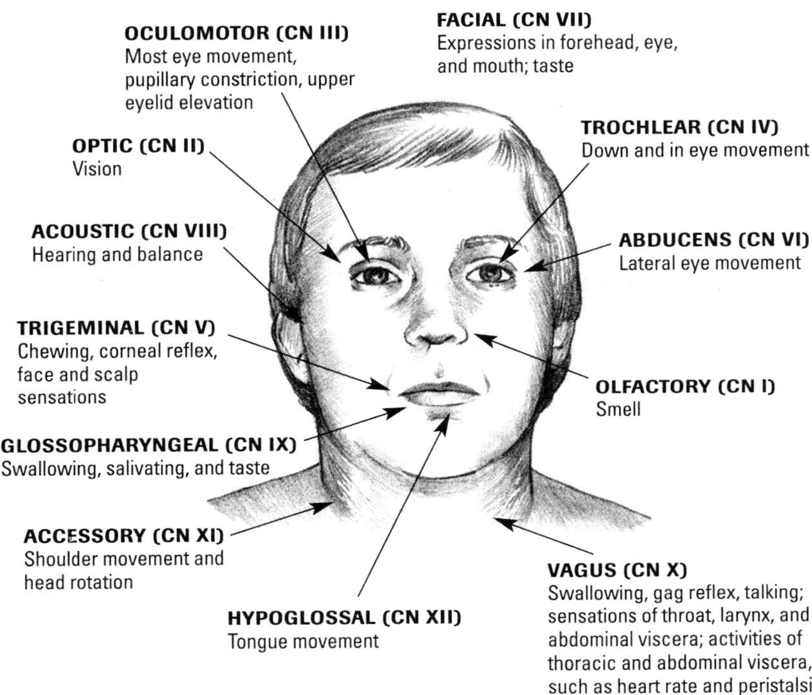

- The CNS is covered and protected by the meninges, which comprise three membranous layers
  - Dura mater
  - Pia mater
  - Arachnoid membrane
- Four ventricles produce and circulate CSF
  - CSF surrounds and protects the brain and spinal cord
  - CSF exchanges nutrients and wastes at the cellular level

Peripheral nervous system (PNS)

- The PNS and the CNS together constitute the nervous system
- The PNS comprises 12 pairs of cranial nerves, 31 pairs of spinal nerves, and the autonomic nervous system (ANS)
  - The cranial nerves consist of the olfactory, optic, oculomotor, trochlear, trigeminal, abducent, facial, acoustic, glossopharyngeal, vagus, accessory, and hypoglossal nerves (see *Identifying cranial nerves*)
  - Spinal nerves carry mixed impulses (motor and sensory) to and from the spinal cord

Cranial nerves and functions

- CN I: Olfactory
  - Smell
- CN II: Optic
  - Vision
- CN III: Oculomotor
  - Most eye movement
  - Pupillary constriction
  - Upper eyelid elevation
- CN IV: Trochlear
  - Down and in eye movement
- CN V: Trigeminal
  - Chewing
  - Corneal reflex
  - Face and scalp sensations
- CN VI: Abducens
  - Lateral eye movement
- CN VII: Facial
  - Expressions in forehead, eye and mouth
  - Taste
- CN VIII: Acoustic
  - Hearing
  - Balance
- CN IX: Glossopharyngeal
  - Swallowing
  - Salivating
  - Taste
- CN X: Vagus
  - Swallowing
  - Gag reflex
  - Talking
  - Sensations of the throat, larynx, and abdominal viscera
  - Activities of the thoracic and abdominal viscera
- CN XI: Accessory
  - Shoulder movement
  - Head rotation
- CN XII: Hypoglossal
  - Tongue movement

Parts of the PNS

- Cranial nerves
- Spinal nerves
- ANS

– The ANS regulates smooth muscle, cardiac muscle, and glands; it comprises the sympathetic and parasympathetic nervous systems
  - Sympathetic activity results in adrenergic responses
  - Parasympathetic activity results in cholinergic responses

What the ANS does

- Regulates smooth muscle, cardiac muscle, and glands
- Comprises the sympathetic and parasympathetic nervous systems

ASSESSMENT FINDINGS

History

- Memory impairment
- Numbness and tingling
- Muscle weakness
- Twitching and spasm
- Ringing in the ears
- Difficulty chewing, swallowing, talking, and walking
- Headache
- Dizziness
- Fainting
- Loss of balance and coordination
- Nausea and vomiting
- Pain
- Mental confusion or excitement
- Blurred or double vision
- Changes in vision
- Change in bowel and bladder patterns
- Sexual dysfunction
- Tremors
- Stiff neck
- Drooping eyelids
- Trauma

Common history assessment findings in a patient with a nervous system disorder

- Memory impairment
- Numbness and tingling
- Muscle weakness
- Twitching and spasm
- Ringing in the ears

Physical examination

- Paresthesia
- Loss of sensation
- Change in level of consciousness (LOC) (see *Glasgow Coma Scale*)
- Ataxic gait
- Dyskinesia
- Tinnitus
- Dysphagia
- Aphasia
- Seizures
- Diplopia
- Papilledema
- Change in visual fields
- Loss of vision
- Abnormal temperature
- Pulse changes
- Abnormal respirations
- Hypertension

Key physical assessment findings in a patient with a nervous system disorder

- Change in LOC
- Abnormal pupil size and reaction
- Abnormal reflexes: Babinski's, plantar response
- Loss of cough, gag, corneal, oculocephalic, and oculovestibular reflexes

Glasgow Coma Scale

To assess a patient's level of consciousness quickly and to uncover baseline changes, use the Glasgow Coma Scale. This assessment tool grades consciousness in relation to eye opening and motor and verbal responses. A decreased reaction score in one or more categories warns of an impending neurologic crisis. A patient scoring 7 or less is comatose and probably has severe neurologic damage.

TEST	PATIENT'S REACTION	SCORE
Best eye opening response	Open spontaneously	4
	Open to verbal command	3
	Open to pain	2
	No response	1
Best motor response	Obeys verbal command	6
	Localizes painful stimuli	5
	Flexion-withdrawal	4
	Flexion-abnormal (decorticate rigidity)	3
	Extension (decerebrate rigidity)	2
	No response	1
Best verbal response	Oriented and converses	5
	Disoriented and converses	4
	Inappropriate words	3
	Incomprehensive sounds	2
	No response	1
Total		3 to 15

- Change in muscle reflexes
- Weakness
- Spasticity, rigidity, flaccidity
- Abnormal pupil size and reaction
- Abnormal reflexes: Babinski's, plantar response
- Loss of cough, gag, corneal, oculocephalic, and oculovestibular reflexes
- Ptosis

DIAGNOSTIC TESTS AND PROCEDURES

EEG

- Definition and purpose
  - Noninvasive test of the brain
  - Graphic representation of the brain's electrical activity
- Nursing interventions before the procedure
  - Determine the patient's ability to lie still
  - Reassure the patient that electrical shock won't occur
  - Explain that the patient will be subjected to stimuli, such as lights and sounds
  - Withhold medications and caffeine for 8 hours before the procedure

Glasgow Coma Scale

- Provides a quick, standardized account of neurologic status
- Assesses eye opening response, motor response, and verbal response
- A score of 7 or less indicates severe neurologic damage

EEG

- Noninvasive test
- Graphic representation of the brain's electrical activity
- Interventions:
- Determine the patient's ability to lie still
- Explain that the patient will be subjected to stimuli, such as lights and sounds
- Withhold medications and caffeine 8 hours before the procedure

CT scan

- Noninvasive test in which contrast dye may be used
- Allows for visualization of the brain and its structures
- Intervention: note the patient's allergies before the procedure

MRI

- Noninvasive test
- Allows for visualization of the brain and its structures
- Interventions:
- Be aware that patients with pacemakers, surgical and orthopedic clips, bullet fragments, or shrapnel shouldn't be scanned
- Assess for history of claustrophobia
- Remove jewelry and metal objects from the patient

Cerebral angiogram

- Invasive procedure using a radiopaque dye
- Allows for examination of the cerebral arteries
- Intervention: note the patient's allergies before the procedure

Computerized tomography (CT) scan

- Definition and purpose
  - Noninvasive scan
  - Contrast dye may be used
  - Visualization of the brain and its structures
- Nursing interventions before the procedure
  - **Note the patient's allergies to iodine, seafood, and radiopaque dyes, if a dye will be used**
  - Allay the patient's anxiety and administer sedation, as ordered
  - Inform the patient about possible throat irritation and flushing of the face, if dye is used
  - Tell the patient that he must lie still during the test
  - Tell the patient to remove hairpins

Magnetic resonance imaging (MRI)

- Definition and purpose
  - Noninvasive scan using magnetic and radio waves
  - Visualization of the brain and its structures
- Nursing interventions before the procedure
  - Be aware that a patient with a pacemaker, surgical or orthopedic clip, bullet fragments, or shrapnel shouldn't be scanned
  - Assess for history of claustrophobia
  - Remove jewelry and metal objects from the patient
  - Determine the patient's ability to lie still
  - Administer sedation, as prescribed

Cerebral angiogram

- Definition and purpose
  - Fluoroscopic procedure using a radiopaque dye
  - Examination of the cerebral arteries
- Nursing interventions before the procedure
  - **Note the patient's allergies to iodine, seafood, or radiopaque dyes**
  - Inform the patient about possible throat irritation and flushing of the face
- Nursing interventions after the procedure
  - Monitor vital signs
  - Allay the patient's anxiety
  - Check the insertion site for bleeding
  - Maintain affected extremity in straight alignment for 6 hours, or as ordered
  - Check pulses in affected extremity
  - Provide adequate hydration orally or I.V., as indicated
  - Monitor neurovital signs (see *Understanding neurovital signs*)

Lumbar puncture (LP)

- Definition and purpose
  - Invasive procedure

Understanding neurovital signs

Neurologic vital signs supplement the routine measurement of temperature, pulse rate, and respirations by evaluating the patient's level of consciousness (LOC), pupillary activity, and orientation to place, time, date, and person. They provide a simple, indispensable tool for quickly checking the patient's neurologic status.

LOC, a measure of environmental awareness and self-awareness, reflects cortical function and usually provides the first sign of central nervous system (CNS) deterioration. Changes in pupillary activity (pupil size, shape, equality, and response to light) may signal increased intracranial pressure associated with a space-occupying lesion. Evaluating muscle strength and tone, reflexes, and posture also may help identify CNS damage.

Changes in vital signs alone rarely indicate neurologic compromise; therefore, evaluate any changes in light of a complete neurologic assessment. Because vital signs are controlled at the medullary level, changes related to neurologic compromise are ominous.

- Collection of CSF from the lumbar subarachnoid space, measurement of CSF pressure, and injection of radiopaque dye for myelogram

- Nursing interventions before the procedure
  - Determine the patient's ability to lie still in a flexed, lateral, recumbent position
  - Explain the procedure to the patient
  - **Know that the presence of increased intracranial pressure (ICP) is a contraindication for having the test**
- Nursing interventions after the procedure
  - Keep the patient flat in bed for 6 to 24 hours
  - Administer analgesics, as prescribed
  - Check the puncture site for bleeding
  - Monitor neurovital signs
  - Encourage fluids to offset CSF leakage
  - Monitor for headache when rising

CSF analysis

- Definition and purpose
  - Laboratory test of CSF obtained via LP
  - Microscopic examination of CSF for blood, white blood cells (WBCs), immunoglobulins, bacteria, protein, glucose, specific gravity, pH, and electrolytes
- Nursing interventions
  - Label specimens properly and send to the laboratory immediately
  - Adhere to nursing interventions after an LP

Electromyography (EMG)

- Definition and purpose
  - Noninvasive test of muscles

Components of neurovital signs

- LOC
- Pupillary activity
- Orientation to place, time, date, and person

Lumbar puncture

- Invasive test
- Purposes:
  - Collection of CSF from lumbar subarachnoid
  - Measurement of CSF pressure
  - Injection of radiopaque dye for myelogram
- Intervention: know that the procedure is contraindicated in the presence of increased ICP

CSF analysis

- Laboratory test of CSF
- Microscopic examination of CSF
- Intervention: label specimens properly and send to the laboratory immediately

EMG
- Noninvasive test
- Graphic recording of the electrical activity of a muscle
- Intervention: administer analgesics, as prescribed, after the procedure

Myleogram
- Invasive test involving an injection of dye via LP
- Allows for visualization of the subarachnoid space, spinal cord, and vertebrae
- Intervention: note the patient's allergies before the procedure

Brain scan
- Invasive test involving injection of a radiopaque dye
- Provides visual imaging of blood flow and distribution and brain structures
- Intervention: note the patient's allergies before the procedure

Skull X-rays
- Noninvasive test
- Radiographic picture of head and neck bones
- Intervention: determine the patient's ability to lie still during the procedure

  - Graphic recording of the electrical activity of a muscle at rest and during contraction
- Nursing interventions
  - Explain that the patient must flex and relax his muscles during the procedure
  - Stress the importance of cooperation during the procedure
  - Explain that the patient will feel some discomfort, but not pain
  - Administer analgesics, as prescribed, after the procedure

Myelogram
- Definition and purpose
  - Injection of radiopaque water- or oil-based dye by LP
  - Visualization of the subarachnoid space, spinal cord, and vertebrae under fluoroscopy
- Nursing interventions before the procedure
  - **Note the patient's allergies to iodine, seafood, and radiopaque dyes**
  - Inform the patient about possible throat irritation and flushing of the face
- Nursing interventions after the procedure
  - Keep the patient flat in bed, as directed
  - Follow postprocedural management for specific dye used
  - Check the puncture site for bleeding
  - Monitor neurovital signs
  - Encourage fluids

Brain scan
- Definition and purpose
  - Procedure that involves injection of a radiopaque dye
  - Visual imaging of blood flow and distribution and brain structures
- Nursing interventions before the procedure
  - **Note the patient's allergies to iodine, seafood, and radiopaque dyes**
  - Inform the patient about possible throat irritation and flushing of the face
  - Determine the patient's ability to lie still during the procedure

Skull X-rays
- Definition and purpose
  - Noninvasive examination
  - Radiographic picture of head and neck bones
- Nursing interventions before the procedure
  - Determine the patient's ability to lie still during the procedure
  - Explain the events that will occur during the procedure

Positron emission tomography (PET) scan
- Definition and purpose
  - Imaging that involves injection of a radioisotope
  - Visualization of oxygen uptake, blood flow, and glucose metabolism

- Nursing interventions
  - Determine the patient's ability to lie still during the procedure
  - Withhold alcohol, tobacco, and caffeine for 24 hours before the procedure
  - Withhold medications, as directed, before the procedure
  - Check the injection site for bleeding after the procedure

Blood chemistry

- Definition and purpose
  - Laboratory test of a blood sample
  - Analysis for potassium, sodium, calcium, phosphorus, protein, albumin, osmolality, glucose, bicarbonate, blood urea nitrogen (BUN), and creatinine
- Nursing interventions
  - Withhold food and fluids before the procedure
  - Monitor the site for bleeding after the procedure

Hematologic studies

- Definition and purpose
  - Laboratory test of a blood sample
  - Analysis for WBCs, red blood cells (RBCs), erythrocyte sedimentation rate, prothrombin time (PT), partial thromboplastin time (PTT), platelets, hemoglobin (Hb), and hematocrit (HCT)
- Nursing interventions
  - Note current drug therapy before the procedure
  - Check the venipuncture site for bleeding after the procedure

PSYCHOSOCIAL IMPACT OF NERVOUS SYSTEM DISORDERS

Developmental impact

- Changes in body image
- Loss of control over body functions
- Fear of rejection
- Embarrassment from changes in body structure and function
- Decreased self-esteem
- Fear of dying
- Dependence

Economic impact

- Disruption or loss of employment to patient or caregiver
- Cost of hospitalizations
- Cost of home health care
- Cost of special equipment

Occupational and recreational impact

- Restrictions in work activity
- Changes in leisure activity
- Restrictions in physical activity
- Need for vocational retraining

PET scan

- Invasive test that involves injection of a radioisotope
- Provides visualization of oxygen uptake, blood flow, and glucose metabolism
- Intervention: withhold alcohol, tobacco, and caffeine for 24 hours before the procedure

Blood chemistry

- Laboratory test of a blood sample
- Analysis for potassium, sodium, calcium, phosphorus, protein, albumin, osmolality, glucose, bicarbonate, BUN, and creatinine
- Intervention: monitor the site for bleeding after the procedure

Hematologic studies

- Laboratory test of a blood sample
- Analysis for WBCs, RBCs, erythrocyte sedimentation rate, PT, PTT, Hb, and HCT
- Intervention: check the venipuncture site for bleeding after the procedure

Psychosocial impact of nervous system disorders

- Change in body image
- Cost of hospitalizations, home health care, special equipment
- Disruption or loss of employment to patient or caregiver
- Restrictions or changes in activity

Modifiable risk factors for a nervous system disorder

- Exposure to chemical or environmental pollutants
- Substance abuse
- Smoking
- Alcohol
- Participation in contact sports
- Hypertension

Nonmodifiable risk factors for a nervous system disorder

- Aging
- Family history of neurologic disease
- History of cardiac disease
- History of head injury
- Exposure to viral or bacterial infection

Key probable nursing diagnoses for a nervous system disorder

- Impaired physical mobility
- Feeding self-care deficit; hygiene self-care deficit; toileting self-care deficit
- Disturbed sensory perception
- Disturbed thought processes

Social impact
- Changes in eating modes
- Changes in elimination patterns and modes
- Social isolation
- Changes in sexual function
- Changes in role performance

RISK FACTORS

Modifiable risk factors
- Exposure to chemical or environmental pollutants
- Substance abuse
- Smoking
- Alcohol
- Participation in contact sports
- Hypertension

Nonmodifiable risk factors
- Aging
- Family history of neurologic disease
- History of cardiac disease
- History of head injury
- Exposure to viral or bacterial infection

NURSING DIAGNOSES

Probable nursing diagnoses
- Impaired physical mobility
- Feeding self-care deficit
- Bathing or hygiene self-care deficit
- Dressing or grooming self-care deficit
- Toileting self-care deficit
- Disturbed sensory perception (visual)
- Disturbed sensory perception (tactile)
- Disturbed thought processes
- Social isolation
- Impaired home maintenance
- Unilateral neglect
- Disturbed body image
- Situational low self-esteem
- Autonomic dysreflexia

Possible nursing diagnoses
- Sexual dysfunction
- Impaired urinary elimination
- Impaired verbal communication
- Bowel incontinence
- Imbalanced nutrition: Less than body requirements
- Ineffective airway clearance

- Ineffective coping
- Risk for injury
- Ineffective tissue perfusion (cerebral)
- Powerlessness
- Risk for self-directed violence
- Disturbed sleep pattern
- Risk for aspiration
- Dysfunctional grieving

CRANIOTOMY

Description

- Surgical opening in the skull to excise a tumor, evacuate a blood clot, relieve ICP, or repair an aneurysm
- Classified as supratentorial or infratentorial

Preoperative nursing interventions

- Complete patient and family preoperative teaching
  - Determine the patient's understanding of the procedure
  - Describe the operating room, postanesthesia care unit (PACU), and preoperative and postoperative routines; demonstrate postoperative turning, coughing, deep breathing, splinting, and range-of-motion (ROM) exercises
  - Explain the postoperative need for drainage tubes, surgical dressings, oxygen therapy, I.V. therapy, and pain control
- Complete a preoperative checklist
- Administer preoperative medications, as prescribed
- Allay the patient's and his family's anxiety about surgery
- Document the patient's history and physical assessment database
- Administer antibiotics, as prescribed
- Explain that the patient's head will be shaved

Postoperative nursing interventions

- Assess cardiac, respiratory, and neurologic status, including LOC
- Assess pain and administer postoperative analgesics, as prescribed
- Assess for return of peristalsis; give solid foods and liquids, as tolerated
- Administer I.V. fluids and total parenteral nutrition (TPN)
- Keep the patient's head in a neutral position
- Allay the patient's anxiety
- Inspect the surgical dressing and change it, as directed
- Reinforce turning, coughing, and deep breathing
- Keep the patient in semi-Fowler's position
- Encourage incentive spirometry
- Maintain active or passive ROM exercises, as tolerated
- Administer oxygen and maintain endotracheal (ET) tube to ventilator
- Monitor vital signs, urine specific gravity, intake and output (I/O), central venous pressure (CVP), laboratory studies, electrocardiogram (ECG), neu-

Key possible nursing diagnoses for a nervous system disorder

- Sexual dysfunction
- Impaired urinary elimination
- Impaired verbal communication

Craniotomy

- Surgical opening in the skull
- Purposes: to excise a tumor, to evacuate a blood clot, to relieve ICP, or to relieve an aneurysm

Key patient teaching topics before craniotomy

- Describe the operating room, PACU, and preoperative and postoperative routines; demonstrate postoperative turning, coughing, deep breathing, splinting, and ROM exercises.
- Explain the postoperative need for drainage tubes, surgical dressings, oxygen therapy, I.V. therapy, and pain control.

rovital signs, neurovascular checks, ICP, arterial blood gas (ABG) values, and pulse oximetry
- Monitor and maintain the position and patency of drainage tubes: nasogastric (NG), indwelling urinary catheter, and wound drainage
- Assess cough and gag reflexes
- Encourage the patient to express his feelings about changes in his body image or a fear of dying
- Check for signs of diabetes insipidus
- Provide eye care and cold compresses, as indicated
- Allow a rest period between each nursing activity
- **Observe for signs of increasing ICP**
- Administer corticosteroids, as prescribed
- Administer anticonvulsants, as prescribed
- Administer laxatives, as prescribed
- Administer antacids, as prescribed
- Administer osmotic diuretics, as prescribed
- Maintain seizure precautions
- Individualize home care instructions
  - Recognize the signs and symptoms of infection
  - Monitor for neurologic changes, including LOC
  - Demonstrate safety measures during seizure activity

Possible surgical complications
- Increased ICP
- Brain herniation
- Seizures
- Respiratory distress
- Diabetes insipidus
- Motor and sensory deficits
- Infection
- Meningitis

ENDARTERECTOMY

Description
- Surgical removal of atheromas from arteries and a patch graft repair of the vessel

Preoperative nursing interventions
- Complete patient and family preoperative teaching
  - Determine the patient's understanding of the procedure
  - Describe the operating room, PACU, and preoperative and postoperative routines
  - Demonstrate postoperative turning, coughing, deep breathing, splinting, and ROM exercises
  - Explain the postoperative need for drainage tubes, surgical dressings, oxygen therapy, I.V. therapy, and pain control
- Complete a preoperative checklist

Key nursing interventions after craniotomy

- Assess cardiac, respiratory, and neurologic status, including LOC.
- Assess pain and administer postoperative analgesics, as prescribed.
- Keep the patient's head in a neutral position.
- Reinforce turning, coughing, and deep breathing.
- Keep the patient in semi-Fowler's position.
- Monitor vital signs, urine specific gravity, I/O, CVP, laboratory studies, ECG, neurovital signs, neurovascular checks, ICP, ABG values, and pulse oximetry.
- Assess cough and gag reflexes.
- Check for signs of diabetes insipidus.
- Provide eye care and cold compresses, as indicated.
- Observe for signs of increasing ICP.
- Administer anticonvulsants, as prescribed.
- Administer osmotic diuretics, as prescribed.
- Maintain seizure precautions.

Endarterectomy

- Removal of atheromas from arteries
- Patch graft repair of the vessel

- Administer preoperative medications, as prescribed
- Allay the patient's and his family's anxiety about surgery
- Document the patient's history and physical assessment database
- Administer antibiotics, as prescribed
- Protect the surgical site from trauma
- Obtain a preoperative vascular assessment

Postoperative nursing interventions

- Assess cardiac, respiratory, and neurologic status
- Assess pain and administer postoperative analgesics, as prescribed
- Assess for return of peristalsis; give solid foods and liquids, as tolerated
- Administer I.V. fluids
- Allay the patient's anxiety
- Inspect the surgical dressing and change it, as directed
- Reinforce turning, coughing, and deep breathing
- Keep the patient in semi-Fowler's position
- Maintain the patient's head in a neutral position
- Provide incentive spirometry
- Maintain activity: active or passive ROM and isometric exercises, as tolerated
- Administer oxygen
- Monitor vital signs, I/O, laboratory studies, neurovital signs, neurovascular checks, and pulse oximetry
- Monitor and maintain the position and patency of drainage tubes: NG, indwelling urinary catheter, and wound drainage
- Check the surgical site for bleeding
- Maintain a pressure dressing
- Provide special care for carotid endarterectomy
  - Check neck edema
  - Assess ability to swallow
- Administer anticoagulants
- Individualize home care instructions
  - Recognize the signs and symptoms of infection
  - Monitor for motor and sensory deficits

Possible surgical complications

- Bleeding
- Embolism
- Thrombosis
- Neurologic deficits
- Infection

PARKINSON'S DISEASE

Definition

- Progressive degenerative disease of the extrapyramidal system associated with dopamine deficiency

Key nursing steps before endarterectomy

- Demonstrate postoperative turning, coughing, deep breathing, splinting, and ROM exercises.
- Administer antibiotics, as prescribed.
- Obtain a preoperative vascular assessment.

Key nursing steps after endarterectomy

- Assess cardiac, respiratory, and neurologic status.
- Inspect the surgical dressing and change it, as directed.
- Reinforce turning, coughing, and deep breathing.
- Maintain the patient's head in a neutral position.
- Monitor vital signs, I/O, laboratory studies, neurovital signs, neurovascular checks, and pulse oximetry.
- Check the surgical site for bleeding.
- Provide special care for carotid endarterectomy.
- Administer anticoagulants.

Parkinson's disease defined

- Progressive degenerative disease of the extrapyramidal system
- Associated with dopamine deficiency

Pathophysiology of Parkinson's disease

- Nerve cells in the basal ganglia are destroyed, resulting in impaired muscular function
- Dopamine degenerates
- Lack of dopamine results in decreased inhibition of the synaptic transmitter

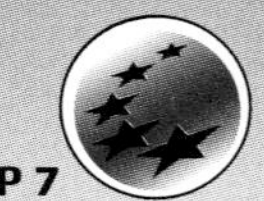

TOP 7

Assessment findings in Parkinson's disease

1. "Pill rolling" tremors
2. Shuffling gait
3. Stiff joints
4. Masklike facial expression
5. Dyskinesia
6. "Cogwheel" rigidity
7. Stooped posture

Possible test findings for Parkinson's disease

- EEG: minimal slowing
- CT scan: normal

Causes

- Unknown
- Imbalance of dopamine and acetylcholine in basal ganglia
- Cerebrovascular disease
- Drug-induced: phentolamine (Regitine), reserpine (Serpasil), methyldopa (Aldomet)
- Dopamine deficiency

Pathophysiology

- Nerve cells in the basal ganglia are destroyed, resulting in impaired muscular function
- Dopamine in the substantia nigra degenerates
- Lack of dopamine results in decreased inhibition of the synaptic transmitter for muscle tone and coordination

Assessment findings

- "Pill rolling" tremors
- Shuffling gait
- Stiff joints
- Masklike facial expression
- Dyskinesia
- Dysphagia
- Drooling
- "Cogwheel" rigidity
- Fatigue
- General weakness
- Stooped posture
- Tremors at rest
- Small handwriting
- Difficulty in initiating voluntary activity
- Visual deficits
- Constipation
- Urinary hesitancy
- Orthostatic hypotension

Diagnostic test findings

- EEG: minimal slowing
- CT scan: normal

Medical management

- Diet: high-residue, high-calorie, and high-protein; soft foods
- Physical therapy
- Activity: as tolerated
- Monitoring: vital signs, I/O, and neurovital signs
- Anticholinergics: benztropine (Cogentin), trihexyphenidyl (Artane)
- Antiparkinsonian agents: levodopa (Larodopa), carbidopa-levodopa (Sinemet), benztropine (Cogentin)
- Antispasmodic: procyclidine (Kemadrin)
- Antidepressant: amitriptyline (Elavil)

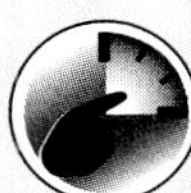

TIME-OUT FOR TEACHING

Patients with nervous system disorders

Be sure to include the following topics in your teaching plan when caring for patients with neurologic disorders.

- Smoking cessation
- Optimal weight maintenance
- Regular exercise
- Medication therapy, including action, adverse effects, and scheduling of medications
- Dietary recommendations and restrictions
- Stress-reduction strategies
- Rest and activity patterns
- Frequent blood pressure monitoring
- Environmental safety
- Community resources
- Self-monitoring for infection
- Avoidance of alcohol
- Danger signs, including changes in mentation and level of consciousness
- Rehabilitation, including adaptive and assistive devices
- Coping mechanisms

- Antiviral: amantadine (Symmetrel)
- Monoamine oxidase-B inhibitor: selegiline (Eldepryl)
- Dopamine receptor agonists: pergolide (Permax), bromocriptine (Parlodel)

Nursing interventions

- Maintain the patient's diet
- Assess neurovascular and respiratory status
- Position the patient to prevent contractures
- Monitor and record vital signs and I/O
- Administer medications, as prescribed
- Encourage the patient to express his feelings about changes in his body image
- Promote daily ambulation
- Promote measures to prevent falls
- Change the patient's position slowly
- Maintain a patent airway
- Provide active and passive ROM exercises
- Provide skin care daily
- Provide oral hygiene
- Reinforce gait training
- Reinforce independence in care
- Provide information about the American Parkinson's Disease Association, Inc.; the Parkinson Disease Foundation; and the National Parkinson's Foundation
- Individualize home care instructions (for more information about patient teaching, see *Patients with nervous system disorders*)
  - Recognize the signs and symptoms of respiratory distress
  - Alternate rest periods with activity
  - Promote a safe environment and prevent falls
  - Take measures to prevent choking
    - Cut food into small pieces

Key teaching topics for a patient with a nervous system disorder

- Smoking cessation
- Regular exercise
- Medication therapy
- Stress-reduction strategies
- Self-monitoring for infection
- Danger signs

Key ways to manage Parkinson's disease

- High-residue, high-calorie, and high-protein diet; soft foods
- Anticholinergics
- Antiparkinsonian agents
- Antispasmodics
- Antidepressants
- Dopamine receptor agonists

Key nursing interventions for a patient with Parkinson's disease

- Assess neurovascular and respiratory status.
- Promote measures to prevent falls.
- Maintain a patent airway.
- Reinforce gait training.
- Reinforce independence in care.

    - Suction the mouth frequently
    - Offer only soft foods
  - Increase intake of roughage and fluids to prevent constipation
  - Monitor weight

Decreasing choking hazards for a patient with Parkinson's disease

- Cut food into small pieces.
- Suction the mouth frequently.
- Offer only soft foods.

Complications

- Depression
- Corneal ulceration
- Injury
- Aspiration
- Constipation
- Psychosis

Possible surgical intervention

- Stereotaxic thalamotomy to relieve tremor and rigidity

MULTIPLE SCLEROSIS (MS)

Definition

- Progressive demyelinating disease of motor and sensory neurons that has periods of remissions and exacerbation

MS highlights

- Progressive demyelinating disease of motor and sensory neurons
- Results in impaired conduction of motor nerve impulses
- Has periods of remissions and exacerbation

Causes

- Unknown
- Autoimmune disease
- Viral

Pathophysiology

- Scattered demyelination occurs in the brain and spinal cord (see *Demyelination in multiple sclerosis*)
- Degeneration of myelin sheath results in patches of sclerotic tissue and impaired conduction of motor nerve impulses

Assessment findings

Key assessment findings in MS

- Weakness
- Nystagmus
- Diplopia
- Paresthesia
- Blurred vision
- Impaired sensation
- Paralysis
- Optic neuritis

- Weakness
- Nystagmus
- Scanning speech
- Ataxia
- Diplopia
- Paresthesia
- Blurred vision
- Impaired sensation
- Feelings of euphoria
- Depression
- Paralysis
- Bowel or bladder dysfunction
- Intention tremor
- Inability to sense or gauge body position
- Optic neuritis
- Intolerance to heat
- Exacerbation and remission of symptoms

Demyelination in multiple sclerosis

Transverse section of cervical spine shows partial loss of myelin, characteristic of multiple sclerosis (MS). This degenerative process is called *demyelination.*

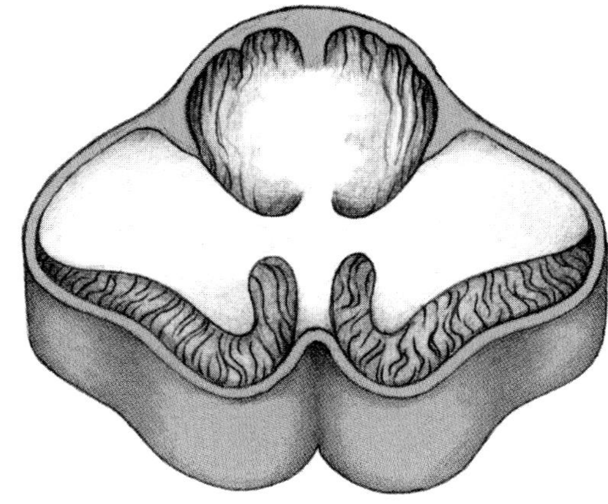

In this illustration, the loss of myelin is nearly complete. Clinical features of MS depend on the extent of demyelination.

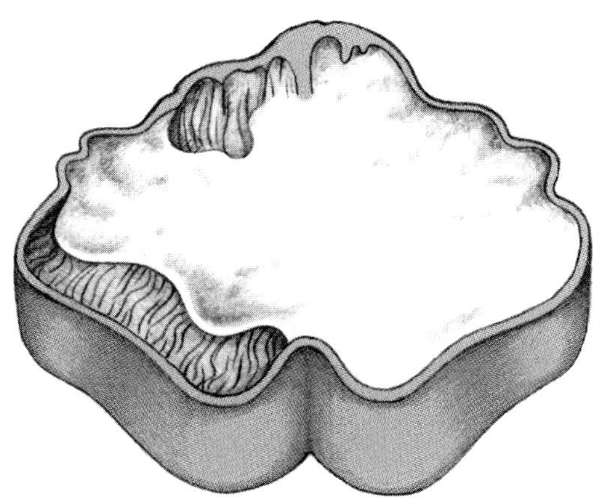

Diagnostic test findings

- CSF analysis: increased immunoglobulin G (IgG), protein, WBCs
- CT scan: normal except in chronic illness, when atrophy is found
- MRI: normal except in chronic illness, when atrophy is found
- Evoked potentials: slowing of nerve conduction
- Oligoclonal banding: positive
- EMG: abnormal

Medical management

- Diet: high-calorie, high-protein, and high-vitamin; gluten-free; low-fat
- Activity: as tolerated
- Monitoring: vital signs, I/O, and neurovital signs

Key diagnostic findings for MS

- CT scan: normal except in chronic illness, when atrophy is found
- MRI: normal except in chronic illness, when atrophy is found

- Speech therapy
- Plasmapheresis
- Muscle relaxant: baclofen (Lioresal)
- Physical therapy
- Glucocorticoids: prednisone (Deltasone), dexamethasone (Decadron), corticotropin (ACTH)
- Antacids: magnesium and aluminum hydroxide (Maalox), aluminum hydroxide gel (AlternaGEL)
- Fluids: increased intake
- Antineoplastic: cyclophosphamide (Cytoxan)
- Immunosuppressant: azathioprine (Imuran)
- Skeletal muscle relaxant: quinine sulfate (Quinamm)

Main therapies for managing MS

- Plasmapheresis
- Muscle relaxant
- Glucocorticoids
- Immunosuppressants
- Skeletal muscle relaxants

Nursing interventions

- Maintain the patient's diet
- Encourage fluids
- Assess neurologic status
- Monitor and record vital signs, I/O, and neurovital signs
- Administer medications, as prescribed
- Encourage the patient to express his feelings about changes in his body image
- Maintain active and passive ROM exercises
- Establish bowel and bladder program
- Maintain activity, as tolerated
- Assist in managing self-care deficits
- Protect the patient from falls
- Maintain a stress-free environment
- Provide information about the National Multiple Sclerosis Society
- Individualize home care instructions
  - Identify ways to reduce stress
  - Recognize the signs and symptoms of exacerbation
  - Avoid exposure to people with infections
  - Alternate rest periods with activity
  - Maintain a safe, quiet environment
  - Use assistive devices in activities of daily living (ADLs), such as specialized eating utensils and wheelchair ramps
  - Reinforce independence
  - Avoid temperature extremes

Key nursing interventions for a patient with MS

- Assess neurologic status.
- Encourage the patient to express his feelings about changes in his body image.
- Maintain active and passive ROM exercises.
- Establish bowel and bladder program.

Key home care instructions for a patient with MS

- Alternate rest periods with activity.
- Avoid temperature extremes.

Complications

- Urinary tract infection (UTI)
- Respiratory tract infection
- Contractures
- Depression
- Paraplegia
- Quadriplegia

Possible surgical intervention

- Contralateral thalamotomy

MYASTHENIA GRAVIS

Definition
- Neuromuscular disorder that results in weakness of voluntary muscles

Causes
- Insufficient acetylcholine
- Autoimmune disease
- Excessive cholinesterase

Pathophysiology
- Disturbance occurs in transmission of nerve impulses at the myoneural junction
- Transmission defect results from deficiency in release of acetylcholine or deficient number of acetylcholine receptor sites
- Thymus gland may remain active, triggering autoimmune reaction

Assessment findings
- Muscle weakness that increases with activity and decreases with rest
- Dysphagia
- Diplopia
- Dysarthria
- Ptosis
- Strabismus
- Impaired speech
- Respiratory distress
- Masklike expression
- Drooling

Diagnostic test findings
- Neostigmine (Prostigmin) or edrophonium (Tensilon) test: relief from symptoms after medication administration
- EMG: decreased amplitude of evoked potentials
- Thymus scan: hyperplasia or thymoma

Medical management
- Diet: high-calorie; soft foods
- Activity: as tolerated
- Monitoring: vital signs, I/O, and neurovital signs
- Glucocorticoids: prednisone (Deltasone), dexamethasone (Decadron), corticotropin (ACTH)
- Antacids: magnesium and aluminum hydroxide (Maalox), aluminum hydroxide gel (AlternaGEL)
- Anticholinesterases: neostigmine (Prostigmin), pyridostigmine (Mestinon), ambenonium (Mytelase)
- Plasmapheresis
- Immunosuppressant: azathioprine (Imuran)
- Antineoplastic: cyclophosphamide (Cytoxan)

Nursing interventions
- Maintain the patient's diet; encourage small, frequent meals

Myasthenia gravis
- Neuromuscular disorder
- Results in weakness of voluntary muscles

Key myasthenia gravis assessment finding
- Muscle weakness that increases with activity and decreases with rest

Possible test findings for myasthenia gravis
- Neostigmine or edrophonium test: relief from symptoms after medication administration
- EMG: decreased amplitude of evoked potentials

Key medications for myasthenia gravis
- Glucocorticoids
- Anticholinesterases
- Immunosuppressants
- Antineoplastics

- Assess neurologic and respiratory status, including vital capacity and tidal volume
- Assess swallow and gag reflexes
- Monitor and record vital signs, I/O, and neurovital signs
- Administer medications, as prescribed, before meals to maximize muscles for swallowing
- Encourage the patient to express his feelings about changes in his body image and about difficulty in communicating verbally
- Determine the patient's activity tolerance
- Provide rest periods
- Provide oral hygiene
- Protect the patient from falls
- Watch the patient for choking while eating
- Provide information about the Myasthenia Gravis Foundation
- Individualize home care instructions
  - Identify ways to reduce stress
  - Recognize the signs and symptoms of respiratory distress
  - Recognize the signs and symptoms of myasthenic crisis
  - Adhere to activity limitations
  - Avoid hot foods and tonic preparations containing quinine

Complications

- Myasthenic crisis
  - Increased symptoms of muscular weakness from undermedication or stress
  - Symptoms improve with edrophonium (Tensilon)
- Cholinergic crisis
  - Increased symptoms of muscular weakness and adverse effects of anticholinesterase medications from overmedication with cholinergic drugs
  - Symptoms worsen with edrophonium (Tensilon)

Possible surgical intervention

- Thymectomy

Key nursing interventions for a patient with myasthenia gravis

- Assess neurologic and respiratory status, including vital capacity and tidal volume.
- Assess swallow and gag reflexes.
- Administer medications, as prescribed, before meals to maximize muscles for swallowing.
- Watch the patient for choking while eating.

Complications of myasthenia gravis

- Myasthenic crisis:
  - Increased symptoms of muscular weakness from undermedication or stress
  - Symptoms improve with edrophonium
- Cholinergic crisis:
  - Increased symptoms of muscular weakness and adverse effects of anticholinesterase medications from overmedication with cholinergic drugs
  - Symptoms worsen with edrophonium

GUILLAIN-BARRÉ SYNDROME (ACUTE INFECTIOUS POLYNEURITIS, POLYRADICULITIS)

Definition

- Peripheral polyneuritis characterized by ascending paralysis

Causes

- Unknown
- Virus
- Infection
- Autoimmune disease

Pathophysiology

- Preceding infection synthesizes lymphocytes, which attack the myelin sheath, causing demyelination

Guillain-Barré syndrome defined

- Peripheral polyneuritis
- Characterized by ascending paralysis

- Demyelination is followed by inflammation around nerve roots, veins, and capillaries
- Inflammatory process compresses nerve roots

Assessment findings

- Acute onset of paresthesia and pain
- Generalized weakness
- Paralysis that starts in the legs
- Ascending paralysis
- Respiratory paralysis
- Tachycardia
- Hypertension
- Increased temperature
- Ptosis
- Facial weakness
- Dysphagia
- Dysarthria

Diagnostic test findings

- CSF analysis: increased protein
- EMG: slowed nerve conduction

Medical management

- Diet: high-calorie, high-protein
- Position: semi-Fowler's
- Activity: bed rest, active and passive ROM and isometric exercises
- Monitoring: vital signs, I/O, vital capacity, and neurovital signs
- Plasmapheresis
- Nutritional support: gastrostomy feedings, NG tube feedings
- Intubation and mechanical ventilation
- Physical therapy
- Indwelling urinary catheter, chest physiotherapy, postural drainage, and suction
- Antibiotics: amoxicillin (Amoxil), ampicillin (Omnipen), gentamicin (Garamycin)
- Glucocorticoids: prednisone (Deltasone), dexamethasone (Decadron), corticotropin (ACTH)
- Antacids: magnesium and aluminum hydroxide (Maalox), aluminum hydroxide gel (AlternaGEL)
- IgG antibody: immune globulin I.V. (Gammagard)
- Pulse oximetry

Nursing interventions

- Maintain the patient's diet
- Administer oxygen
- Provide suction and turning; encourgage coughing and deep breathing
- Assess respiratory and neurologic status
- Maintain the position and patency of NG and ET tubes
- Keep the patient in semi-Fowler's position

Key signs and symptoms of Guillain-Barré syndrome

- Generalized weakness
- Paralysis that starts in the legs
- Ascending paralysis
- Respiratory paralysis

Diagnostic findings in Guillain-Barré syndrome

- CSF analysis: increased protein
- EMG: slowed nerve conduction

Key ways to manage Guillain-Barré syndrome

- Plasmapheresis
- Nutritional support: gastrostomy feedings, NG tube feedings
- Intubation and mechanical ventilation
- Glucocorticoids

Key nursing interventions for a patient with Guillain-Barré syndrome

- Assess respiratory and neurologic status.
- Maintain the position and patency of NG and ET tubes.
- Monitor and record vital signs, I/O, vital capacity, neurovital signs, and pulse oximetry.
- Assess muscle strength.
- Assess gag and swallow reflexes.
- Assess for Homans' sign.
- Apply antiembolism stockings.
- Turn the patient every 2 hours.

Key home care instructions for a patient with Guillain-Barré syndrome

- Maintain a safe, quiet environment.
- Exercise hands, arms, and legs regularly.

Seizure disorders

- Involuntary muscle contractions caused by abnormal discharge of electrical impulses from nerve cells
- May involve abnormal movements, abnormal sensations, and a change in LOC

- Monitor and record vital signs, I/O, vital capacity, neurovital signs, and pulse oximetry
- Administer medications, as prescribed
- Encourage the patient to express his feelings about powerlessness, changes in his body image, and difficulty in communicating verbally
- **Assess muscle strength**
- **Assess gag and swallow reflexes**
- Provide eye and mouth care
- Establish alternate means of communicating with the patient
- Protect the patient from falls
- Prevent skin breakdown
- Provide ROM exercises
- Assess for Homans' sign
- Establish a bowel and bladder program
- Apply antiembolism stockings
- Turn the patient every 2 hours
- Provide information about the Guillain-Barré Foundation
- Individualize home care instructions
  - Identify ways to reduce stress
  - Maintain a safe, quiet environment
  - Minimize environmental stress
  - Exercise hands, arms, and legs regularly

Complications
- Respiratory failure
- Contractures
- Aspiration
- Pneumonia

Possible surgical interventions
- None

SEIZURE DISORDERS

Definition
- Involuntary muscle contractions caused by abnormal discharge of electrical impulses from nerve cells
- Classification of seizures (see *Classifying seizures*)
  - Generalized seizures
    - Generalized absence (petit mal)
    - Generalized tonic-clonic (grand mal)
    - Myoclonic
    - Atonic
  - Partial seizures (focal seizures)
    - Simple partial
    - Complex partial
  - Unclassified seizures

Classifying seizures

Seizures can take various forms depending on their origin and whether they're localized to one area of the brain, as occurs in partial seizures, or occur in both hemispheres, as happens in generalized seizures. This chart describes each type of seizure and lists common signs and symptoms.

TYPE	DESCRIPTION	SIGNS AND SYMPTOMS
Partial		
Simple partial	Symptoms confined to one hemisphere	May have motor (change in posture), sensory (hallucinations), or autonomic (flushing, tachycardia) symptoms; no loss of consciousness
Complex partial	Begins in one focal area, but spreads to both hemispheres (more common in adults)	Loss of consciousness; aura of visual disturbances; postictal symptoms
Generalized		
Absence (petit mal)	Sudden onset; lasts 5 to 10 seconds; can have 100 daily; precipitated by stress, hyperventilation, hypoglycemia, fatigue; differentiated from daydreaming	Loss of responsiveness, but continued ability to maintain posture control and not fall; twitching eyelids; lip smacking; no postictal symptoms
Myoclonic	Movement disorder (not a seizure); seen as child awakens or falls asleep; may be precipitated by touch or visual stimuli; focal or generalized; symmetrical or asymmetrical	No loss of consciousness; sudden, brief, shocklike involuntary contraction of one muscle group
Clonic	Opposing muscles contract and relax alternately in rhythmic pattern; may occur in one limb more than others	Mucus production
Tonic	Muscles are maintained in continuous contracted state (rigid posture)	Variable loss of consciousness; pupils dilate; eyes roll up; glottis closes; possible incontinence; may foam at mouth
Tonic-clonic (grand mal, major motor)	Violent total body seizure	Aura; tonic first (20 to 40 seconds); clonic next; postictal symptoms
Atonic	Drop and fall attack; needs to wear protective helmet	Loss of posture tone
Akinetic	Sudden brief loss of muscle tone or posture	Temporary loss of consciousness

(continued)

Types of partial seizures

- Simple partial: symptoms confined to one hemisphere
- Complex partial: begins in one focal area; spreads to both hemispheres

Types of generalized seizures

- Absence (petit mal): loss of responsiveness, but continued ability to maintain posture control and not fall
- Myoclonic: movement disorder (not a seizure)
- Clonic: opposing muscles contract and relax alternately in rhythmic pattern
- Tonic: muscles are maintained in continuous contracted state (rigid posture)
- Tonic-clonic (grand mal, major motor): violent total body seizure
- Atonic: drop and fall attack
- Akinetic: sudden brief loss of muscle tone or posture

Causes

- Idiopathic origin
- Head injury
- Hypoglycemia
- Brain tumor

Unclassified seizures

- Febrile: seizure threshold lowered by elevated temperature
- Status epilepticus: prolonged or frequent repetition of seizures without interruption

Key symptoms of a seizure

- Aura
- Loss of consciousness

Key test findings in seizure disorders

- EEG: abnormal wave patterns
- MRI: pathologic changes

Common treatments for seizure disorders

- Special care: Seizure precautions
- Anticonvulsants
- Diazepam for status epilepticus

Classifying seizures *(continued)*

TYPE	DESCRIPTION	SIGNS AND SYMPTOMS
Unclassified		
Febrile	Seizure threshold lowered by elevated temperature; only one seizure per fever; common in 4% of population under age 5; occurs when temperature is rapidly rising	Lasts less than 5 minutes; generalized, transient, and nonprogressive; doesn't generally result in brain damage; EEG is normal after 2 weeks
Status epilepticus	Prolonged or frequent repetition of seizures without interruption; results in anoxia and cardiac and respiratory arrest	Consciousness not regained between seizures; lasts more than 30 minutes

- Infection
- Anoxia

Pathophysiology

- Many neurons fire in a synchronous pattern, resulting in a transient physiologic disturbance
- Physiologic disturbances include abnormal movements, abnormal sensations, and a change in LOC

Assessment findings

- Aura
- Loss of consciousness
- Dyspnea
- Fixed and dilated pupils
- Incontinence

Diagnostic test findings

- EEG: abnormal wave patterns, focus of seizure activity
- CT scan: a space-occupying lesion
- MRI: pathologic changes
- Brain mapping: identification of seizure areas

Medical management

- Diet: ketogenic
- I.V. therapy: saline lock
- Activity: bed rest
- Monitoring: vital signs, I/O, and neurovital signs
- Laboratory studies: glucose, potassium, and anticonvulsant drug levels, if applicable
- Special care: seizure precautions
- Anticonvulsants: phenytoin (Dilantin), ethosuximide (Zarontin), phenobarbital (Luminal), carbamazepine (Tegretol), valproic acid (Depakote), gabapentin (Neurontin), lamotrigine (Lamictal), topiramate (Topamax)
- Diazepam (Valium), for status epilepticus

Nursing interventions
- Maintain the patient's diet
- Assess neurologic and respiratory status
- Monitor and record vital signs, I/O, neurovital signs, and laboratory studies
- Administer medications, as prescribed
- Encourage the patient to express his feelings about powerlessness
- Maintain seizure precautions
- Protect the patient from injury during seizure activity
- Observe and record seizure activity
  - Initial movement
  - Respiratory pattern
  - Duration of seizure
  - Loss of consciousness
  - Aura
  - Incontinence
  - Pupillary changes
- Assess postictal state
- Maintain a patent airway
- Protect the patient from falls
- Provide information about the Epilepsy Foundation of America; the National Epilepsy League, Inc.; and the National Association to Control Epilepsy
- Individualize home care instructions
  - Recognize the signs and symptoms of seizure activity
  - Avoid drinking alcohol
  - Promote a safe environment
  - Wear a medical identification bracelet
  - Identify and time seizure activity
  - Prevent injury during seizure activity

Complications
- Musculoskeletal injury
- Hypoxia
- Status epilepticus

Possible surgical intervention
- Excision of epileptogenic area (rare)

INCREASED INTRACRANIAL PRESSURE

Definition
- Elevated ICP beyond the normal pressure exerted by blood, brain, and CSF within the skull

Causes
- Tumor
- Abscess
- Space-occupying lesion
- Edema
- Hemorrhage

What to observe during seizure activity
- Initial movement
- Respiratory pattern
- Duration of seizure
- Loss of consciousness
- Aura
- Incontinence
- Pupillary changes

Important precautions for a patient with seizures
- Wear a medical identification bracelet.
- Recognize the signs and symptoms of seizure activity.
- Prevent injury during seizure activity.

Increased ICP
- Elevated ICP beyond the normal pressure exerted by blood, brain, and CSF within the skull
- Results in decreased cerebral circulation and anoxia
- May lead to permanent brain damage

- Hydrocephalus
- Head injury
- Infection
- Congenital abnormality

Pathophysiology

- Because the skull can't expand, an increase in brain tissue, CSF, or blood results in increased ICP
- Increased ICP results in decreased cerebral circulation and anoxia, which can lead to permanent brain damage

Assessment findings

- Restlessness
- Hypertension
- Bradycardia
- Pupillary changes
  - Sluggish reaction
  - Dilation
- Weakness
- Decreased LOC
- Widening pulse pressure
- Abnormal posturing
  - Decortication
  - Decerebration
- Headache
- Vomiting
- Papilledema

Diagnostic test findings

- ICP measurement via ventriculostomy, epidural sensor, and subarachnoid screw: increased pressure
- LP: contraindicated

Medical management

- Diet: withhold food and fluids, as ordered
- I.V. therapy: electrolyte replacement, saline lock
- Oxygen therapy
- Intubation and mechanical ventilation with hyperventilation
- GI decompression: NG tube
- Position: semi-Fowler's
- Activity: bed rest, passive ROM exercises
- Monitoring: vital signs, I/O, ECG, ICP, neurovital signs, cerebral perfusion pressure (CPP), and arterial pressure
- Laboratory studies: potassium, sodium, glucose, osmolality, BUN, serum osmolarity, and creatinine levels
- Indwelling urinary catheter
- ICP monitoring: ventriculostomy, subarachnoid screw, epidural sensor
- Diuretics: mannitol (Osmitrol), furosemide (Lasix)
- Antacids: magnesium and aluminum hydroxide (Maalox)
- CSF drainage via ventriculostomy

Key assessment findings in ICP

- Restlessness
- Hypertension
- Bradycardia
- Pupillary changes
- Decreased LOC
- Widening pulse pressure
- Abnormal posturing

ICP test findings

- ICP measurement via ventriculostomy, epidural sensor, and subarachnoid screw: increased pressure
- LP: contraindicated

Common steps in managing ICP

- Oxygen therapy
- Intubation and mechanical ventilation with hyperventilation
- Position: semi-Fowler's
- Monitoring: vital signs, I/O, ECG, ICP, neurovital signs, CPP, and arterial pressure
- Laboratory studies: potassium, sodium, glucose, osmolality, BUN, serum osmolarity, and creatinine levels
- Diuretics
- CSF drainage via ventriculostomy
- Anticonvulsants
- Glucocorticoids
- Seizure precautions

- Anticonvulsant: phenytoin (Dilantin)
- Glucocorticoid: dexamethasone (Decadron)
- Histamine antagonists: cimetidine (Tagamet), ranitidine (Zantac)
- Barbiturate-induced coma or sedation
- Seizure precautions
- Pulse oximetry
- Mucosal barrier fortifier: sucralfate (Carafate)

Nursing interventions

- Maintain fluid restrictions
- Administer I.V. fluids
- Administer oxygen
- Suction only as needed
- Assist with turning, coughing, and deep breathing
- Assess neurologic and respiratory status
- Maintain the position and patency of the NG tube; provide low suctioning
- Maintain the position and patency of the ET tube and indwelling urinary catheter
- Keep the patient in semi-Fowler's position
- Maintain a quiet and dimly lit room
- Monitor and record vital signs, I/O, ICP, neurovital signs, laboratory studies, CPP, and pulse oximetry
- Administer medications, as prescribed
- Allay the patient's anxiety
- Maintain neutral alignment of the patient's neck with his body
- Turn the patient every 2 hours
- Prevent jugular vein constriction
- Allow a period of rest between each nursing activity
- Maintain a quiet environment
- Continue bed rest
- Prevent Valsalva's maneuver
- Provide mouth and skin care
- Provide appropriate sensory input and stimuli with frequent reorientation
- Assist with ADLs; make referrals to appropriate community agencies
- Maintain seizure precautions
- Individualize home care instructions
  - Recognize the signs and symptoms of decreased LOC
  - Recognize the signs and symptoms of seizures
  - Minimize environmental stress
  - Set limits for impulsive behavior
  - Continue fluid restrictions

Complications

- Brain herniation
- Coma
- Seizure
- Death

Possible surgical intervention

- Craniotomy for surgical decompression

Key nursing interventions for a patient with ICP

- Maintain fluid restrictions.
- Suction only as needed.
- Assess neurologic and respiratory status.
- Keep the patient in semi-Fowler's position.
- Monitor and record vital signs, I/O, ICP, neurovital signs, laboratory studies, CPP, and pulse oximetry.
- Maintain neutral alignment of the patient's neck with his body.
- Prevent jugular vein constriction.
- Maintain seizure precautions.

Home care instructions for a patient with increased ICP

- Recognize the signs and symptoms of decreased LOC.
- Recognize the signs and symptoms of seizures.
- Minimize environmental stress.
- Set limits for impulsive behavior.
- Continue fluid restrictions.

HEAD INJURY

Definition
- Classified by the type of fracture, hemorrhage, or trauma to the brain
- Fractures
  - Depressed
  - Comminuted
  - Linear
  - Basal skull fracture
- Hemorrhages
  - Epidural
  - Subdural
  - Intracerebral
  - Subarachnoid
- Trauma
  - Concussion
  - Contusion

3 types of head injuries
- Fracture
- Hemorrhage
- Trauma

Causes
- Auto accidents
- Falls
- Assaults
- Blunt trauma
- Penetrating trauma

Pathophysiology
- Brain injury or bleeding within the brain results in edema and hypoxia

Most common signs of head injury
- Disorientation to time, place, or person
- Decreased LOC
- Unequal pupil size

Assessment findings
- Disorientation to time, place, or person
- Paresthesia
- Positive Babinski's reflex
- Decreased LOC
- Otorrhea
- Rhinorrhea
- Unequal pupil size
- Loss of pupil reaction

Key test findings for head injury
- Skull X-ray: skull fracture
- CT scan: hemorrhage, cerebral edema, or shift of midline structures

Diagnostic test findings
- Skull X-ray: skull fracture
- CT scan: hemorrhage, cerebral edema, or shift of midline structures
- MRI: hemorrhage, cerebral edema, or shift of midline structures
- Cerebral angiography: intracerebral, subdural, epidural hematoma
- Echoencephalogram: shift of midline structures

Medical management
- Diet: restricted fluids
- I.V. therapy: electrolyte replacement, saline lock
- Oxygen therapy
- Intubation and mechanical ventilation with hyperventilation
- GI decompression: NG tube

- Position: semi-Fowler's
- Activity: bed rest, active and passive ROM exercises
- Monitoring: vital signs, I/O, ECG, hemodynamic variables, ICP, CVP, neurovital signs, and arterial line
- Laboratory studies: potassium, sodium, osmolality, ABG analysis, Hb, and HCT
- Indwelling urinary catheter
- Analgesic: codeine (Paveral)
- Diuretics: mannitol (Osmitrol), furosemide (Lasix)
- Antacids: magnesium and aluminum hydroxide (Maalox), aluminum hydroxide gel (AlternaGEL)
- Anticonvulsant: phenytoin (Dilantin)
- Glucocorticoid: dexamethasone (Decadron)
- Histamine antagonists: cimetidine (Tagamet), ranitidine (Zantac)
- Cervical collar
- Reflex checks: oculocephalic, oculovestibular, corneal, cough, and gag
- Mucosal barrier fortifier: sucralfate (Carafate)
- Pulse oximetry

Nursing interventions

- Restrict fluids
- Administer I.V. fluids
- Administer oxygen
- Provide suction and turning; encourage coughing and deep breathing
- Assess neurologic and respiratory status
- Maintain position, patency, and low suction of NG tube
- Maintain position and patency of ET tube and indwelling urinary catheter
- Elevate the head of the bed to reduce cerebral edema
- Monitor and record vital signs, I/O, hemodynamic variables, ICP, CVP, specific gravity, urine glucose and ketones, laboratory studies, and pulse oximetry
- Maintain seizure precautions
- Administer medications, as prescribed
- Encourage the patient to express feelings about changes in body image
- Assess for CSF leak: otorrhea, rhinorrhea
- Assess pain
- Check for signs of diabetes insipidus
- Check cough and gag reflexes
- Provide appropriate sensory input and stimuli with frequent reorientation
- Provide means of communication
- Observe for signs of increasing ICP
- Provide eye, skin, and mouth care
- Turn the patient every 2 hours
- Assist with ADLs
- Provide information about the National Head Injury Foundation
- Individualize home care instructions
  - Recognize the signs and symptoms of decreased LOC
  - Recognize the signs and symptoms of seizures

Main treatment options for head injury

- Diet: restricted fluids
- I.V. therapy: electrolyte replacement, saline lock
- Intubation and mechanical ventilation with hyperventilation
- Position: semi-Fowler's
- Monitoring: vital signs, I/O, ECG, hemodynamic variables, ICP, CVP, neurovital signs, and arterial line
- Laboratory studies: potassium, sodium, osmolality, ABG analysis, Hb, and HCT
- Diuretics
- Anticonvulsants
- Glucocorticoids
- Cervical collar

Key steps in nursing care for a patient with a head injury

- Administer oxygen.
- Assess neurologic and respiratory status.
- Elevate the head of the bed to reduce cerebral edema.
- Maintain seizure precautions.
- Assess for CSF leak: otorrhea, rhinorrhea.
- Check for signs of diabetes insipidus.
- Check cough and gag reflexes.
- Observe for signs of increasing ICP.

– Set limits for impulsive behavior
– Adhere to fluid restrictions

Complications
- Shock
- Meningitis
- Increased ICP
- Stress ulcer
- Diabetes insipidus
- Infection

Possible surgical intervention
- Craniotomy for evacuation of hematomas

STROKE

Definition
- Disruption of cerebral circulation that results in motor and sensory deficits

Causes
- Cerebral arteriosclerosis
- Syphilis
- Trauma
- Hypertension
- Thrombosis
- Embolism
- Hemorrhage
- Vasospasm

Pathophysiology
- Disruption of cerebral blood flow causes cerebral anoxia
- Cerebral anoxia results in cerebral infarction
- Infarction results in edema

Assessment findings
- Syncope
- Change in LOC
- Paresthesia
- Headache
- Aphasia
- Seizures
- Labile emotional responses
- Paralysis
- Weakness
- Ataxia

Diagnostic test findings
- LP: increased pressure, bloody CSF
- CT scan: intracranial bleeding, infarct, or shift of midline structures
- EEG: focal slowing in area of lesion

Stroke defined
- Disruption of cerebral circulation
- Results in motor and sensory deficits

Key stroke assessment findings
- Change in LOC
- Paresthesia
- Aphasia
- Paralysis
- Weakness

Key test findings in stroke
- CT scan: intracranial bleeding, infarct, or shift of midline structures
- MRI: intracranial bleeding, infarct, or shift of midline structures
- Digital subtraction angiography: occlusion or narrowing of vessels

- MRI: intracranial bleeding, infarct, or shift of midline structures
- Brain scan: decreased perfusion
- Digital subtraction angiography: occlusion or narrowing of vessels

Medical management

- Diet: low-sodium, increased potassium
- I.V. therapy: saline lock
- Oxygen therapy
- Intubation and mechanical ventilation
- GI decompression: NG tube
- Position: semi-Fowler's
- Activity: bed rest, active and passive ROM and isometric exercises
- Monitoring: vital signs, I/O, ECG, ICP, and neurovital signs
- Laboratory studies: sodium, potassium, glucose, ABG analysis, PT, and PTT
- Nutritional support: TPN
- Indwelling urinary catheter, incentive spirometry
- Seizure precautions
- Analgesic: codeine (Paveral)
- Diuretics: mannitol (Osmitrol), furosemide (Lasix)
- Antacids: magnesium and aluminum hydroxide (Maalox), aluminum hydroxide gel (AlternaGEL)
- Anticonvulsant: phenytoin (Dilantin)
- Glucocorticoid: dexamethasone (Decadron)
- Histamine antagonists: cimetidine (Tagamet), ranitidine (Zantac)
- Antihypertensive: diazoxide (Hyperstat)
- Anticoagulants: warfarin (Coumadin), heparin
- Pulse oximetry
- Physical therapy

Nursing interventions

- Maintain the patient's diet
- Administer I.V. fluids
- Administer oxygen
- Provide suction and turning; encourage coughing and deep breathing
- Assess neurovascular, cardiac, and respiratory status
- Maintain position, patency, and low suction of NG tube
- Keep the patient in semi-Fowler's position
- Monitor and record vital signs, I/O, ICP, neurovital signs, laboratory studies, and pulse oximetry
- Administer TPN
- Administer medications, as prescribed
- Encourage the patient to express his feelings about changes in his body image and about difficulty in communicating verbally
- Maintain a quiet environment
- Assess for receptive and expressive aphasia
- Assess for hemianopsia
- Protect the patient from falls and injury
- Apply antiembolism stockings

Key management options for strokes

- Semi-Fowler's position
- Monitor vital signs, I/O, ECG, ICP, and neurovital signs
- Anticonvulsants
- Glucocorticoids
- Anticoagulants

Monitoring parameters for stroke

- Vital signs
- I/O
- ICP
- Neurovital signs
- Laboratory studies
- Pulse oximetry

Key nursing interventions for a patient with stroke

- Assess neurovascular, cardiac, and respiratory status.
- Keep the patient in semi-Fowler's position.
- Protect the patient from falls and injury.
- Maintain seizure precautions.

Problems caused by immobility due to stroke

- Thrombophlebitis
- Pulmonary embolism
- Osteoporosis
- Urinary stasis

Key facts about cerebral aneurysm

- Dilation or localized weakness of the middle layer of an artery
- Three types: saccular (berry), fusiform, and mycotic

- Maintain seizure precautions
- Provide passive ROM exercises
- Turn and position the patient every 2 hours
- Provide a means of communication
- Provide skin and mouth care
- Provide information about the American Heart Association and the National Stroke Foundation
- Individualize home care instructions
  - Identify ways to reduce stress
  - Recognize the signs and symptoms of seizures
  - Minimize environmental stress
  - Reinforce established methods of communication (aphasic patient)
  - Monitor blood pressure
  - Use assistive devices in ADLs
  - Teach scanning

Complications

- Cerebral edema
- Vasospasm
- Pneumonia
- Increased ICP
- Problems from immobility
  - Thrombophlebitis
  - Pulmonary embolism
  - Osteoporosis
  - Urinary stasis

Possible surgical interventions

- Carotid endarterectomy
- Craniotomy for evacuation of a clot or for superior temporal artery—middle cerebral artery anastomosis

CEREBRAL ANEURYSM

Definition

- Dilation or localized weakness of the middle layer of an artery (see *Most common sites of cerebral aneurysm*)
- Classified by aneurysm type
  - Saccular (berry)
  - Fusiform
  - Mycotic

Causes

- Atherosclerosis
- Trauma
- Congenital weakness
- Syphilis

Most common sites of cerebral aneurysm

Cerebral aneurysms usually arise at arterial bifurcations in the Circle of Willis and its branches. The illustration below shows the most common aneurysm sites around this circle.

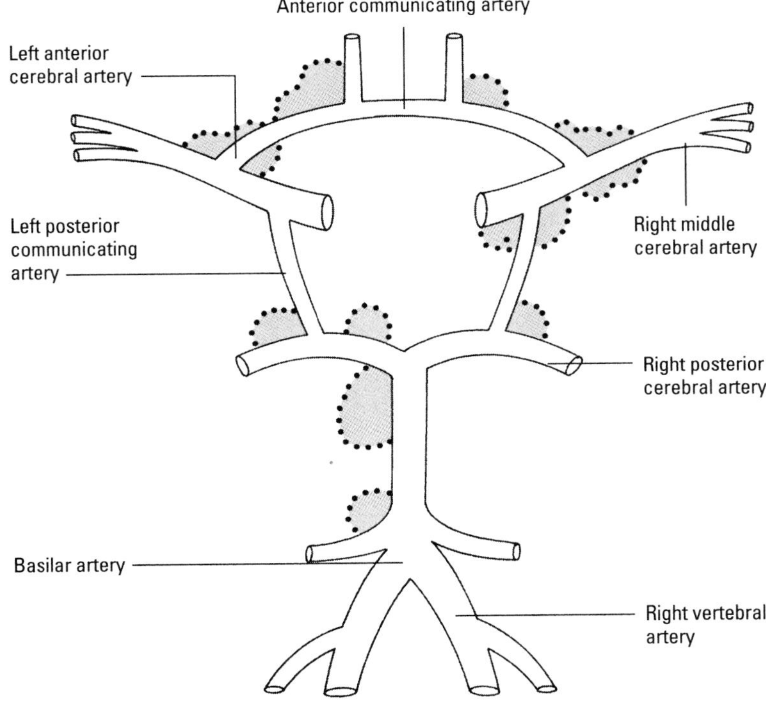

Pathophysiology

- Enlargement of aneurysm compresses nerves
- Enlargement of the aneurysm finally results in dissolution of the wall and rupture of the aneurysm
- Rupture of the aneurysm results in subarachnoid hemorrhage
- Release of serotonin, prostaglandins, and catecholamines from blood precipitates vasospasm

Assessment findings

- Diplopia
- Ptosis
- Severe headache
- Hemiparesis
- Nuchal rigidity
- Decreased LOC
- Seizure activity

Where cerebral aneurysms arise

- Arterial bifurcations in the Circle of Willis and its branches

Key assessment findings in cerebral aneurysm

- Severe headache
- Decreased LOC
- Vomiting

- Blurred vision
- Vomiting

Diagnostic test findings

- CT scan: shift of intracranial midline structures, blood in subarachnoid space
- MRI: shift of intracranial midline structures, blood in subarachnoid space
- Cerebral angiogram: identification of vasospasm and vasculature associated with aneurysm
- LP (contraindicated with increased ICP): increased pressure, protein, WBCs; bloody and xanthochromic CSF

Medical management

- I.V. therapy: saline lock
- Oxygen therapy
- Position: semi-Fowler's
- Activity: bed rest, passive ROM exercises
- Monitoring: vital signs, I/O (fluid restrictions), ICP, neurovital signs, and arterial line
- Precautions: aneurysm and seizure
- Antacids: magnesium and aluminum hydroxide (Maalox), aluminum hydroxide gel (AlternaGEL)
- Anticonvulsant: phenytoin (Dilantin)
- Glucocorticoid: dexamethasone (Decadron)
- Histamine antagonists: cimetidine (Tagamet), ranitidine (Zantac)
- Stool softener: docusate (Colace)
- Antifibrinolytic: aminocaproic acid (Amicar)
- Antihypertensives: methyldopa (Aldomet), hydralazine (Apresoline)
- Ergot alkaloid: methysergide (Sansert)
- Calcium channel blocker: nimodipine (Nimotop)
- Intubation and mechanical ventilation
- Pulse oximetry
- Mucosal barrier fortifier: sucralfate (Carafate)

Nursing interventions

- Restrict fluids
- Administer oxygen
- Assess neurologic status
- Keep the patient in semi-Fowler's position
- Monitor and record vital signs, I/O, ICP, and pulse oximetry
- Administer medication, as prescribed
- Encourage the patient to express his feelings about a fear of dying
- Allay the patient's anxiety
- Maintain a quiet, darkened environment
- Assess pain
- Allow a rest period between nursing activities
- Maintain bed rest
- Prevent Valsalva's maneuver
- Assess for signs of increased ICP

Key diagnostic test findings in cerebral aneurysm

- CT scan: shift of intracranial midline structures, blood in subarachnoid space
- Cerebral angiogram: identification of vasospasm and vasculature associated with aneurysm

Common medications used to treat cerebral aneurysm

- Anticonvulsants
- Glucocorticoids
- Histamine antagonists
- Stool softeners
- Calcium channel blockers

Key nursing interventions for a patient with a cerebral aneurysm

- Keep the patient in semi-Fowler's position.
- Maintain a quiet, darkened environment.
- Assess pain.
- Assess for signs of increased ICP.
- Maintain seizure and aneurysm precautions.
- Prevent constipation.
- Assess for meningeal irritation.

- Maintain seizure and aneurysm precautions
- Provide passive ROM exercises
- Limit visitors
- Provide skin care
- Assist with ADLs
- Prevent constipation
- Assess for meningeal irritation
- Individualize home care instructions
  - Recognize the signs and symptoms of decreasing LOC
  - Minimize environmental stress
  - Alter ADLs to compensate for neurologic deficits
  - Prevent constipation

Complications
- Vasospasm
- Rebleeding of the aneurysm
- Increased ICP
- Rupture of the aneurysm
- Hydrocephalus
- Brain herniation

Possible surgical interventions
- Craniotomy for clipping or wrapping of an aneurysm or for evacuation of hematomas
- Guglielmi coils

Surgical option for cerebral aneurysm — craniotomy
- For clipping or wrapping of an aneurysm
- For evacuation of hematomas

BRAIN TUMOR

Definition
- Malignant or benign tumor of the brain that may be primary or metastatic

Causes
- Genetic
- Environmental

Pathophysiology
- Unregulated cell growth and uncontrolled cell division result in the development of a neoplasm
- Tumors are classified according to tissue of origin
  - Gliomas
  - Meningiomas
  - Neuromas
  - Metastatic lesions
  - Developmental (congenital) tumors
- Tumors can be infiltrative and destroy surrounding tissue or be encapsulated and displace brain tissue
- Presence of lesion and compression of blood vessels produces ischemia, edema, and increased ICP

Key facts about a brain tumor
- Malignant or benign tumor of the brain
- May be primary or metastatic

Classifications of tumors
- Gliomas
- Meningiomas
- Neuromas
- Metastatic lesions
- Developmental (congenital) tumors

General symptoms of a brain tumor

- Headache
- Vomiting
- Papilledema

Key diagnostic test findings for a brain tumor

- EEG: seizure activity
- MRI or CT scan: location and size of tumor
- Skull X-ray: location and size of tumor

Common ways to manage a brain tumor

- Radiation therapy
- Antineoplastics
- Diuretics
- Anticonvulsants
- Glucocorticoids
- Seizure precautions

Assessment findings

- Tumor in any brain area
  - Headache
  - Vomiting
  - Papilledema
- Tumor in the frontal lobe
  - Personality changes
  - Aphasia (expressive)
  - Memory loss
- Tumor in the temporal lobe
  - Seizures
  - Aphasia (receptive)
- Tumor in the parietal lobe
  - Motor seizures
  - Sensory impairment
- Tumor in the occipital lobe
  - Visual impairment
  - Homonymous hemianopia
  - Visual hallucinations
- Tumor in the cerebellum
  - Impaired equilibrium
  - Impaired coordination

Diagnostic test findings

- EEG: seizure activity
- MRI or CT scan: location and size of tumor
- Skull X-ray: location and size of tumor
- Angiography: location and size of tumor
- LP (contraindicated with increased ICP): increased protein

Medical management

- Diet: high-protein, high-calorie
- I.V. therapy: saline lock
- Oxygen therapy
- Position: semi-Fowler's
- Activity: bed rest
- Monitoring: vital signs, I/O, ICP, and neurovital signs
- Laboratory studies: sodium, potassium, and glucose levels
- Nutritional support: TPN
- Radiation therapy
- Antineoplastics: vincristine (Oncovin), lomustine (CeeNU), carmustine (BiCNU)
- Diuretics: mannitol (Osmitrol), furosemide (Lasix)
- Antacids: magnesium and aluminum hydroxide (Maalox), aluminum hydroxide gel (AlternaGEL)
- Anticonvulsant: phenytoin (Dilantin)
- Glucocorticoid: dexamethasone (Decadron)
- Histamine antagonists: cimetidine (Tagamet), ranitidine (Zantac)

- Seizure precautions
- Chemotherapy
- Stereotaxic brachytherapy
- Stereotaxic radiosurgery (Roentgen knife)
- Mucosal barrier fortifier: sucralfate (Carafate)

Nursing interventions

- Maintain the patient's diet
- Encourage the patient to drink fluids
- Administer I.V. fluids
- Administer oxygen
- Assess neurologic and respiratory status
- Keep the patient in semi-Fowler's position
- Monitor and record vital signs, I/O, ICP, neurovital signs, and laboratory studies
- Administer TPN
- Administer medications, as prescribed
- Encourage the patient to express his feelings about changes in his body image and a fear of dying
- Assess pain
- Assess for increased ICP
- Provide oral hygiene
- Provide postchemotherapeutic and postradiation nursing care
  - Provide prophylactic skin and mouth care
  - Monitor dietary intake
  - Administer antiemetics and antidiarrheals, as prescribed
  - Monitor the patient for bleeding, infection, and electrolyte imbalance
  - Provide rest periods
- Maintain seizure precautions
- Provide information about the National Head Injury Foundation and the Association for Brain Tumor Research
- Individualize home care instructions
  - Recognize the signs and symptoms of change in LOC
  - Maintain a safe, quiet environment
  - Respect quality-of-life decisions
  - Make referrals for hospice care

Complications

- Increased ICP
- Brain herniation
- Seizures

Possible surgical intervention

- Craniotomy for surgical excision of a tumor

Key nursing interventions for a patient with a brain tumor

- Assess neurologic and respiratory status.
- Keep the patient in semi-Fowler's position.
- Assess for increased ICP.
- Maintain seizure precautions.

Postchemotherapeutic and postradiation care for a patient with a brain tumor

- Administer antiemetics and antidiarrheals, as prescribed.
- Monitor the patient for bleeding, infection, and electrolyte imbalance.

Spinal cord injury highlights

- Traumatic injury to spinal cord
- Edema and hemorrhage cause ischemia
- Necrosis and scar tissue form
- Results in sensory and motor deficits

Types of spinal cord injury

- Paraplegia: paralysis of the legs
- Quadriplegia: paralysis of all four extremities

Common assessment findings in spinal cord injury

- Paralysis below the level of the injury
- Paresthesia below the level of the injury
- Loss of bowel and bladder control

Diagnostic test findings for spinal cord injury

- CT scan: spinal cord edema, vertebral fracture, spinal cord compression
- MRI: spinal cord edema, vertebral fracture, spinal cord compression

SPINAL CORD INJURY

Definition

- Traumatic injury to the spinal cord that results in sensory and motor deficits
- Two types of spinal cord injury
  - Paraplegia: paralysis of the legs
  - Quadriplegia: paralysis of all four extremities

Causes

- Car accidents
- Falls
- Gunshot wounds
- Stab wounds
- Diving into shallow water
- Infections
- Tumors
- Congenital anomalies

Pathophysiology

- Injury may result in complete transection of the spinal cord
- Associated edema and hemorrhage from the injury cause ischemia
- Necrosis and scar tissue form in the area of the traumatized cord
- Injury may result in paraplegia or quadriplegia

Assessment findings

- Paralysis below the level of the injury
- Paresthesia below the level of the injury
- Neck pain
- Loss of bowel and bladder control
- Respiratory distress
- Numbness and tingling
- Flaccid muscle
- Absence of reflexes below the level of the injury
- Loss of perspiration below level of the injury

Diagnostic test findings

- Spinal X-rays: vertebral fracture
- CT scan: spinal cord edema, vertebral fracture, spinal cord compression
- MRI: spinal cord edema, vertebral fracture, spinal cord compression

Medical management

- Diet: low-calcium, high-protein
- I.V. therapy: saline lock
- Oxygen therapy
- Intubation and mechanical ventilation
- GI decompression: NG tube
- **Position: flat, neck immobilized**
- Activity: bed rest, passive ROM exercises
- Monitoring: vital signs, I/O, ECG, ICP, and neurovital signs

- Laboratory studies: sodium, potassium, and glucose levels and WBC count
- Indwelling urinary catheter
- Antacids: magnesium and aluminum hydroxide (Maalox), aluminum hydroxide gel (AlternaGEL)
- Anticonvulsant: phenytoin (Dilantin)
- Glucocorticoid: dexamethasone (Decadron), methylprednisolone sodium succinate (Solu-Medrol)
- Histamine antagonists: cimetidine (Tagamet), ranitidine (Zantac)
- Cervical collar
- Maintenance of vertebral alignment: Stryker turning frame, Crutchfield tongs, Halo brace
- Laxative: bisacodyl (Dulcolax)
- Antianxiety agent: diazepam (Valium)
- Antihypertensives: diazoxide (Hyperstat), hydralazine (Apresoline)
- Muscle relaxant: dantrolene (Dantrium)
- Pulse oximetry
- Specialized bed: rotation (Rotorest, Tilt and Turn, Paragon)
- Mucosal barrier fortifier: sucralfate (Carafate)

Nursing interventions

- Maintain the patient's diet
- Encourage fluids
- Administer I.V. fluids
- Administer oxygen
- Provide suction and turning; encourage coughing and deep breathing
- Assess neurologic and respiratory status
- Keep the patient flat
- Monitor and record vital signs, I/O, laboratory studies, and pulse oximetry
- Administer medications, as prescribed
- Encourage the patient to express his feelings about changes in his body image, changes in sexual expression and function, and altered mobility
- Turn the patient every 2 hours using the logrolling technique
- Maintain body alignment
- Initiate bowel and bladder retraining
- Provide sexual counseling
- Provide passive ROM exercises
- **Check for autonomic dysreflexia**
- **Assess for spinal shock**
- Provide skin care
- Provide heel and elbow protectors and sheepskin
- Apply antiembolism stockings
- Provide information about the National Spinal Cord Injury Association
- Individualize home care instructions
  - Exercise regularly to strengthen muscles
  - Recognize the signs and symptoms of autonomic dysreflexia, UTI, and upper respiratory infection
  - Continue bowel and bladder program
  - Maintain acidic urine with cranberry juice

Key ways to manage spinal cord injury

- Position: flat, neck immobilized
- Glucocorticoids
- Histamine antagonists
- Cervical collar
- Maintenance of vertebral alignment: Stryker turning frame, Crutchfield tongs, Halo brace
- Muscle relaxants
- Specialized bed: rotation (Rotorest, Tilt and Turn, Paragon)

Key nursing interventions for a patient with spinal cord injury

- Assess neurologic and respiratory status.
- Keep the patient flat.
- Monitor and record vital signs, I/O, laboratory studies, and pulse oximetry.
- Turn the patient every 2 hours using the logrolling technique.
- Check for autonomic dysreflexia.
- Assess for spinal shock.
- Provide skin care.

Key home care instructions for a patient with spinal cord injury

- Exercise regularly to strengthen muscles.
- Recognize the signs and symptoms of autonomic dysreflexia, UTI, and upper respiratory infection.
- Continue bowel and bladder program.
- Maintain skin integrity.
- Reinforce independence.

– Consume adequate fluids: 3 L/day
– Use assistive devices for ADLs
– Maintain skin integrity
– Stay mobile using a wheelchair
– Reinforce independence

Complications
- Spinal shock
- Autonomic dysreflexia
- Respiratory distress
- Osteomyelitis
- Pressure ulcers

Possible surgical interventions
- Laminectomy
- Spinal fusion

AMYOTROPHIC LATERAL SCLEROSIS (ALS)—LOU GEHRIG DISEASE

ALS highlights
- Progressive degenerative neurologic disease
- Results in decreased motor function in the upper and lower motor neuron systems

Definition
- Progressive degenerative neurologic disease resulting in decreased motor function in the upper and lower motor neuron systems (see *Motor neuron disease*)

Causes
- Unknown cause
- Genetic predisposition
- Viral infection
- Excess of glutamate

Pathophysiology
- Myelin sheaths are destroyed and replaced with scar tissue, resulting in distorted or blocked nerve impulses
- Nerve cells die and muscle fibers have atrophic changes

Key signs of ALS
- Fatigue
- Awkwardness of fine finger movements
- Dysphagia
- Muscle weakness of hands and arms

Assessment findings
- Fatigue
- Awkwardness of fine finger movements
- Dysphagia
- Muscle weakness of hands and arms
- Fasciculations of face
- Nasal quality of speech
- Spasticity
- Atrophy of tongue

Testing for ALS
- No one specific diagnostic test used
- Diagnosis based on assessment findings

Diagnostic test findings
- EMG: decreased amplitude of evoked potentials
- Laboratory values: elevated creatine kinase (CK)
- No one specific diagnostic test used
- Diagnosis based on assessment findings

Motor neuron disease

In its final stages, motor neuron disease affects both upper and lower motor neuron cells. However, the site of initial cell damage varies according to the specific disease.

- *Progressive bulbar palsy:* degeneration of upper motor neurons in the medulla oblongata
- *Progressive muscular atrophy:* degeneration of lower motor neurons in the spinal cord
- *Amyotrophic lateral sclerosis:* Degeneration of upper motor neurons in the medulla oblongata and lower motor neurons in the spinal cord.

Medical management

- Focused on symptomatic relief
- Activity: as tolerated
- Monitoring: vital signs, I/O, neurovital signs
- Mechanical ventilation: negative-pressure ventilators
- NG tube feedings
- Gastrostomy tube feedings
- Antispasmodics: baclofen (Lioresal), diazepam (Valium)
- Muscle cramps: Quinine therapy
- Investigational: thyrotropin-releasing hormone, interferon

Nursing interventions

- Maintain the patient's diet
- Assess neurologic and respiratory status
- Assess swallow and gag reflexes
- Monitor and record vital signs, I/O, and neurovital signs
- Administer medications, as prescribed
- Encourage the patient to complete advanced directives or a "living will"
- Monitor for choking while eating
- Suction oral pharynx, as necessary
- Assist the patient to maintain as much independence as possible
- Provide psychological support for the patient and his family
- Provide information about the ALS Foundation
- Individualize home care instructions
  - Teach the patient to maintain tucked chin position while eating or drinking
  - Teach the patient to use tonsillar suction tip to clear oral pharynx
  - Inform the patient about prosthetic devices to assist with ADLs

Complications

- Respiratory failure
- Pneumonia
- Death

Possible surgical intervention

- None

Types of motor neuron disease

- Progressive bulbar palsy
- Progressive muscular atrophy
- Amyotrophic lateral sclerosis

Main treatment options for ALS

- Focus on symptomatic relief
- Antispasmodics

Key nursing interventions for a patient with ALS

- Assess swallow and gag reflexes.
- Monitor for choking while eating.
- Suction oral pharynx, as necessary.

INTERVERTEBRAL DISK HERNIATION

Definition
- All or part of the nucleus pulposus is forced through the disk's outer ring (annulus fibrosus)

Causes
- Degenerative disk changes
- Trauma
- Physical stress
- Scoliosis/kyphosis

Pathophysiology
- The extruded disk may impinge on spinal nerve roots as they exit from the spinal canal or on the spinal cord itself
- The result is back pain and other signs of nerve root irritation

Assessment findings
- In lumbosacral area
  - Acute, intermittent pain in the lower back radiating across the buttock and down the leg
  - Pain on ambulation
  - Weakness, numbness, and tingling of the foot and leg
  - Diminished reflexes of the affected extremity
- In cervical area
  - Weakness of the affected upper extremity
  - Neck pain that radiates down the arm to the hand
  - Sensory loss of the hand
  - Diminished or absent reflexes of the arm
- In thoracic area
  - Bandlike pain around chest

Diagnostic test findings
- MRI: herniation of affected area of spine, degenerative changes, and condition of the canal and nerve root
- Myelogram: degree of injury and level of herniation
- CT scan: outlines bone and soft tissue structures
- Lasegue's sign and straight-leg-raising test: positive

Medical management
- Diet: increased fiber and fluids
- Position: bed rest in semi-Fowler's position with hip and knee flexion and passive ROM exercises, as indicated
- Monitoring: vital signs, I/O, laboratory studies, and neurovascular checks
- Nonsteroidal anti-inflammatory drugs: indomethacin (Indocin), ibuprofen (Motrin), sulindac (Clinoril), piroxicam (Feldene), flurbiprofen (Ansaid), diclofenac (Voltaren), naproxen (Naprosyn), diflunisal (Dolobid)
- Muscle relaxants: diazepam (Valium), cyclobenzaprine (Flexeril), methocarbamol (Robaxin), metaxalone (Skelaxin)
- Corticosteroids: oral or epidural

Key facts about intervertebral disk herniation
- All or part of the nucleus pulposus is forced through the disk's outer ring
- Results in back pain and other signs of nerve root irritation

Key assessment findings in intervertebral disk herniation
- Lumbosacral:
  - Acute, intermittent pain in the lower back
  - Pain on ambulation
  - Weakness, numbness, and tingling of the foot and leg
- Cervical:
  - Weakness of the affected upper extremity
  - Neck pain that radiates down the arm to the hand
- Thoracic:
  - Bandlike pain around chest

Key diagnostic test findings in intervertebral disk herniation
- MRI: herniation of spine and degenerative changes
- Myelogram: degree of injury and level of herniation

- Analgesics: propoxyphene (Darvon), oxycodone (Tylox), hydrocodone (Vicodin), oxycodone hydrochloride (OxyContin)
- Stool softener: docusate (Colace)
- Heating pad and moist, warm compresses
- Orthopedic devices, including back brace or cervical collar
- Traction
- Transcutaneous electrical nerve stimulation, ultrasound

Nursing interventions

- Maintain the patient's diet
- Encourage fluids
- Maintain bed rest with proper body alignment
- Monitor neurovascular status, vital signs, I/O, and laboratory values
- Assess level of pain and administer analgesics, as necessary
- Administer medications, as prescribed
- Encourage the patient to express his feelings about changes in his body image and about fears of disability
- Provide back and skin care
- Turn the patient every 2 hours using the logrolling technique
- Maintain traction, braces, and cervical collar
- Promote independence in ADLs
- Provide information about Back School
- Individualize home care instruction
  - Exercise regularly, according to physician's guidelines, to strengthen and stretch the muscles
  - Avoid heavy lifting
  - Avoid flexion, extension, or rotation of the neck, if cervical
  - Use a back brace or cervical collar
  - Practice relaxation techniques
  - Use proper body mechanics

Complications

- Persistent neurologic deficits
- Bowel and bladder dysfunction

Possible surgical intervention

- Microdiscectomy
- Percutaneous discectomy
- Laminotomy or discectomy, with or without the use of instrumentation

MENINGITIS

Definition

- Inflammation of the brain and spinal cord meninges

Causes

- Bacterial infection, such as *Neisseria meningitides* and *Streptococcus pneumoniae,* most common cause
- *Haemophilus influenzae* is a common bacterial cause in children ages 2 months to 7 years

Key treatment options for intervertebral disk herniation

- Nonsteroidal anti-inflammatory drugs
- Corticosteroids
- Analgesics
- Stool softener
- Orthopedic devices, including back brace or cervical collar
- Traction

Key nursing interventions for a patient with intervertebral disk herniation

- Maintain bed rest with proper body alignment.
- Monitor neurovascular status, vital signs, I/O, and laboratory values.
- Assess level of pain and administer analgesics, as necessary.
- Turn the patient every 2 hours using the logrolling technique.
- Maintain traction, braces, and cervical collar.

Meningitis defined

- Inflammation of the brain and spinal cord meninges
- Most commonly caused by a bacterial infection

- Beta-hemolytic streptococci and *Listeria monocytogenes* are common causes in infants
- Enteroviruses, mumps, and herpes simplex are common causes of viral meningitis (aseptic meningitis)
- Cryptococcosis, candidiasis, histoplasmosis, and coccidioidomycosis are common causes of fungal meningitis
- TB meningitis is a bacterial infection caused by *Mycobacterium tuberculosis*

Key symptoms of systemic infection

- Fever
- Chills
- Tachycardia
- Petechial rash

Pathophysiology

- Infecting organisms gain entry through basilar skull fractures with dural tears, chronic otitis media or sinusitis, neurosurgical contamination, penetrating head wounds, or septicemia
- Infecting organisms produce an inflammatory response
- Exudate formation causes meningeal irritation and increased ICP

Assessment findings

- Systemic infection
  - Fever
  - Tachycardia
  - Chills
  - Petechial rash
- Meningeal signs
  - Severe throbbing headache
  - Photophobia
  - Nuchal rigidity
  - Positive Kernig's sign (see *Important signs of meningitis*)
  - Positive Brudzinski's sign
- Neurologic findings
  - Decreased LOC
  - Cranial nerve palsies, most commonly ptosis, diplopia, facial weakness, tinnitus, vertigo, and deafness
  - Focal motor weakness
  - Ataxia
  - Seizures

Key meningeal symptoms

- Severe throbbing headache
- Photophobia
- Nuchal rigidity
- Positive Kernig's sign
- Positive Brudzinski's sign

Key neurologic findings

- Decreased LOC
- Ataxia
- Seizures

Diagnostic test findings

- Cultures: identify source of infection in blood, urine, and nose and throat secretions
- X-rays: assesses for fractures, abscesses, or signs of infection in chest, skull, and sinuses
- LP: elevated CSF pressure; cloudy, turbid, or clear in appearance; normal or increased protein; glucose decreased or normal; culture and sensitivity tests identify bacteria, unless viral cause
- WBC count: elevated

Key diagnostic test findings in meningitis

- Cultures: identify source of infection in blood, urine, and nose and throat secretions
- LP: elevated CSF pressure; cloudy, turbid, or clear in appearance; normal or increased protein; glucose decreased or normal; culture and sensitivity tests identify bacteria, unless viral cause

Medical management

- Diet: withhold food and fluids, as ordered; enteral or parenteral feeding, as indicated
- I.V. therapy: electrolyte replacement, saline lock
- Oxygen therapy

Important signs of meningitis

Brudzinski's sign: Place the patient in a dorsal recumbent position, put your hands behind her neck, and bend it forward. Pain and resistance may indicate meningeal inflammation, neck injury, or arthritis. If the patient also flexes her hips and knees in response to this manipulation, chances are she has meningitis.

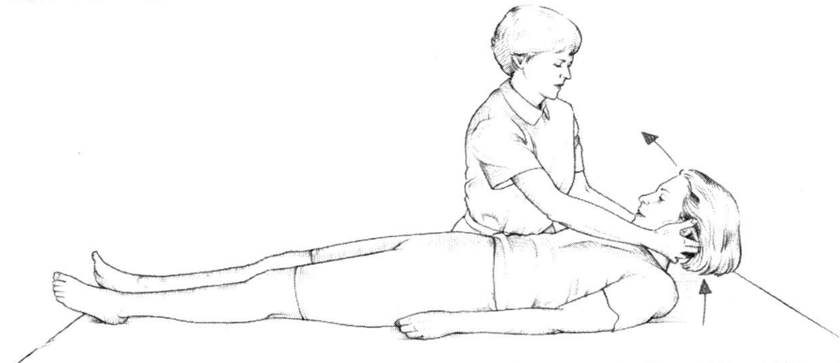

Kernig's sign: Place the patient in a supine position. Flex her leg at the hip and knee and then straighten the knee. Pain or resistance points to meningitis.

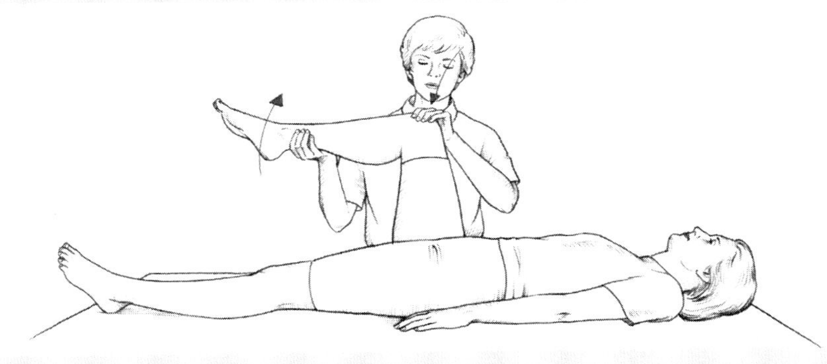

- Position: semi-Fowler's
- Activity: bed rest in darkened room
- Monitoring: vital signs, I/O, ECG, ICP, neurovital signs, pulse oximetry, and laboratory values
- Antibiotics: penicillin, ampicillin (Omnipen), or chloramphenicol (Chloromycetin) or one of the cephalosporins (ceftriaxone [Rocephin], cefotaxime [Claforan]); vancomycin (Vancocin) alone or in combination with rifampin (Rifadin), for resistant strains
- Antipyretics/analgesics: aspirin, acetaminophen (Tylenol)
- Anticonvulsants: phenytoin (Dilantin), phenobarbital (Luminal)
- Glucocorticoid: dexamethasone (Decadron)
- Diuretic: mannitol (Osmitrol)
- Isolation
- Seizure precautions

Important meningitis signs

- Brudzinski's sign
- Kernig's sign

Key treatments for meningitis

- I.V. therapy: electrolyte replacement, saline lock
- Oxygen therapy
- Antibiotics
- Anticonvulsants
- Diuretics

Key nursing interventions for a patient with meningitis

- Assess neurologic, cardiovascular, and respiratory status.
- Maintain a quiet, dimly lit environment.
- Implement isolation techniques, if necessary.
- Report meningococcal meningitis to local health authorities.

Key home care instructions for a patient with meningitis

- Prevent meningitis from recurring by seeking proper medical treatment for chronic sinusitis or other chronic infections.
- Recognize signs and symptoms of meningitis and ICP.

Alzheimer's disease key characteristics

- Irreversible, degenerative disorder of the cerebral cortex
- Characterized by a progressive dementia

Nursing interventions

- Administer I.V. fluids
- Administer oxygen
- Assess neurologic, cardiovascular, and respiratory status
- Keep the patient on bed rest in the semi-Fowler's position
- Monitor and record vital signs, I/O, ICP, neurovital signs, laboratory studies, and pulse oximetry
- Administer medications, as ordered
- Allay the patient's anxiety
- Turn the patient every 2 hours; provide ROM exercises
- Maintain a quiet, dimly lit environment
- **Maintain seizure precautions**
- Use a cooling blanket or tepid bath to control temperature
- Assess for headache and administer analgesics, as appropriate
- Provide nutrition, as appropriate
- Provide skin care
- **Implement isolation techniques, if necessary**
- **Report meningococcal meningitis to local health authorities**
- Refer the patient for rehabilitation, if appropriate
- Individualize home care instruction
  - Recognize signs and symptoms of meningitis
  - Recognize signs and symptoms of ICP
  - Prevent meningitis from recurring by seeking proper medical treatment for chronic sinusitis or other chronic infections
  - Reduce risk of spread of disease

Complications

- Visual impairment
- Optic neuritis
- Deafness
- Personality changes
- Headache
- Seizures
- Paresis
- Death

Possible surgical intervention

- None

ALZHEIMER'S DISEASE

Definition

- Irreversible, degenerative disorder of the cerebral cortex characterized by progressive dementia

Causes

- Exact cause unknown
- Neurotransmitter deficiencies
- Virus

Stages of Alzheimer's disease

EARLY STAGE	INTERMEDIATE STAGE	END STAGE
• Recent memory loss • Inability to learn and retain new information • Difficulty finding words • Personality changes and mood swings • Progressive difficulty performing activities of daily living (ADLs)	• Inability to learn and recall new information • Reduced ability to remember past events • Increased need for assistance with ADLs • Wandering • Agitation, hostility, or physical aggressiveness • Lack of orientation to time and place • Bladder and bowel incontinence	• Inability to walk • Total incontinence • No recent or remote memory • Inability to swallow and eat • No intelligible speech

- Trauma
- Genetics

Pathophysiology

- Neurofibrillary tangles, which are a twisting and distortion of the protein in the neuron
- Neuritic plaques that represent areas of degeneration and granulovascular changes
- Senile plaques, which are the result of dying nerve cells that accumulate around protein

Assessment findings

- Altered behavior and memory may include recent memory loss and impaired judgment (see *Stages of Alzheimer's disease*)
- Muscle rigidity, myoclonic jerks, and restlessness
- Obsessive behaviors
- Anomia (inability to remember one's name)
- Aphasia (impaired ability to communicate verbally or in writing)
- Loss of self-care skills (late finding)
- Loss of speech (late finding)
- Loss of voluntary movement (late finding)

Diagnostic test findings

- Diagnosed when other dementia-producing conditions have been ruled out; diagnosis confirmed at autopsy
- EEG: may be normal early in disease
- MRI: structural and neurologic changes; decrease in size of hippocampus occurs in late stages
- PET scan: Evaluates metabolic activity of the brain; may identify the disease earlier
- Neuropsychologic testing: a series of tests to evaluate cognitive status

Stages of Alzheimer's disease

- Early stage
- Intermediate stage
- End stage

Abnormal structures involved in the development of Alzheimer's disease

- Neurofibrillary tangles
- Neuritic plaques
- Senile plaques

Most common assessment findings in Alzheimer's disease

- Altered behavior and memory
- Restlessness
- Loss of self-care skills (late)

Diagnosing Alzheimer's disease

- Diagnosed when other dementia-producing conditions have been ruled out
- Diagnosis confirmed at autopsy

Chief treatments for Alzheimer's disease

- Anticholinesterase agents
- Maintain patient safety

Key nursing interventions for a patient with Alzheimer's disease

- Monitor neurologic status, including emotional state, mental status, and motor function.
- Provide for repetitive activity and exercise.
- Approach the patient in a calm, slow manner.
- Provide a safe environment.
- Refer family members or caregivers to local support groups.

Medical management

- Diet: individualized according to the patient's needs
- Provide hydration, I.V. or orally
- Activity, as tolerated
- Monitor: vital signs, I/O, and laboratory values
- Anticholinesterase agents: tacrine (Cognex), donepezil (Aricept), rivastigmine (Exelon), and galantamine (Reminyl)
- Maintain patient safety

Nursing interventions

- Maintain the patient's diet
- Provide small, frequent feedings and stay with the patient to encourage him to eat
- Serve finger foods or semi-soft or pureed foods, as appropriate
- Assess ability to swallow
- Use feeding aids, when necessary
- Encourage fluid intake
- Monitor and record vital signs, I/O, and laboratory values
- Administer medications, as ordered
- Monitor neurologic status, including emotional state, mental status, and motor function
- Provide skin and mouth care
- Provide for repetitive activity and exercise
- Approach the patient in a calm, slow manner
- Allow sufficient time for interaction
- Assess ability to perform self-care and assist when necessary
- Obtain physical and occupational therapy consults
- **Provide a safe environment**
- Provide information about the Alzheimer's Association
- Individualize home care instructions
  - Refer family members or caregivers to local support groups
  - Discuss power of attorney with family
  - Review safety concerns
  - Learn stress-relief measures

Complications

- Malnutrition or dehydration
- Pressure ulcers
- Muscle contractions
- Physical injuries
- Abuse
- Infection
- Death

Possible surgical interventions

- None

BELL'S PALSY

Definition

- Disease of the seventh cranial nerve that produces unilateral facial weakness or paralysis

Causes

- Infection
- Hemorrhage
- Tumor
- Meningitis
- Local trauma

Pathophysiology

- The seventh cranial nerve, which is responsible for motor innervation of the muscles of the face, is blocked
- The conduction block is due to an inflammatory reaction around the nerve (usually at the internal auditory meatus)

Assessment findings

- Eye rolls upward and tears excessively when the patient attempts to close it
- Inability to close eye completely on the affected side
- Pain around the jaw or ear
- Ringing in the ears
- Taste distortion on the affected anterior portion of the tongue
- Unilateral facial weakness

Diagnostic test findings

- Based on clinical presentation
- EMG: predicts level of expected recovery

Medical management

- Diet: soft, nutritionally balanced
- I.V. therapy: saline lock
- Position: semi-Fowler's
- Activity: ad lib, as tolerated
- Monitoring: vital signs, I/O
- Corticosteroids: prednisone (Deltasone)
- Electrotherapy
- Moist heat
- Physical therapy

Nursing interventions

- Maintain the patient's diet
- Avoid hot foods and fluids
- Arrange for privacy at mealtimes to avoid embarrassment
- Apply facial sling to improve lip alignment
- Provide frequent mouth care
- Administer medication, as ordered
- Provide massage therapy

Bell's palsy

- Blocked seventh cranial nerve
- Results in unilateral facial weakness or paralysis

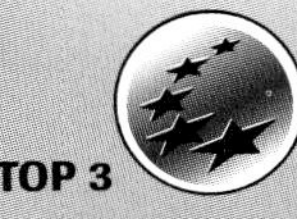

TOP 3

Bell's palsy signs and symptoms

1. Inability to close eye completely on the affected side
2. Pain around the jaw or ear
3. Unilateral facial weakness

Diagnosing Bell's palsy

- No specific diagnostic test
- EMG predicts level of expected recovery

Key treatments for Bell's palsy

- Corticosteroids
- Moist heat

Key nursing interventions for a patient with Bell's palsy

- Arrange for privacy at mealtimes to avoid embarrassment.
- Provide massage therapy.
- Protect eye with patch, as indicated.
- Apply moist heat to affected side of face to reduce pain.

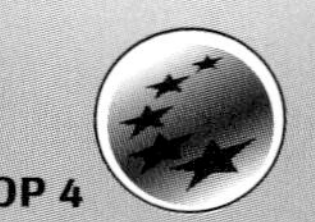

TOP 4

Items to study for your next test on the nervous system

1. Structures and functions of the brain and spinal cord
2. The 12 cranial nerves and their functions
3. How the Glasgow Coma Scale is used
4. Common disorders of the nervous system, such as Parkinson's disease, MS, seizure disorders, stroke, and Alzheimer's disease

- Encourage active facial exercises
- Protect eye with patch, as indicated
- Apply moist heat to affected side of face to reduce pain
- Encourage the patient to verbalize feelings of altered body image
- Individualize home care instructions
  - Perform facial exercise
  - Use moist heat to relieve pain
  - Perform massage and facial exercise
  - Take corticosteroids, as instructed
  - Chew on unaffected side of mouth
  - Protect eye with patch

Complications

- Facial contractures
- Facial paralysis

Possible surgical interventions

- None

NCLEX CHECKS

It's never too soon to begin your NCLEX preparation. Now that you've reviewed this chapter, carefully read each of the following questions and choose the best answer. Then compare your responses to the correct answers.

1. Brudzinski's sign and Kernig's sign are two tests that help diagnose which of the following neurologic disorders?

☐ **A.** Alzheimer's disease
☐ **B.** Epilepsy
☐ **C.** Stroke
☐ **D.** Meningitis

2. The nurse is caring for a comatose patient who has suffered a closed head injury. Which intervention should the nurse implement to prevent an increase in intracranial pressure (ICP)?

☐ **A.** Suctioning the airway every hour
☐ **B.** Elevating the head of the bed 15 to 40 degrees
☐ **C.** Turning the patient and changing his position every 2 hours
☐ **D.** Maintaining a well-lit room

3. The nurse explains to the patient's family that which of the following disorders is characterized by progressive degeneration of the cerebral cortex?

☐ **A.** Alzheimer's disease
☐ **B.** Epilepsy
☐ **C.** Guillain-Barré syndrome
☐ **D.** Stroke

4. To encourage adequate nutritional intake for a patient with Alzheimer's disease, the nurse should:

- ☐ **A.** stay with the patient and encourage him to eat.
- ☐ **B.** help the patient fill out his menu.
- ☐ **C.** give the patient privacy during meals.
- ☐ **D.** fill out the menu for the patient.

5. The nurse is teaching a patient and his family about dietary practices related to Parkinson's disease. A priority for the nurse to address is the risk of:

- ☐ **A.** fluid overload and drooling.
- ☐ **B.** aspiration and anorexia.
- ☐ **C.** choking and diarrhea.
- ☐ **D.** dysphagia and constipation.

6. The nurse is assessing a patient with a brain tumor in the occipital lobe. She should expect which of the following possible assessment findings? (Select all that apply.)

- ☐ **A.** Visual impairment
- ☐ **B.** Memory loss
- ☐ **C.** Aphasia
- ☐ **D.** Visual hallucinations
- ☐ **E.** Homonymous hemianopia
- ☐ **F.** Personality changes

7. A patient undergoes a lumbar puncture (LP) for a myelogram. Shortly after the procedure, he reports a severe headache. What should the nurse do?

- ☐ **A.** Increase the patient's fluid intake.
- ☐ **B.** Administer prescribed antihypertensives.
- ☐ **C.** Dim the lights in the room.
- ☐ **D.** Place cool packs over the LP site.

8. The nurse is caring for a patient with increased intracranial pressure (ICP). Which procedure is contraindicated in this case?

- ☐ **A.** EEG
- ☐ **B.** Skull X-rays
- ☐ **C.** Lumbar puncture (LP)
- ☐ **D.** Computed tomography (CT) scan

ANSWERS AND RATIONALES

1. CORRECT ANSWER: D

A positive response to one or both of these tests indicates meningeal irritation. Brudzinski's sign and Kernig's sign aren't used in the diagnosis of Alzheimer's disease, epilepsy, or stroke.

2. CORRECT ANSWER: B

To facilitate venous drainage and avoid jugular compression, the nurse should elevate the head of the bed to 15 to 40 degrees. The patient with increased ICP tolerates suctioning poorly and shouldn't be suctioned on a regular basis. Turning from side to side increases the risk of jugular compression and increased ICP. The room should be kept quiet and dimly lit.

3. CORRECT ANSWER: A
Alzheimer's disease is characterized by progressive degeneration of the cerebral cortex leading to symptoms ranging from recent memory loss to debilitating dementia. Epilepsy is characterized by involuntary muscle contractions caused by abnormal discharge of electrical impulses from nerve cells. Guillain-Barré syndrome is characterized by ascending paralysis caused by demyelination and inflammation. Stroke is characterized by sensory and motor deficits caused by a disruption of cerebral circulation.

4. CORRECT ANSWER: A
Staying with the patient and encouraging him to feed himself will ensure adequate food intake. A patient with Alzheimer's disease can forget to eat. Filling out the patient's menu, helping the patient to fill out his menu, or allowing privacy during meals doesn't ensure adequate nutritional intake.

5. CORRECT ANSWER: D
Eating problems associated with Parkinson's disease include aspiration, choking, constipation, and dysphagia. Fluid overload isn't specifically related to Parkinson's disease and, although drooling occurs with Parkinson's disease, it doesn't take priority. Anorexia and diarrhea aren't specifically associated with Parkinson's disease.

6. CORRECT ANSWER: A, D, E
Because the occipital lobe is the site of vision, a brain tumor in that area may cause such visual disturbances as visual impairment, visual hallucinations, and homonymous hemianopia. Memory loss, aphasia, and personality changes typically occur in patients with tumors in the frontal lobe, the site of personality, motor speech, and intellectual functioning. Aphasia may also occur with tumors in the temporal lobe, the site of hearing, taste, smell, and speech.

7. CORRECT ANSWER: A
Headache following an LP is usually caused by a cerebrospinal fluid (CSF) leak. Increased fluid intake will help restore CSF volume. Antihypertensives don't address the problem. Dimming the lights and putting ice packs on the site don't address the problem of reduced CSF volume, which caused the headache.

8. CORRECT ANSWER: C
An LP, the removal of cerebrospinal fluid (CSF) from the subarachnoid space in the lumbar region, is contraindicated in the presence of increased ICP. Removing CSF could decrease pressure within the spinal column, causing the patient's brain to herniate downward. ICP isn't affected by an EEG, skull X-rays, or a CT scan.

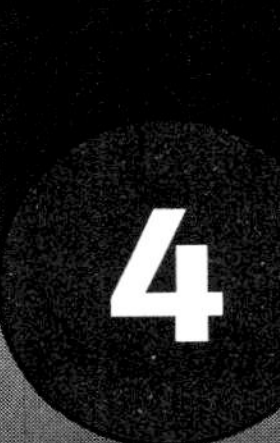

4 Sensory system: Eyes and ears

LEARNING OBJECTIVES

After studying this chapter, you should be able to:

- Describe the psychosocial impact of sensory disorders.
- Differentiate between the modifiable and nonmodifiable risk factors in the development of a sensory disorder.
- List three probable and three possible nursing diagnoses for a patient with a sensory disorder.
- Identify nursing interventions for a patient with a sensory disorder.
- Identify three teaching topics for a patient with a sensory disorder.

CHAPTER OVERVIEW

Caring for the patient with a sensory disorder requires a sound understanding of eye and ear anatomy and physiology as well as the psychological impact of sight and hearing loss. A thorough assessment is essential to planning and implementing appropriate patient care. The assessment includes a complete history, physical examination, diagnostic testing, identification of modifiable and nonmodifiable risk factors, and information related to the psychosocial impact of the disorder on the patient.

Nursing diagnoses focus primarily on sensory and perceptual disturbances, social isolation, and deficient knowledge. The goal of nursing interventions is to improve the patient's safety and decrease his anxiety about body image changes. Patient teaching — a crucial nursing activity — involves instructing the patient

External structures of the eyes

- Eyelids
- Palpebral fissure
- Conjunctiva
- Extraocular muscles
- Eyeball

Internal structures of the eyes

- Sclera
- Choroid
- Iris
- Ciliary body
- Schlemm's canal
- Pupil
- Lens
- Vitreous humor
- Retina
- Lens zonules
- Retinal cones
- Retinal rods
- Macula lutea
- Optic nerve
- Optic disk

about medical follow-up, medication regimens, signs and symptoms of complications, and how to reduce modifiable risk factors by taking safety precautions to protect the eyes and ears.

ANATOMY AND PHYSIOLOGY REVIEW

Eyes

- External structures
  - Eyelids — two movable, musculofibrous folds that protect the eye by opening and closing; distribute tears across the eyelid when blinking
  - Palpebral fissure — space between the open lids
  - Conjunctiva — thin transparent mucous membrane that lines the lid
  - Extraocular muscles — focus muscles abduct, adduct, elevate, or depress; two muscles direct the eye laterally, inferiorly, or superiorly
  - Eyeball — spherical organ surrounded by orbital fat and positioned in orbit; three layers include the sclera, uvea, and retina
- Internal structures (see *Cross section of the eye*)
  - Sclera — dense, white, fibrous protective coating of eye; optic nerve and central retinal vessel pass through posterior opening; anterior opening serves as refracting window; provides structural strength to front of eye
  - Choroid — highly vascular posterior portion of uveal tract that nourishes retina
  - Iris — thin, circular, pigmented muscular structure in eye; gives color to eye; divides space between cornea and lens into anterior and posterior chamber; peripheral border attaches to ciliary body
  - Ciliary body — muscular fibers in middle pigmented layer of eye that contract and relax the lens zonules; maintain intraocular pressure (IOP) by secreting aqueous humor
  - Schlemm's canal — system of channels responsible for drainage of aqueous humor
  - Pupil — circulation aperture in iris that changes size as iris adapts to amount of light entering eye
  - Lens — biconvex, avascular, colorless, and transparent structure suspended behind the iris by the zonules
  - Vitreous humor — clear, transparent, avascular, gelatinous fluid that fills the space in the posterior portion of the eye; bounded by the lens, retina, and optic disk; maintains transparency and form of the eye
  - Retina — thin, semitransparent layer of nerve tissue that lines the eye wall; rods and cones respond to light energy and initiate the neural response that's interpreted in the brain
  - Lens zonules — suspend lens; contraction and relaxation of zonules changes shape of lens and allows it to focus light on the retina
  - Retinal cones — responsible for visual acuity and color discrimination
  - Retinal rods — responsible for peripheral vision under decreased light conditions

Cross section of the eye

This cross section details important anatomic structures of the eye.

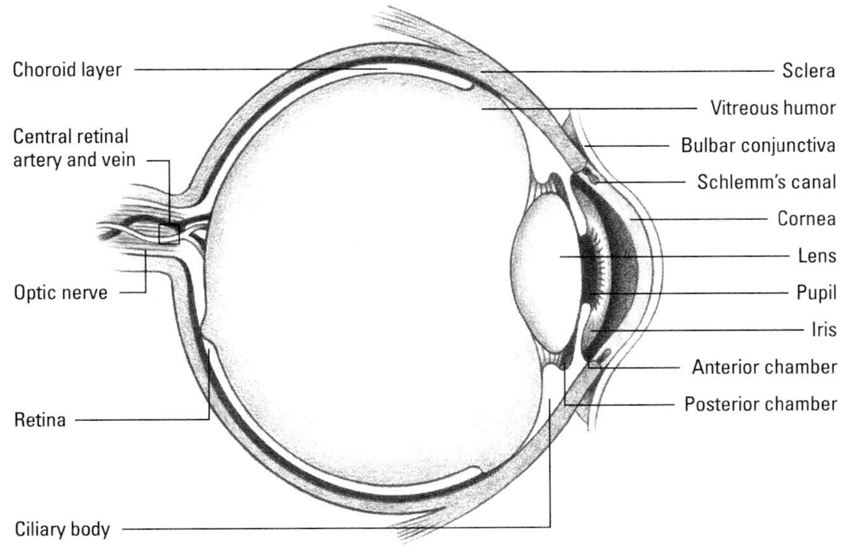

- Macula lutea — center of posterior retina with fovea centralis for acute vision, color vision, and resolution of image
- Optic nerve — convergence of nerve fibers of retina
- Optic disk — head of the optic nerve known as the blind spot

- Image formation
  - Light rays enter the eye through the cornea and pass through the pupil, lens, and vitreous body to the retina
  - Light rays stimulate the retinal sensory receptors to send impulses through the optic nerve to the occipital cortex, where the impulses are registered as visual sensations
- Aqueous humor formation
  - Watery, transparent liquid that flows through the anterior and posterior chambers and exits through Schlemm's canal
  - Serves circulatory function for avascular tissues of eye
  - Responsible for maintaining IOP
- Accommodation — the process of contraction and relaxation of the lens zonules that changes the shape of lens and allows it to focus light on the retina

Ears

- External ear
  - Portion of ear that includes the pinna (auricle) and external auditory canal (see *A close look at the ear,* page 172)

The retina's functions

- Lines the eye wall
- Rods and cones respond to light energy and initiate the neural response that's interpreted in the brain

The difference between rods and cones

- Rods are responsible for peripheral vision under decreased light conditions.
- Cones are responsible for visual acuity and color discrimination.

How an image is formed

- Light rays enter the eye through the cornea and pass through the pupil, lens, and vitreous humor to the retina.
- Light rays stimulate the retinal sensory receptors to send impulses through the optic nerve to the occipital cortex, where the impulses are registered as visual sensations.

External ear structures
- External auditory canal
- Auricle
- Helix
- Anthelix
- Concha
- Antitragus
- Lobule

Middle ear structures
- Malleus
- Incus
- Stapes
- Tympanic membrane

Inner ear structures
- Vestibule
- Cochlea
- Semicircular canals
- Eustachian tube
- Acoustic nerve branches

A close look at the ear

Use this illustration to review the structures of the ear.

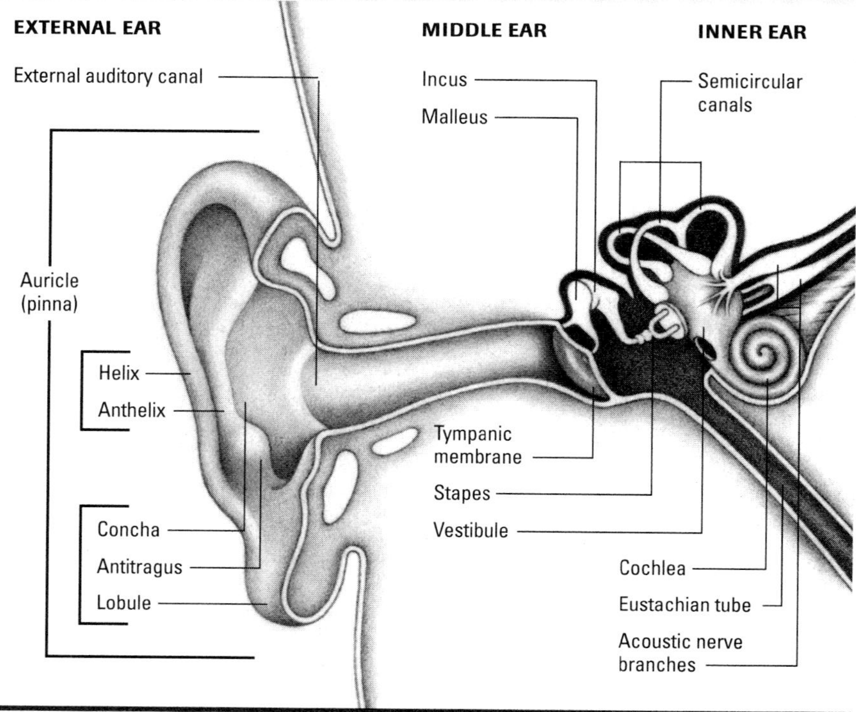

  - Separated from the middle ear by the tympanic membrane
- Middle ear
  - Air-filled cavity in the temporal bone
  - Contains three small bones (malleus, incus, and stapes)
  - Opens to the eustachian tube or auditory tube, which connects to the nasopharynx
- Inner ear
  - Portion of the ear that consists of the cochlea, vestibule, and semicircular canals
  - Also known as the labyrinth
- Sound transmission — airborne vibrations are transformed to sound through mechanical stimulation of the endolymphatic fluids
- Equilibrium — Position changes of the head are detected by maculae or cristae

ASSESSMENT FINDINGS

History
- Eyes
  - Blurred distance vision
  - Difficulty watching television or reading

  - Headaches
  - Dizziness
  - Eye or brow pain
  - Eye weeping
  - Scratchy or itchy eye
  - Inflamed eye
  - Watery eye
  - Puffy eyelids
  - Crossed eyes
  - Unequal pupils
  - Squinting
  - Increased blinking
  - Rubbing eye
  - Encrusted eye
  - Burning sensation in the eye
  - Double vision
  - Spots before the eye
  - Difficulty differentiating colors
  - Difficulty driving at night
  - Flashes of light
  - Sensation of veil or curtain across the field of vision
  - Sudden change in vision
- Ears
  - Tinnitus
  - Decreased ability to hear at group meetings
  - Need to turn up volume on television and radio
  - Social withdrawal
  - Fatigue
  - Indifference
  - Insecurity
  - Suspiciousness

Physical examination

- Eyes
  - Visual acuity changes
  - Vertigo
  - Discharge from eye
  - Sty
  - Presbyopia
  - Ptosis
  - Nystagmus
  - Optic atrophy
  - Myopia
  - Hyperopia
  - Anisometropia
  - Astigmatism
  - Loss of red reflex

Key warning signs for eyes

- Eye or brow pain
- Unequal pupils
- Spots before the eye
- Flashes of light
- Sensation of veil or curtain across the field of vision
- Sudden change in vision

Key warning signs for ears

- Tinnitus
- Decreased ability to hear at group meetings
- Need to turn up volume on television and radio

Key eye examination findings

- Visual acuity changes
- Loss of red reflex

- Ears
  - Speech deterioration
  - Ear pain
  - Ear deformities
  - Ear lesions
  - Ear canal discharge
  - Mastoid pain
  - Pressure of cerumen
  - Ear canal inflammation
  - Foreign body in ear canal
  - Change in landmarks and color of tympanic membrane

Key ear examination findings

- Speech deterioration
- Ear pain
- Change in landmarks and color of tympanic membrane

DIAGNOSTIC TESTS AND PROCEDURES

Visual acuity

- Definition and purpose
  - A screening test of central vision
  - Tests clarity of vision using letter chart (Snellen) placed 20′ (6.1 m) from the patient (see *Visual acuity charts*)
  - Expressed in a ratio
    - Top number (20) is the distance between the patient and the chart
    - Bottom number is the distance from which a person with normal vision could read the line
- Nursing interventions
  - Explain the testing procedure to the patient
  - Answer the patient's questions
  - Remind the patient to bring eyeglasses or contact lenses, if presently prescribed
  - Advise the examiner if the patient can't read alphabet letters
  - Advise the examiner if the patient has difficulty hearing or following directions
  - Test each eye separately, then together

Visual acuity testing

- A screening test of central vision
- Tests clarity of vision using letter chart placed 20′ from the patient
- Intervention: remind the patient to bring eyeglasses or contact lenses, if presently prescribed

Extraocular eye muscle testing

- Definition and purpose
  - Tests parallel alignment of the eyes and integrity of nervous control of eye muscles (cranial nerves III [oculomotor], IV [trochlear], and VI [abducens])
  - Correlated action of the extraocular muscles results in parallel gaze
- Nursing interventions
  - Explain the testing procedure to the patient
  - The patient follows a pencil or finger as it moves in the shape of the letter "H"
  - Advise the examiner if the patient has difficulty hearing or following directions

Extraocular eye muscle testing

- Tests parallel alignment of the eyes
- Tests integrity of the nervous control of eye muscles (cranial nerves III, IV, and VI)
- Intervention: the patient follows a pencil or finger as it moves in the shape of the letter "H"

Visual field testing

- Definition and purpose

Visual acuity charts

The most commonly used charts for testing vision are the Snellen alphabet chart (left) and the Snellen E chart (right) – the latter of which is used for young children and adults who can't read. Both charts are used to test distance vision and measure visual acuity. The patient reads each chart at a distance of 20′ (6.1 m).

RECORDING RESULTS

Visual acuity is recorded as a fraction. The top number (20) is the distance between the patient and the chart. The bottom number is the distance from which a person with normal vision could read the line. The larger the bottom number is, the poorer the patient's vision.

AGE DIFFERENCES

In adults and children age 6 and older, normal vision is measured as 20/20. For children younger than age 6, normal vision varies. For children age 3 and younger, normal vision is 20/50; for children age 4, 20/40; and for children age 5, 20/30.

SNELLEN ALPHABET CHART

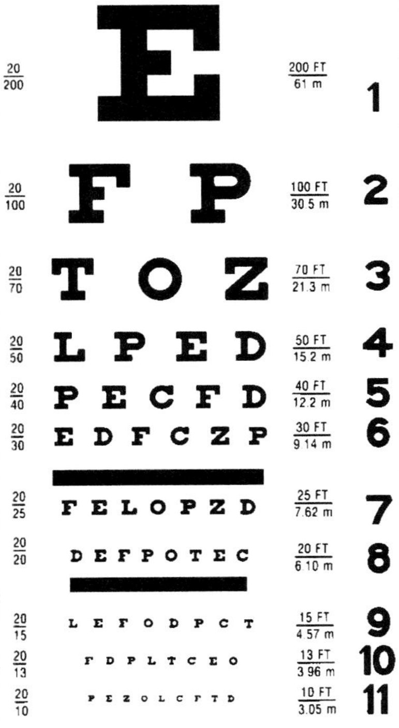

20/200	E	200 FT / 61 m	1
20/100	F P	100 FT / 30.5 m	2
20/70	T O Z	70 FT / 21.3 m	3
20/50	L P E D	50 FT / 15.2 m	4
20/40	P E C F D	40 FT / 12.2 m	5
20/30	E D F C Z P	30 FT / 9.14 m	6
20/25	F E L O P Z D	25 FT / 7.62 m	7
20/20	D E F P O T E C	20 FT / 6.10 m	8
20/15	L E F O D P C T	15 FT / 4.57 m	9
20/13	F D P L T C E O	13 FT / 3.96 m	10
20/10	F E Z O L C F T D	10 FT / 3.05 m	11

SNELLEN E CHART

20/200	200 FT / 61 M
20/100	100 FT / 30.5 M
20/70	70 FT / 21.7 M
20/50	50 FT / 15.2 M
20/30	30 FT / 9.1 M
20/20	20 FT / 6.1 M
20/15	15 FT / 4.6 M

Types of visual acuity charts

- Snellen alphabet chart
- Snellen E chart

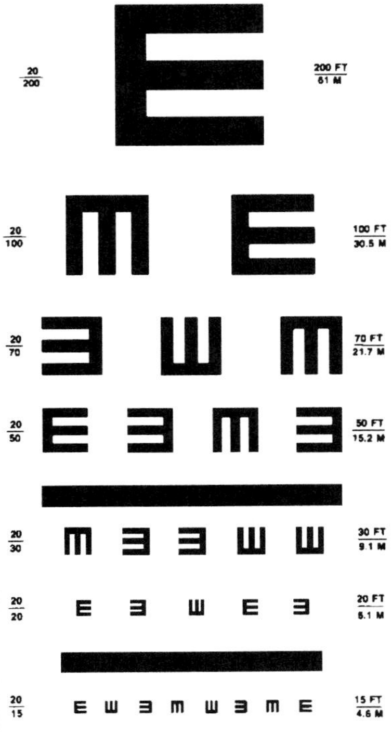

How to record visual acuity

- Record as a fraction
- Top number is the distance between the patient and the chart (20)
- Bottom number is the distance from which a person with normal vision can read the line

Normal vision measurement by age group

- Adults and children age 6 and older: 20/20
- Children age 5: 20/30
- Children age 4: 20/40
- Children age 3 and younger: 20/50

– A test of the entire area seen by an eye
– Tests degree of peripheral vision of each eye by confrontation
– Examiner and patient sit 2′ apart, directly facing each other; patient covers one eye while looking directly at examiner's nose; examiner covers one eye; examiner moves an object along a horizontal plane

Visual field testing

- Test of the entire area seen by an eye
- Tests degree of peripheral vision of each eye by confrontation
- Intervention: advise the examiner if the patient has difficulty hearing or following directions

Tonometry

- Test used to measure IOP
- When performing, ask the patient to remain still
- Intervention: advise that a puff of air may be felt touching the eye

Endothelial cell counter

- Test used to observe endothelial cell morphology on the cornea
- Uses photographic instrument
- Intervention: advise the patient to remain still

Ultrasound of the eye

- Test used to detect tumors or lesions of the eye
- High-frequency pulses of ultrasound are emitted from a small probe placed on the eye
- Intervention: advise the patient not to rub his eye

Otoscopic examination

- Test used to visualize the tympanic membrane
- Uses otoscope
- Intervention: explain to the patient that he'll feel a gentle pull and slight pressure in his ear

into central view from peripheral points about one-half distance between them

- Nursing interventions
  - Explain the testing procedure to the patient
  - Answer the patient's questions
  - Advise the examiner if the patient has difficulty hearing or following directions

Tonometry

- Definition and purpose
  - Test to measure IOP
  - Examiner uses contact or noncontact tonometer
- Nursing interventions
  - Ask the patient to remain still
  - Depending on the method of examination, advise the patient that a puff of air or the instrument may be felt touching the eye

Endothelial cell counter

- Definition and purpose
  - Test to observe high-resolution details of endothelial cell morphology on the cornea
  - Photographic instrument is attached to a slit lamp
- Nursing interventions
  - Explain the testing procedure to the patient
  - Answer the patient's questions
  - Advise the patient to remain still

Ultrasound of the eye

- Definition and purpose
  - Test to detect tumors or lesions of the eye
  - High-frequency pulses of ultrasound are emitted from a small probe placed on the eye
- Nursing interventions before the procedure
  - Explain the testing procedure to the patient
  - Answer the patient's questions
  - Administer topical anesthetic eyedrops
- Nursing interventions after the procedure
  - Advise the patient not to rub his eyes
  - Place the patient on eye rest

Otoscopic examination

- Definition and purpose
  - Test used to visualize the tympanic membrane (color, contour, and landmarks)
  - Examiner uses otoscope
- Nursing interventions
  - Advise the patient to hold still
  - Explain to the patient that he'll feel a gentle pull on his auricle and a slight pressure in his ear

Audiometry
- Definition and purpose
  - Test to measure the degree of hearing of different sound frequencies
  - Examiner uses pure-tone or speech methods
- Nursing interventions
  - Explain to the patient that he needs to wear earphones for the procedure
  - Explain to the patient that he needs to signal when he hears a tone while sitting in a soundproof room

Auditory acuity
- Definition and purpose
  - General estimation of the patient's hearing
  - Assesses the patient's ability to hear a whispered phrase or ticking watch
- Nursing interventions
  - Explain the testing procedure to the patient
  - Answer the patient's questions
  - Advise the examiner if the patient has difficulty following directions

PSYCHOSOCIAL IMPACT OF SENSORY DISORDERS

Developmental impact
- Failing in school
- Changes in body image
- Fear of rejection
- Decreased self-esteem
- Potential developmental delays

Economic impact
- Cost of adaptive equipment
- Disruption or loss of job
- Cost of hospitalization and follow-up care
- Cost of medications

Occupational and recreational impact
- Limited job opportunities
- Changes in leisure activity
- Restrictions in physical activity

Social impact
- Social isolation
- Changes in role performance

RISK FACTORS

Modifiable risk factors
- Eyes
  - Work setting

Audiometry
- Test to measure the degree of hearing of different sound frequencies
- Examiner uses pure-tone or speech methods
- Intervention: explain to the patient that he must signal when he hears a tone while sitting in a soundproof room

Auditory acuity
- Assesses patient's ability to hear a whispered phrase or ticking watch
- Provides a general estimate of the patient's hearing
- Intervention: advise the examiner if the patient has difficulty following directions

Developmental impact of sensory disorders
- Failing in school
- Changes in body image
- Fear of rejection
- Decreased self-esteem
- Potential developmental delays

Nonmodifiable risk factors for eye disorders

- Glaucoma
- Diabetes
- Hypertension
- Eye trauma
- Eye surgery
- Family history
- Cataracts
- Aging

Probable nursing diagnoses for eye disorders

- Disturbed sensory perception: visual
- Fear
- Anxiety
- Deficient knowledge (specify)
- Disturbed body image

Probable nursing diagnoses for ear disorders

- Disturbed sensory perception: auditory
- Social isolation
- Deficient knowledge (specify)
- Anxiety
- Acute pain

    - Leisure activities
    - Sports activities
    - Exposure to airborne irritants
    - Work activities
    - Sun exposure
- Ears
    - Exposure to loud noises
    - Use of ototoxic drugs, such as streptomycin, neomycin, or aspirin

Nonmodifiable risk factors

- Eyes
    - Glaucoma
    - Diabetes
    - Hypertension
    - Eye trauma
    - Eye surgery
    - Family history: glaucoma, blindness, hypertension, cataracts, diabetes, eye infections
    - Cataracts
    - Aging
- Ears
    - Diabetes
    - Aging
    - Congenital or genetic abnormalities

NURSING DIAGNOSES

Probable nursing diagnoses

- Eyes
    - Disturbed sensory perception: visual
    - Fear
    - Anxiety
    - Deficient knowledge (specify)
    - Disturbed body image
- Ears
    - Disturbed sensory perception: auditory
    - Social isolation
    - Deficient knowledge (specify)
    - Anxiety
    - Acute pain

Possible nursing diagnoses

- Eyes
    - Dressing or grooming self-care deficit
    - Acute pain
    - Social isolation
    - Risk for injury
- Ears
    - Risk for injury

– Risk for infection

EYE SURGERIES

Description

- Cataract surgery
  - Removal of an opacified lens, which is then replaced with an implanted intraocular lens
  - Intracapsular — removal of the entire intact lens as a unit using a cryoprobe
  - Extracapsular — removal of the anterior capsule by expressing the lens nucleus and aspirating the remaining soft and cortical fragments with the use of a special irrigation aspiration machine
- Corneal transplantation — microsurgical, full-thickness replacement of the cornea with tissue from a deceased donor
- Retinal reattachment — transscleral cryotherapy (scleral buckling) is applied around the retinal tear, producing a chorioretinal adhesion that seals the break so that liquid vitreous can no longer pass through the subretinal space

Preoperative nursing interventions

- Complete patient and family preoperative teaching
  - Determine the patient's understanding of the procedure
  - Describe the operating room, postanesthesia care unit (PACU), and preoperative and postoperative routines
  - Demonstrate postoperative turning and deep breathing
  - Explain the postoperative need for surgical eye bandages, oxygen therapy, I.V. therapy, and pain control
  - Explain that most surgeries are outpatient; patient is usually discharged within 2 hours of the procedure
- Complete the preoperative checklist
- Administer the preoperative medications, as prescribed
- Allay the patient's and his family's anxiety about surgery
- Document the patient's history and physical assessment data
- Confirm that patient has a ride home after surgery

Postoperative nursing interventions

- Assess the patient's pain level and administer postoperative analgesics, as prescribed
- Administer I.V. fluids, as prescribed
- Allay the patient's anxiety
- Provide incentive spirometry for prolonged general anesthesia or extensive smoking history
- Monitor and record vital signs
- Assess cardiac and respiratory status
- Inspect the surgical eye bandages and change them, as directed
- Encourage the patient to express his feelings about the potential for loss of sight

3 types of eye surgery

- Cataract surgery
  - Removal of opacified lens; replacement with an implanted intraocular lens
  - Intracapsular: removal of the entire intact lens as a unit using a cryoprobe
  - Extracapsular: removal of the anterior capsule by expressing the lens nucleus and aspirating the remaining soft and cortical fragments with the use of a special irrigation aspiration machine
- Corneal transplantation
  - Microsurgical procedure
  - Full-thickness replacement of the cornea with tissue from a deceased donor
- Retinal reattachment
  - Transscleral cryotherapy is applied around the retinal tear
  - Chorioretinal adhesion is produced

Key nursing interventions after eye surgery

- Inspect the surgical eye bandages and change them, as directed.
- Provide for the patient's safety.
- Administer antibiotics, as prescribed.
- Assess the eye for drainage, redness, swelling, cloudy vision, halos around lights, and impaired vision.
- Don't administer morphine because it causes miosis.

Home care instructions after eye surgery

- Use an eye shield or patch, as prescribed, such as during sleep.
- Use dark glasses in strong light.
- Avoid reading and close-up vision.
- Avoid coughing, sneezing, lifting, constipation, squeezing eyes shut, and fast head movements.

Key complications after cataract surgery

- Corneal endothelial damage
- Pupillary block
- Glaucoma

Key complications after corneal transplant surgery

- Hemorrhage
- Epithelial defects
- Wound leaks

- Assess the patient's ability to complete activities of daily living (ADLs) and self-care
- Provide for patient safety
- Administer antibiotics, as prescribed
- Orient the patient to time, place, and surroundings
- Assess the patient's eye for drainage, redness, swelling, cloudy vision, halos around lights, and impaired vision
- **Don't administer morphine because it causes miosis**
- Individualize home care instructions
  - Encourage eye rest
  - Use an eye shield or patch, as prescribed, such as during sleep
  - Use dark glasses in strong light
  - Avoid reading and close-up vision
  - Apply cold or warm compresses, as prescribed
  - Don't rub or wipe eyes
  - Label medication bottles with large letters
  - Wash hands before instilling eye drops
  - Assess the patient's home for safety to prevent falls
  - Adapt lighting to the patient's needs
  - Listen to a radio for diversion
  - Administer eye medications, as prescribed
  - Avoid coughing, sneezing, lifting, constipation, squeezing eyes shut, and fast head movements
  - Avoid smoking

Possible surgical complications

- Cataract surgery
  - Corneal endothelial damage
  - Pupillary block
  - Glaucoma
  - Hemorrhage
  - Wound fistula
  - Choroidal detachment
  - Uveitis
- Corneal transplant
  - Hemorrhage
  - Epithelial defects
  - Wound leaks
  - Glaucoma
  - Graft rejection
- Retinal reattachment
  - Increased IOP
  - Glaucoma
  - Infection
  - Choroidal detachment
  - Diplopia

EAR SURGERIES

Description

- Tympanoplasty — surgery to cure or repair inflammatory process or restore function in the middle ear
- Cochlear implant
  - Placement of auditory prosthesis for a patient who's profoundly deaf and designated as untreatable by other methods
  - Helps patient detect environmental sounds, but doesn't restore normal hearing

Preoperative nursing interventions

- Complete patient and family preoperative teaching
  - Determine the patient's understanding of the procedure
  - Describe preoperative routines
  - Explain the postoperative need for drainage tubes, surgical dressings, oxygen therapy, I.V. therapy, and pain control
- Complete the preoperative checklist
- Administer preoperative medications, as prescribed
- Allay the patient's and his family's anxiety about surgery
- Document the patient's history and physical assessment data

Postoperative nursing interventions

- Assess the patient's pain level and administer postoperative analgesics, as prescribed
- Administer I.V. fluids, as prescribed
- Allay the patient's anxiety
- Provide incentive spirometry and encourage deep breathing with prolonged general anesthesia
- Encourage activity
- Monitor and record vital signs, intake and output (I/O), laboratory studies, and pulse oximetry
- Assess cardiac and respiratory status
- Inspect the surgical dressing and change it, as directed
- Monitor and maintain the position and patency of wound drainage tubes
- Encourage the patient to express his feelings about a potential loss of hearing
- Assess the patient for dizziness, nystagmus, and nausea
- Administer antibiotics, as prescribed
- Administer antivertigo agent, as prescribed
- Administer antiemetic, as prescribed
- Give solid foods and liquids, as tolerated
- Individualize home care instructions
  - Avoid blowing nose, sneezing, or coughing
  - Avoid shampooing hair or showering
  - Monitor self for mouth dryness, altered taste, facial paralysis, and ear pressure
  - Avoid sudden head movements

Tympanoplasty

- Surgery to repair inflammatory process or restore function in the middle ear

Cochlear implant surgery

- Placement of auditory prosthesis
- Helps patient detect environmental sounds
- Doesn't restore normal hearing

Key nursing interventions after ear surgery

- Assess the patient for dizziness, nystagmus, and nausea.
- Administer antivertigo agent, as prescribed.
- Administer antiemetic, as prescribed.

- Decrease environmental noise
- Have people face the patient directly while speaking slowly and loudly
- Use nonverbal clues when communicating
- Avoid people with colds
- Cover ears when outside
- Change dressing, as directed
- Don't fly, lift, bend, or swim
- Elevate the head of the bed

Key home care instructions after ear surgery

- Avoid blowing nose, sneezing, or coughing.
- Avoid shampooing hair or showering.
- Avoid sudden head movements.
- Don't fly, lift, bend, or swim.

Surgical complications

- Infections
- Tissue rejection of graft or prosthesis
- Facial nerve paralysis

CATARACT

Definition

- Opacification of the normally clear, transparent crystalline lens

Key facts about cataracts

- Opacification of the normally clear, transparent crystalline lens
- Primary cause is aging

Causes

- Aging
- Blunt or penetrating trauma
- Long-term steroid treatment
- Diabetes mellitus
- Hypoparathyroidism
- Radiation exposure
- Anterior uveitis
- Ultraviolet light and sunlight exposure
- Congenital

Pathophysiology

- The nucleus of the lens takes on a yellowish brown hue
- Surrounding opacities are spokelike, white densities anterior and posterior to the nucleus

Assessment findings

- Disabling glare
- Dimmed or blurred vision
- Distorted images
- Poor night vision
- Yellow, gray, or white pupil
- Loss of red reflex

Key assessment findings for cataracts

- Dimmed or blurred vision
- Poor night vision
- Yellow, gray, or white pupil
- Loss of red reflex

Diagnostic test findings

- Endothelial cell counter: 2,000 cells/ml
- A-scan ultrasound: areas of increased density around the nucleus of the lens
- Ophthalmoscopy or slit lamp: reveals a dark area in the normally homogenous red reflex

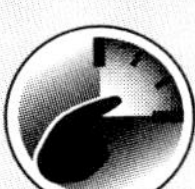

TIME-OUT FOR TEACHING

Patients with a sensory disorder

Be sure to include these topics in your teaching plan for the patient with a sensory disorder.

- Follow-up appointments
- Medication therapy, including the action, adverse effects, and scheduling
- Feelings about changes in lifestyle and activities of daily living (ADLs)
- Signs and symptoms of infection, hearing loss, and decreased vision
- Activity limitations
- Activities that prevent social isolation
- Safe, stress-free environment
- Independence with ADLs and any modifications and assistive devices needed to compensate for limited sensory input
- Community agencies and resources for supportive services

PREVENTIVE CARE

- Eye: protection from injury, bright sun, and chemicals; need for eye rest; work in well-lighted areas
- Ear: wear protective devices during work, leisure, and sports; avoid exposure to high-frequency sounds

Medical management

- No specific medical treatment
- Laboratory studies: IOP, endothelial cell counter, A-scan ultrasound

Nursing interventions

- Assess vision status
- Allay the patient's anxiety
- Encourage the patient to express his feelings about changes in his body image and effect on ADLs
- Provide information about preventing cataracts, cataract progression, and surgery
- Provide for the patient's safety
- Individualize home care instructions (for more information about teaching, see *Patients with a sensory disorder*)
  - Wear dark glasses in bright light
  - Arrange furniture to avoid sitting in direct sunlight
  - Wear wide-brimmed hat while in the sun
  - Lower visor while driving

Complications

- Glaucoma
- Blindness
- Severe vision loss

Possible surgical intervention

- Cataract extraction

Preventive care measures for eyes

- Protect from injury, bright light, and chemicals.
- Rest eyes.
- Work in well-lighted areas.

Preventive care measures for ears

- Wear protective devices during work, leisure, and sports.
- Avoid exposure to high-frequency sounds.

Home care instructions for a patient with cataracts

- Wear dark glasses in bright light.
- Arrange furniture to avoid sitting in direct sunlight.
- Wear a wide-brimmed hat while in the sun.
- Lower visor while driving.

GLAUCOMA

Definition

- A group of diseases that differ in pathophysiology, clinical presentation, and treatment
- Characterized by visual field loss because of damage to the optic nerve caused by increased IOP
- The increased IOP results from pathologic changes that prevent normal circulation and outflow of aqueous humor

Glaucoma defined

- Visual field loss because of damage to the optic nerve caused by increased IOP
- Two types: open-angle glaucoma and acute angle-closure glaucoma

Causes

- Diabetes mellitus
- Black race (increases risk)
- Family history of glaucoma
- Previous eye trauma or surgery
- Long-term steroid treatment
- Uveitis
- Congenital defects

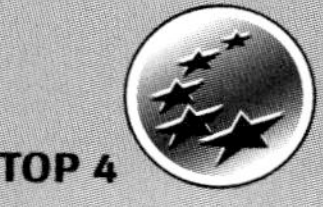

TOP 4 Causes of glaucoma

1. Diabetes mellitus
2. Black race (increases risk)
3. Family history of glaucoma
4. Previous eye trauma or surgery

Pathophysiology

- Open-angle glaucoma: increased IOP is caused by increased resistance to aqueous humor outflow, resulting in neuronal and optic nerve degeneration
- Acute angle-closure glaucoma: increased resistance to aqueous humor flow caused by blockage of trabecular meshwork by peripheral iris

Possible assessment findings

- Open-angle glaucoma
  - Initially asymptomatic
  - Usually bilateral
  - Narrowed field of vision
  - Atrophy and cupping of optic nerve head
  - Increased IOP
  - Mild headaches
  - Halos around lights
- Acute angle-closure glaucoma
  - Typically unilateral
  - Acute eye or facial pain
  - Halo vision
  - Blurred vision
  - Redness in eye
  - Increased IOP
  - Atrophy and cupping of optic nerve head
  - Dilated pupil
  - Abrupt decrease in visual acuity

Key signs of open-angle glaucoma

- Initially asymptomatic
- Increased IOP

Key signs of acute angle-closure glaucoma

- Acute eye or facial pain
- Halo vision
- Blurred vision
- Increased IOP
- Dilated pupil

Diagnostic test findings

- Tonometry: increased IOP
- Perimetry: decreased field of vision

- Gonioscopy: angle open or closed
- Ophthalmoscopy: atrophy and cupping of optic nerve head

Medical management

- Dietary restrictions: sodium and fluid
- Activity: as tolerated
- Monitoring: vital signs and I/O
- Laboratory studies: tonometry, perimetry, ophthalmoscopy
- Primary open-angle glaucoma
  - Beta-adrenergic blocker: timolol (Timoptic)
  - Adrenergic agonist: epinephrine (Epifrin)
  - Carbonic anhydrase inhibitor: acetazolamide (Diamox)
- Acute angle-closure glaucoma
  - Cholinergic agent: pilocarpine (Iopidine)
  - Carbonic anhydrase inhibitor: acetazolamide (Diamox)
  - Avoid such drugs as atropine, anticholinergics, or others with pupil-dilating effects

Nursing interventions

- Maintain the patient's diet restrictions
- Limit fluid intake
- Assess vision status
- Monitor and record vital signs, I/O, and laboratory studies
- Administer medications, as prescribed
- Allay the patient's anxiety
- Encourage the patient to express his feelings about changes in his body image
- Assess eye pain
- Individualize home care instructions
  - Avoid rubbing eye
  - Use hypoallergenic cosmetics
  - Wear goggles while swimming
  - Wear protective glasses while playing sports and working
  - Monitor eye for redness, discharge, watering, blurred or cloudy vision, halos, flashes of light, and floaters
  - Administer eyedrops according to instructions

Complication

- Blindness

Surgical interventions

- Primary open-angle glaucoma
  - Laser or incisional trabeculoplasty with continued medication
  - Laser or incisional trabeculectomy with continued medication
  - Laser or incisional peripheral iridectomy
- Acute angle-closure glaucoma
  - Laser or incisional iridectomy

Key test findings in glaucoma

- Tonometry: increased IOP
- Ophthalmoscopy: atrophy and cupping of optic nerve head

Common ways to treat open-angle glaucoma

- Beta-adrenergic blockers
- Adrenergic agonists
- Carbonic anhydrase inhibitors

Common ways to treat acute angle-closure glaucoma

- Cholinergic agents
- Carbonic anhydrase inhibitors
- Avoid such drugs as atropine, anticholinergics, or others with pupil-dilating effects

RETINAL DETACHMENT

Definition
- Separation of the sensory layers of the retina from the underlying retinal pigment epithelium

Causes
- Aging
- Diabetic neovascularization
- Familial tendency
- Hemorrhage
- Inflammatory process
- Myopia
- Trauma
- Tumor
- Intraocular surgery

Pathophysiology
- Vitreous body traction causes retinal tears or holes
- Vitreous fluid leaks through holes or tears behind the retina
- Retinal separation occurs

Assessment findings
- Floating spots
- Recurrent flashes of light (photopsia)
- With progression of detachment, painless vision loss may be described as veil, curtain, or cobweb that eliminates part of the visual field

Diagnostic tests
- Ophthalmoscopy: gray or opaque retina; in severe detachment, retinal folds and ballooning out of the area
- Indirect ophthalmoscopy: reveals retinal tear or detachment
- Ultrasound: retinal tear or detachment in presence of cataract

Medical management
- Diet: no restrictions
- **Activity: complete bed rest with retinal hole or tear at lowest point of eye**
- **Restrict eye movement until surgical reattachment**

Nursing interventions
- Maintain the patient's diet
- Monitor and record vital signs, I/O, and laboratory studies
- Allay the patient's anxiety
- Provide preoperative care
  - Maintain bed rest with retinal hole or tear in lowest position
  - Apply an eye patch
  - Provide emotional support
  - Explain procedure and what to expect postoperatively
  - Administer preoperative antibiotics, as ordered
  - Wash face with no-tear shampoo

Retinal detachment defined

- Separation of the sensory layers of the retina from the underlying retinal pigment epithelium

Signs of retinal detachment

- Floating spots
- Recurrent flashes of light
- Painless vision loss that may be described as a veil, curtain, or cobweb that eliminates part of the visual field

Key steps in managing retinal detachment

- Complete bed rest with retinal hole or tear at lowest point of eye.
- Restrict eye movement until surgical reattachment.

- Administer cycloplegic-mydriatic eyedrops, as ordered
- Provide postoperative care
  - **Position the patient according to the surgical procedure**
  - **Tell the patient to avoid activities that increase IOP, such as coughing, sneezing, vomiting, lifting, straining during bowel movements, bending from the waist, and rapidly moving the head**
  - Administer antiemetics, as indicated
  - Protect the eye with a shield or glasses
  - Apply cold compresses, as ordered
  - Assess for pain and administer analgesics, as needed
  - Administer cycloplegic and steroid-antibiotic eyedrops, as ordered
- Individualize home care instructions
  - Instill eyedrops, as prescribed
  - Notify the physician if experiencing floaters, flashes of light, blurred vision, or pain unrelieved by analgesics
  - Report fever, yellow or green eye discharge, increased redness or puffiness of the eye, or reduced vision
  - Perform dressing changes
  - Wear an eye shield at night
  - Follow activity restrictions and head positioning

Complications
- Blindness

Surgical interventions
- Cryothermy
- Laser therapy
- Scleral buckling procedure

Key nursing steps after surgery for retinal detachment

- Position the patient according to the surgical procedure.
- Tell the patient to avoid activities that increase IOP.
- Protect the eye with a shield or glasses.
- Administer cycloplegic and steroid-antibiotic eyedrops, as ordered.

MÉNIÈRE'S DISEASE

Definition
- Condition of the inner ear characterized by recurrent and usually progressive symptoms, including vertigo, tinnitus, a sensation of pressure in the ears, and neurosensory hearing loss

Ménière's disease highlights

- Inner ear disorder
- Characterized by vertigo, tinnitus, a sensation of pressure in the ears, and neurosensory hearing loss

Causes
- Exact mechanism unknown
- Possible causes
  - Abnormal hormonal influence on blood flow to the labyrinth
  - Excess labyrinth fluid (endolymph)
  - Allergic response
  - Autoimmune disorder
  - Abnormal metabolites

Possible causes of Ménière's disease

- Abnormal hormonal influence on blood flow to the labyrinth
- Excess labyrinth fluid
- Allergic response
- Autoimmune disorder
- Abnormal metabolites

Pathophysiology
- The labyrinth doesn't function normally (see *Normal vestibular function*, page 188)

Normal vestibular function

- When the head is moved, endolymph inside each of the three ear canals moves in an opposite direction.
- The movement stimulates hair cells that send electrical impulses to the brain.
- Head movement also causes movement of the vestibular otoliths in their gel medium, which tugs on hair cells, initiating electrical-impulse transmission to the brain.

Normal vestibular function

The semicircular canals and vestibule of the inner ear are responsible for equilibrium and balance. Each of the three semicircular canals lies at a 90-degree angle to the others. When the head is moved, endolymph inside each canal moves in an opposite direction. The movement stimulates hair cells, which send electrical impulses to the brain through the vestibular portion of cranial nerve VIII. Head movement also causes movement of the vestibular otoliths (crystals of calcium salts) in their gel medium, which tugs on hair cells, initiating the transmission of electrical impulses to the brain through the vestibular nerve. Together these two organs help detect the body's present position as well as change in direction or motion.

Assessment findings

- Paroxysmal whirling vertigo with nausea and vomiting
- Tinnitus
- Fluctuating unilateral neurosensory hearing loss of low tones
- Sense of pressure in the ear
- Nystagmus
- Ataxia

Chief assessment findings in Ménière's disease

- Tinnitus
- Fluctuating unilateral neurosensory hearing loss of low tones

Diagnostic test findings

- Audiogram: hearing loss
- Magnetic resonance imaging, X-ray, computed tomography scan: negative
- Electronystagmography: labyrinth dysfunction
- Auditory dehydration test: positive audiometric fluctuation

Medical management

- Dietary restrictions: fluid, sodium, caffeine
- Activity: as tolerated
- Monitoring: vital signs and I/O
- Glucocorticoid: dexamethasone (Decadron)
- Benzodiazepine: oxazepam (Serax)
- Anticholinergic: atropine (Atropine)
- Antihistamine: diphenhydramine (Benadryl)
- Diuretic: spironolactone (Aldactone)
- Antiemetic: prochlorperazine (Compazine)
- Vasodilators: nicotinic acid (Nicobid), tolazoline (Priscoline), methantheline (Banthine)

Key ways to manage Ménière's disease

- Dietary restrictions: fluid, sodium, caffeine
- Anticholinergics
- Antihistamines
- Diuretics
- Antiemetics

Nursing interventions

- Maintain the patient's diet
- Limit fluid intake
- Assess hearing status
- Monitor and record vital signs, I/O, and laboratory studies
- Administer medications, as prescribed
- Allay the patient's anxiety
- Provide for the patient's safety

- Individualize home care instructions
  - Have the patient lie down to relieve dizziness
  - Learn to read lips
  - Use hearing aid
  - Use sign language and gestures to communicate

Complication
- Deafness

Possible surgical interventions
- Endolymphatic subarachnoid shunt
- Endolymphatic system—mastoid shunt
- Ultrasonic surgery
- Total labyrinthectomy

Key nursing interventions for a patient with Ménière's disease
- Assess hearing status.
- Provide for the patient's safety.
- Advise the patient to lie down to relieve dizziness.

HEARING LOSS

Definition
- A mechanical or nervous impediment to the transmission of sound waves
- Major forms are classified as conductive loss, sensorineural loss, or mixed loss

Hearing loss defined
- Mechanical or nervous impediment to the transmission of sound waves
- Types: conductive hearing loss, sensorineural hearing loss, and mixed loss

Causes
- Conductive hearing loss
  - Obstruction of the external ear canal, such as from impacted cerumen, edema of the ear canal, neoplasms, or stenosis
  - Congenital malformations
  - Disruption or fixation of the middle ear ossicles
  - Fluid behind eardrum or within middle ear
  - Perforated tympanic membrane
  - Scar tissue in ear canal or eardrum
  - Trauma to tympanic membrane or inner ear
  - Tumors of the tympanic membrane
- Sensorineural hearing loss
  - Congenital factors
  - Hereditary factors
  - Noise trauma
  - Aging (presbycusis)
  - Ménière's disease
  - Ototoxicity
  - Systemic disease, such as certain collagen diseases, diabetes, syphilis, and Paget's disease

Key causes of hearing loss
- Conductive: the interrupted passage of sound from the external ear to the inner ear
- Sensorineural: impaired cochlea or acoustic nerve transmission of sound impulses within the inner ear or brain

Pathophysiology
- Conductive hearing loss results from the interrupted passage of sound from the external ear to the inner ear
- Sensorineural hearing loss is caused by impaired cochlea or acoustic nerve (CN VIII) transmission of sound impulses within the inner ear or brain
- Mixed loss is a combined dysfunction of conduction and sensorineural transmission

Key assessment finding for hearing loss

- Altered hearing at all frequencies and decibel levels

Key test findings for hearing loss

- Rinne test: air conduction greater than bone conduction (sensorineural); bone conduction greater than air conduction (conductive)
- Audiometry: hearing loss

Nursing interventions to aid in communication

- Stand in front of the patient when speaking.
- Speak slowly and distinctly.
- Avoid shouting.
- Develop alternative means of communication.

Assessment findings

- Congenital hearing loss
  - Lack of response to auditory stimulation
  - Impaired speech development
- Gradual hearing loss or following acute infection
  - Altered hearing at all frequencies and decibel levels
- Presbycusis
  - Tinnitus
  - Inability to understand the spoken word
- Hearing loss caused by neoplasm or fluid
  - Feeling of fullness in the ear

Diagnostic test findings

- Whisper test: reduced ability or inability to hear
- Rinne test: air conduction greater than bone conduction in sensorineural hearing loss; bone conduction greater than air conduction suggests conductive loss
- Weber's test: sound lateralizes to the better functioning ear in sensorineural hearing loss; sound lateralizes to the ear with the poorest hearing in conductive hearing loss
- Audiometry: hearing loss
- Tympanometry: impaired compliance

Medical management

- Diet: no restrictions
- Activity: no restrictions
- Rehabilitation: speech and hearing
- Sound amplification: hearing aid, pocket talker

Nursing interventions

- Maintain the patient's diet
- Maintain and use hearing aid or other assistive device
- Assess the patient's degree of hearing loss
- Stand in front of the patient when speaking
- Speak slowly and distinctly
- Avoid shouting
- Approach within the patient's visual range
- Develop alternative means of communication
- Provide emotional support and encourage verbalization of fears
- Prevent isolation
- Individualize home care instructions
  - Maintain hearing aid or assistive device
  - Replace batteries when appropriate
  - Use alternative means of communication
  - Engage in social activities

Possible surgical interventions

- Stapedectomy
- Tympanoplasty

- **Complications**
  - Deafness
  - Speech impairment
  - Developmental delays

NCLEX CHECKS

It's never too soon to begin your NCLEX preparation. Now that you've reviewed this chapter, carefully read each of the following questions and choose the best answer. Then compare your responses to the correct answers.

1. The nurse is teaching a patient being discharged after cataract removal and intraocular lens insertion. Which statement by the patient indicates that further teaching is necessary?

☐ **A.** "I'll rest by reading a book."
☐ **B.** "I'll wear sunglasses when I'm outside during the day."
☐ **C.** "I'll wear an eye shield when I sleep."
☐ **D.** "I'll administer eye drops as I have been instructed."

2. A patient with retinal detachment is most likely to report which of the following symptoms?

☐ **A.** Eye pain, halo vision, and redness in the eye
☐ **B.** Light flashes and floaters
☐ **C.** A recent driving accident while changing lanes
☐ **D.** Disabling glare

3. The nurse is assessing a patient's extraocular eye movements as part of the neurologic examination. Which of the following cranial nerves is the nurse assessing? (Select all that apply.)

☐ **A.** Cranial nerve II
☐ **B.** Cranial nerve III
☐ **C.** Cranial nerve IV
☐ **D.** Cranial nerve V
☐ **E.** Cranial nerve VI
☐ **F.** Cranial nerve VIII

4. The nurse is teaching a patient with early glaucoma. The nurse should instruct the patient to:

☐ **A.** wear an eye patch at night.
☐ **B.** avoid constipation.
☐ **C.** administer eyedrops.
☐ **D.** use cold compresses to relieve eye pain.

5. Which of the following drugs reported during a health history would concern the nurse most about ototoxicity?

☐ **A.** Acetaminophen
☐ **B.** Penicillin
☐ **C.** Aspirin
☐ **D.** Oxycodone

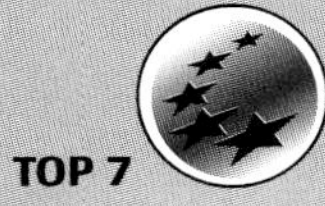

TOP 7

Items to study for your next test on the eyes and ears

1. Structures of the eyes and ears
2. The difference between rods and cones
3. The bones of the middle ear
4. How to record visual acuity using a Snellen chart
5. How to test extraocular eye muscle function
6. Key signs and symptoms of cataracts, glaucoma, and retinal detachment
7. Types of hearing loss

6. A patient has an absence of the red reflex on ophthalmoscopic examination. The nurse knows that this finding is most likely associated with which of the following disorders?

- ☐ **A.** Open-angle glaucoma
- ☐ **B.** Cataract
- ☐ **C.** Retinal detachment
- ☐ **D.** Acute angle-closure glaucoma

ANSWERS AND RATIONALES

1. CORRECT ANSWER: A

Following cataract surgery, the patient shouldn't read until his vision stabilizes. The patient should protect his eyes by wearing sunglasses in sunlight and an eye shield at night. The patient should administer eyedrops as prescribed.

2. CORRECT ANSWER: B

Light flashes and floaters are characteristic of a detached retina. Eye pain, halo vision, and redness in the eye are findings of acute angle-closure glaucoma. Difficulty seeing cars in another lane suggests a loss of peripheral vision, which may indicate glaucoma. Disabling glare is a symptom of cataracts.

3. CORRECT ANSWER: B, C, E

Assessing extraocular eye movements helps evaluate the function of cranial nerves III (oculomotor), IV (trochlear), and VI (abducens). The oculomotor nerve originates in the brainstem and controls the movement of the eyeball up, down, and inward; raises the eyelid; and constricts the pupil. The trochlear nerve rotates the eyeball downward and outward. The abducens nerve originates in the pons and rotates the eyeball laterally. Assessing the patient's vision helps evaluation of cranial nerve II. Cranial nerve V, the trigeminal nerve, has three branches that require assessment: the ophthalmic branch, the maxillary branch, and the mandibular branch. Assessing hearing (cochlear) and balance (vestibular) helps evaluation of cranial nerve VIII, the acoustic nerve.

4. CORRECT ANSWER: C

Administering eyedrops is a critical component of self-care for a patient with glaucoma. An eye patch, avoiding constipation, and applying cold compresses aren't necessary unless the patient has undergone eye surgery.

5. CORRECT ANSWER: C

Aspirin as well as streptomycin and neomycin are associated with ototoxicity. Acetaminophen, penicillin, and oxycodone are not.

6. CORRECT ANSWER: B

A loss of the red reflex, the reflection of light on the vascular retina, is characteristic of a cataract. It isn't associated with open-angle glaucoma, acute angle-closure glaucoma, or retinal detachment.

5

Gastrointestinal system

LEARNING OBJECTIVES

After studying this chapter, you should be able to:

- Describe the psychosocial impact of GI disorders.
- Differentiate between modifiable and nonmodifiable risk factors in the development of a GI disorder.
- List three probable and three possible nursing diagnoses for a patient with a GI disorder.
- Identify nursing interventions for a patient with a GI disorder.
- Identify three teaching topics for a patient with a GI disorder.

CHAPTER OVERVIEW

Caring for the patient with a GI disorder requires a sound understanding of GI anatomy, physiology, and function. A thorough assessment is essential to planning and implementing appropriate patient care. The assessment includes a complete history, physical examination, diagnostic testing, identification of modifiable and nonmodifiable risk factors, and information related to the psychosocial impact of GI dysfunction on the patient.

Nursing diagnoses focus primarily on a change in bowel habits (constipation or diarrhea) and imbalanced nutrition. Patient teaching—a crucial nursing activity—involves instructing patients about medical follow-up, medication regimens, signs and symptoms of possible complications, and reduction of modifiable risk factors (decreased alcohol consumption, diet restrictions, stress management, and smoking cessation). The psychosocial impact of changes in body image and decreased self-esteem is also an important focus for nursing care.

ANATOMY AND PHYSIOLOGY REVIEW

Functions of the mouth

- Where mechanical and chemical digestion originate
- Tongue and teeth are accessory organs of digestion
- Salivary glands secrete saliva

Mouth (see *Parts of the GI system*)
- Mechanical and chemical digestion originate here
- Tongue and teeth are accessory organs of digestion
- Salivary glands secrete saliva, which combines with food during mastication

Function of the esophagus

- Provides for the transfer of food from the oropharynx to the stomach

Esophagus
- This organ provides for the transfer of food from the oropharynx to the stomach
- Closure of the epiglottis prevents food from entering the trachea
- Closure of the cardiac sphincter prevents reflux of gastric contents

Functions of the stomach

- Secretes pepsin, renin, lipase, mucus, and hydrochloric acid for digestion
- Mixes and stores chyme
- Secretes intrinsic factor necessary for absorption of cyanocobalamin

Stomach
- A hollow, 1-qt (1-L) muscular pouch
- Secretes pepsin, renin, lipase, mucus, and hydrochloric acid for digestion
- Mixes and stores chyme
- Secretes intrinsic factor necessary for absorption of cyanocobalamin (vitamin B_{12})

Functions of the intestines

- Small intestine: digests food and absorbs nutrients
- Large intestine: absorbs fluids and electrolytes; synthesizes vitamin K using intestinal bacteria; and stores fecal material

Small intestine
- Consists of duodenum, jejunum, and ileum
  - Chyme, in liquid or semiliquid form, enters the duodenum through the pyloric sphincter
  - Bile and pancreatic secretions enter the duodenum through the common bile duct at the ampulla of Vater
- Digests food
- Absorbs nutrients
- Lined with villi that contain capillaries and lymphatic
- Motor activity includes mixing and peristalsis

Large intestine
- Consists of the cecum, colon, rectum, and anus
- Segments of the colon are the cecum, ascending colon, transverse colon, descending colon, and sigmoid colon
- Chyme enters the cecum through the ileocecal valve
- Has several functions
  - Absorbs fluid and electrolytes
  - Synthesizes vitamin K using intestinal bacteria
  - Stores fecal material
- Chyme becomes more solid as the intestinal wall of the colon absorbs water
- Defecation is the movement of feces from the rectum through the anal sphincter

Parts of the GI system

This illustration shows the GI system's major anatomic structures. Knowing these structures will help you conduct an accurate physical assessment.

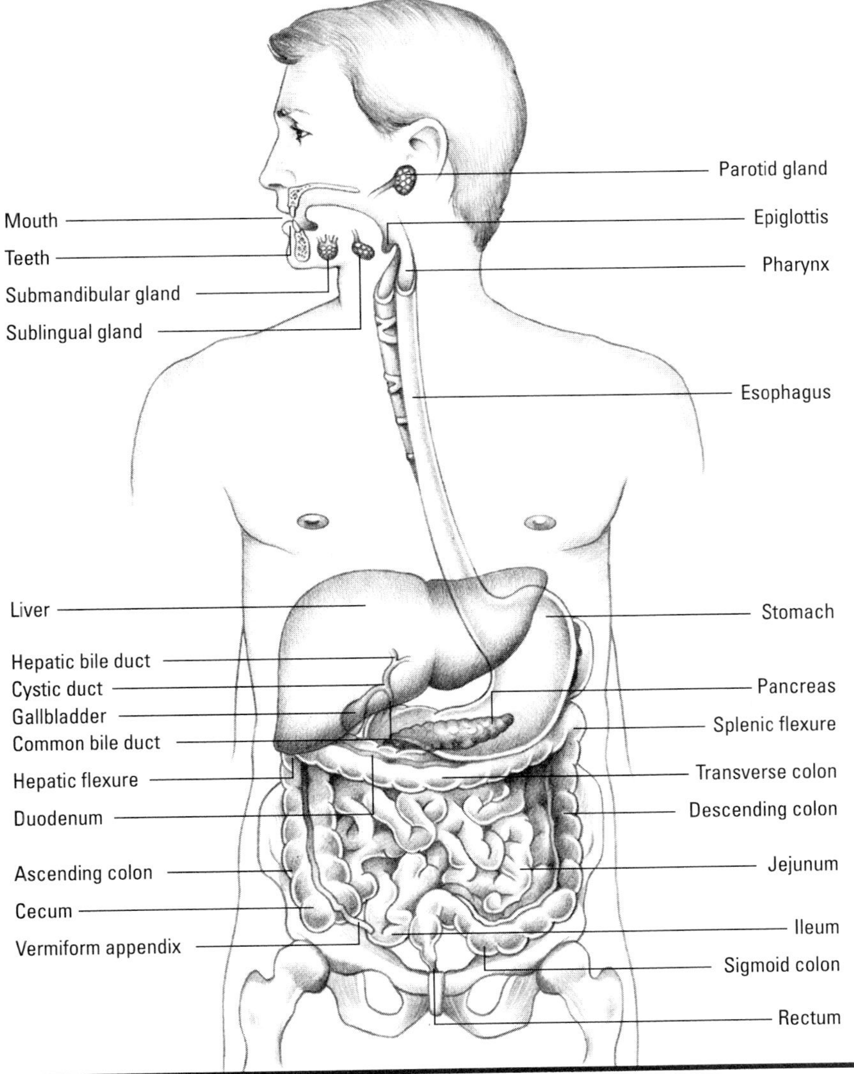

Parts of the GI system

- Parotid gland
- Mouth
- Teeth
- Epiglottis
- Submandibular gland
- Sublingual gland
- Pharynx
- Esophagus
- Liver
- Stomach
- Hepatic bile duct
- Cystic duct
- Gallbladder
- Pancreas
- Common bile duct
- Splenic flexure
- Hepatic flexure
- Transverse colon
- Descending colon
- Duodenum
- Jejunum
- Ascending colon
- Cecum
- Vermiform appendix
- Ileum
- Sigmoid colon
- Rectum

Liver

- Largest organ in the body
- Produces bile (main function), which emulsifies fats and stimulates peristalsis
- Conveys bile from the gallbladder, where it's stored, until it enters the duodenum at Oddi's sphincter through the common bile duct
- Metabolizes carbohydrates, fats, and proteins
- Synthesizes coagulation factors VII, IX, X, and prothrombin

Functions of the liver

- Produces bile
- Conveys bile from the gallbladder
- Metabolizes carbohydrates, fats, and proteins
- Synthesizes coagulation factors VII, IX, X, and prothrombin
- Stores vitamins A, D, E, K, B_{12}, copper, and iron
- Detoxifies chemicals
- Excretes bilirubin
- Obtains dual blood supply from portal vein and hepatic artery
- Produces and stores glycogen
- Promotes erythropoiesis when bone marrow production is insufficient

Gallbladder

- Hollow organ
- Stores and secretes bile

Pancreas

- Accessory gland of digestion
- Secretes large amounts of sodium bicarbonate
- Secretes three digestive enzymes: amylase, lipase, and trypsin

Stool abnormalities associated with GI disorders

- Melena
- Clay-colored stools
- Frothy stools
- Steatorrhea
- Occult blood in stool

- Stores vitamins A, D, E, K, B_{12}, copper, and iron
- Detoxifies chemicals
- Excretes bilirubin
- Obtains dual blood supply from portal vein and hepatic artery
- Produces and stores glycogen
- Promotes erythropoiesis when bone marrow production is insufficient

Gallbladder

- Hollow, pear-shaped organ that stores bile
- Secretes bile via the cystic duct to the common bile duct

Pancreas

- Accessory gland of digestion
- Exocrine function: secretes three digestive enzymes
  - Amylase
  - Lipase
  - Trypsin
- Endocrine function: secretes hormones from the islets of Langerhans
  - Insulin
  - Glucagon
  - Somatostatin
- Main pancreatic duct joins the common bile duct and empties into the duodenum at the ampulla of Vater
- Responsible for secreting large amounts of sodium bicarbonate, which neutralizes acid chyme

ASSESSMENT FINDINGS

History

- Inadequate diet
- **Change in bowel habits**
  - Constipation
  - Diarrhea
  - Flatus
- Complaints of indigestion
- Nausea and vomiting
- Abdominal pain (for more information, see *Abdominal pain: Determining the possible causes,* pages 198 and 199)
- Dysphagia
- Loss of appetite

Objective data associated with GI disorders

- Weight changes
- **Abnormal color and consistency of stool**
  - Melena
  - Clay-colored stools
  - Frothy stools
  - Steatorrhea
  - Occult blood in stool

- Abnormal bowel sounds
- Abdominal distention
- Rectal bleeding
- Jaundice
- Edema
- Hematemesis
- Anorexia

DIAGNOSTIC TESTS AND PROCEDURES

Upper GI series

- Definition and purpose
  - Fluoroscopic procedure using barium as a contrast medium
  - Examination of the esophagus, stomach, duodenum, and other portions of the small bowel after swallowing barium
- Nursing interventions before the procedure
  - Withhold food and fluids
  - Administer fluids, cathartics, and enemas, as prescribed
- Nursing interventions after the procedure
  - Inform the patient that stool will be light-colored for several days
  - Administer cathartics, fluids, and enemas, as prescribed

Lower GI series (barium enema)

- Definition and purpose
  - Fluoroscopic procedure using barium as a contrast medium
  - Examination of the large intestine after administration of barium via an enema
- Nursing interventions before the procedure
  - Withhold food and fluids
  - Encourage the patient to discuss feelings of embarrassment
  - Administer bowel preparation (laxatives and enemas), as prescribed
- Nursing interventions after the procedure
  - Determine if the patient is constipated
  - Encourage fluids, unless contraindicated
  - Administer enemas and laxatives, as prescribed
  - Monitor color and consistency of stool

Endoscopy

- Definition and purpose
  - Procedure using an endoscope
  - Direct visualization of the esophagus and stomach
- Nursing interventions before the procedure
  - Withhold food and fluids for 6 to 12 hours before the test
  - Make sure that an informed consent form has been signed
  - Obtain baseline vital signs
  - Administer sedatives, as prescribed
- Nursing interventions after the procedure
  - **Withhold food and fluids until the gag reflex returns**

(Text continues on page 200.)

Key symptoms of a GI disorder

- Weight changes
- Rectal bleeding
- Jaundice
- Hematemesis

Upper GI series

- Fluoroscopic procedure using barium as a contrast medium
- Allows for examination of the esophagus, stomach, duodenum, and other portions of the small bowel after swallowing barium
- Intervention: before the procedure, administer fluids, cathartics, and enemas, as prescribed

Lower GI series

- Fluoroscopic procedure
- Allows for examination of the large intestine after administration of a barium enema
- Intervention: before the procedure, withhold food and fluids

Endoscopy

- Procedure using an endoscope
- Provides direct visualization of the esophagus and stomach
- Intervention: withhold food and fluids 6 to 12 hours before the test

GO WITH THE FLOW

Abdominal pain: Determining the possible causes

This flowchart highlights the decision-making process used to determine the possible causes of a patient's abdominal pain.

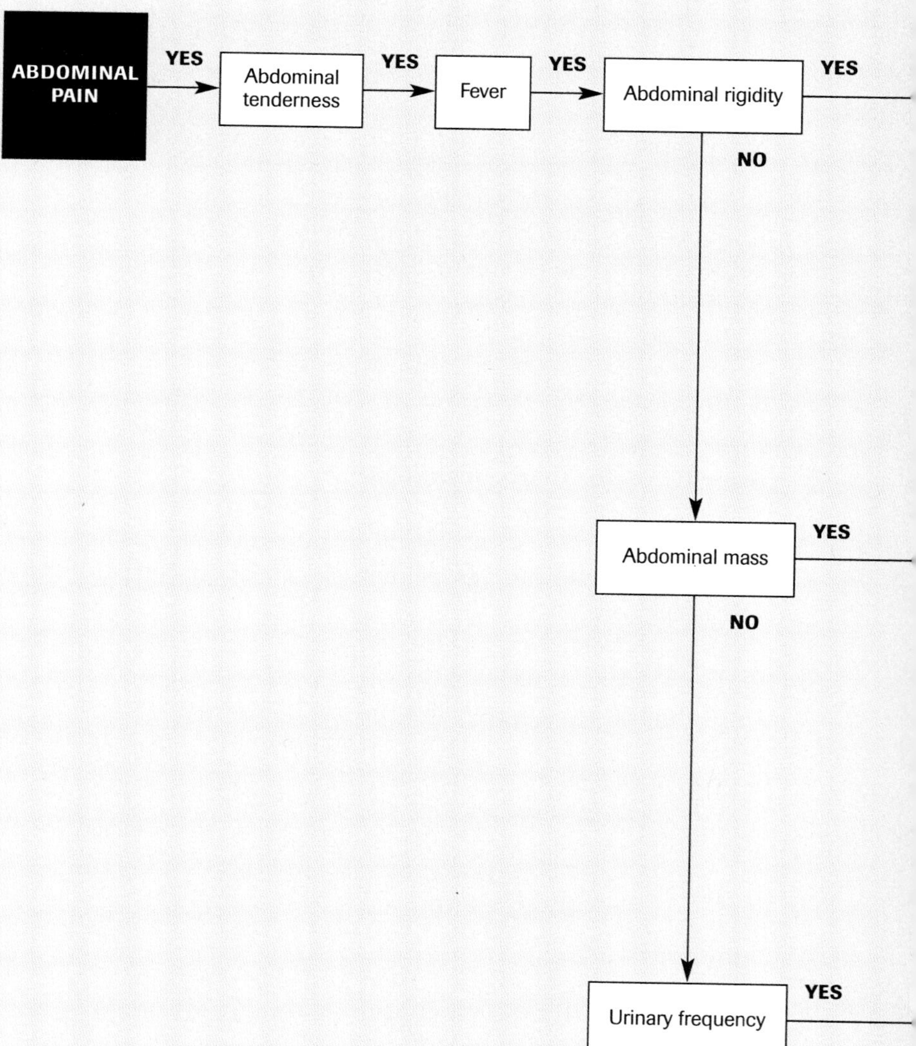

Symptoms of a possible abdominal problem

- Abdominal tenderness
- Fever
- Abdominal rigidity
- Abdominal mass
- Urine frequency
- Anorexia, nausea, vomiting
- Bowel sound changes
- Amenorrhea
- Abdominal distention
- Weight changes
- Weakness
- Costovertebral angle tenderness

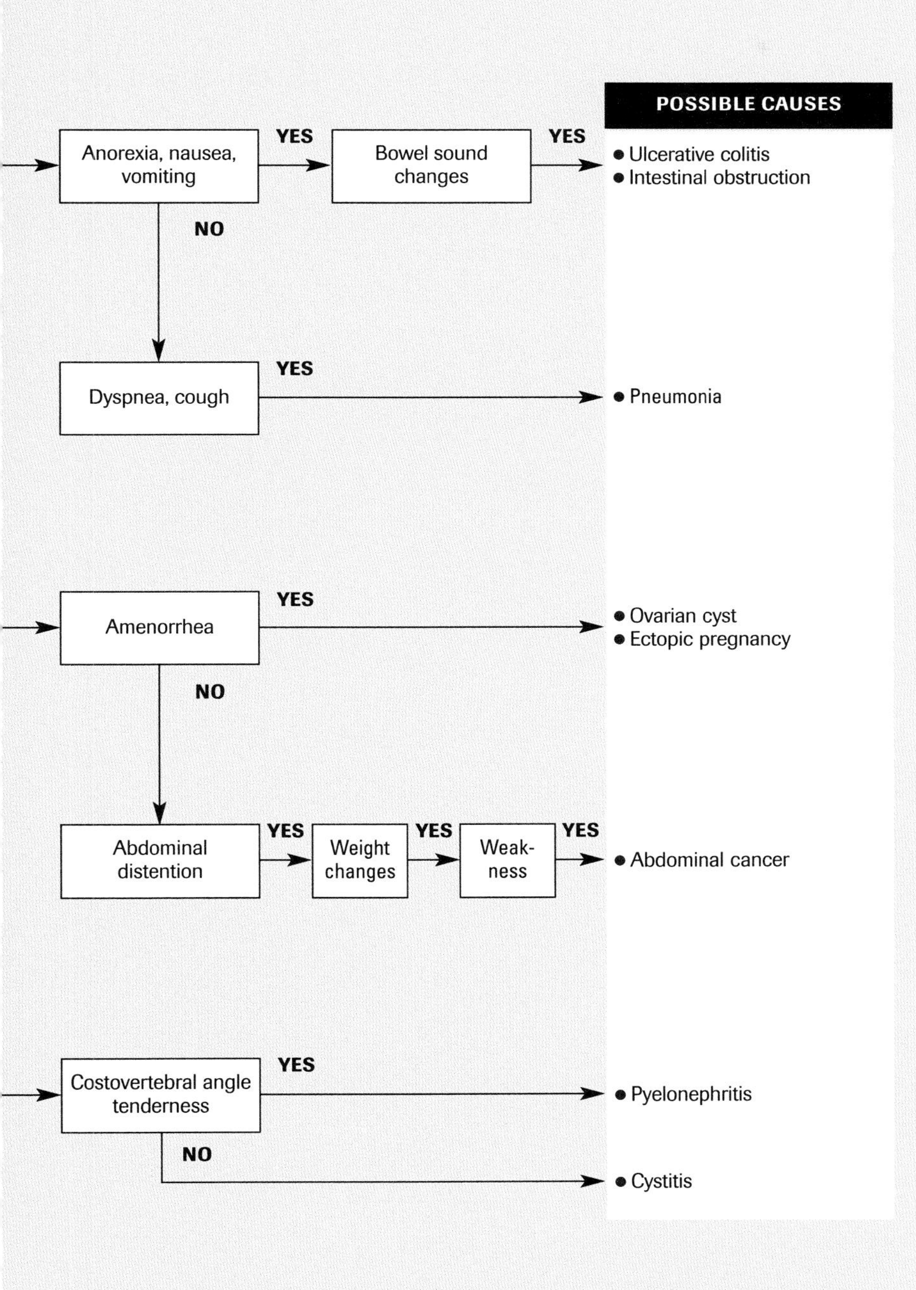

Possible causes of abdominal pain

- Ulcerative colitis
- Intestinal obstruction
- Pneumonia
- Ovarian cyst
- Ectopic pregnancy
- Abdominal cancer
- Pyelonephritis
- Cystitis

- Assess gag and cough reflexes
- Assess vasovagal response

Fecal occult blood test

- Laboratory test using a reagent
- Analysis of stool for blood
- Intervention: advise the patient to avoid red meat, iron, and high fiber for 1 to 3 days prior to the procedure

Fecal occult blood test

- Definition and purpose
  - Laboratory test using a reagent
  - Analysis of stool for blood
- Nursing interventions before the procedure
  - Advise the patient to avoid red meat, iron, and high fiber for 1 to 3 days
  - Document the administration of aspirin, vitamin C, and anti-inflammatory drugs

Fecal fat test

- Laboratory test using a stain
- Analysis of stool for fat
- Intervention: advise the patient to restrict alcohol intake and maintain a high-fat diet for 72 hours before examination

Fecal fat test

- Definition and purpose
  - Laboratory test using a stain
  - Analysis of stool for fat
- Nursing interventions before the procedure
  - Advise the patient to restrict alcohol intake and maintain a high-fat diet 72 hours before the examination
  - Refrigerate specimen
  - Document current medications

Proctosigmoidoscopy

- Procedure using a lighted scope
- Provides direct visualization for the sigmoid colon, rectum, and anal canal
- Intervention: check the patient for bleeding after the procedure

Proctosigmoidoscopy

- Definition and purpose
  - Procedure using a lighted scope
  - Direct visualization of the sigmoid colon, rectum, and anal canal
- Nursing interventions before the procedure
  - Encourage the patient to discuss feelings of embarrassment
  - Inform the patient that the procedure requires a side-lying position
  - Administer bowel preparation, as prescribed
  - Place obtained written informed consent in the patient's chart
  - Document iron intake
- Nursing interventions after the procedure
  - Check the patient for bleeding
  - Monitor the patient's vital signs

Barium swallow

- Fluoroscopic procedure using barium as a contrast medium
- Allows for examination of the pharynx and esophagus after administration of barium
- Intervention: after the procedure, encourage fluids, unless contraindicated

Barium swallow

- Definition and purpose
  - Procedure using barium as a contrast medium
  - Fluoroscopic examination of the pharynx and esophagus after administration of barium
- Nursing interventions before the procedure
  - Withhold food and fluids
  - Explain the procedure to the patient
- Nursing interventions after the procedure
  - Determine if the patient is constipated
  - Encourage fluids, unless contraindicated
  - Administer laxatives, as prescribed

Cholangiography

- Definition and purpose
  - Procedure using an injection of a radiopaque dye through a catheter
  - Radiographic examination of the biliary duct system
- Nursing interventions before the procedure
  - Encourage a low-residue, high-simple fat diet 1 day before the examination
  - Withhold food and fluids after midnight
  - **Note the patient's allergies to iodine, seafood, and radiopaque dyes**
  - Inform the patient about possible throat irritation and flushing of the face
- Nursing interventions after the procedure
  - Check the injection site for bleeding
  - Monitor the patient's vital signs

Liver scan

- Definition and purpose
  - Procedure using an I.V. injection of a radioisotope
  - Visual imaging of the distribution of blood flow in the liver
- Nursing interventions before the procedure
  - Determine the patient's ability to lie still during the procedure
  - Check the patient for possible allergies
- Nursing interventions after the procedure
  - Assess the I.V. insertion site for bleeding, bruising, or hematoma
  - **Assess the patient for signs of delayed allergic reaction to the radioisotope, such as itching and hives**

Gastric analysis

- Definition and purpose
  - Procedure that aspirates the contents of the stomach through a nasogastric (NG) tube
  - Fasting analysis to measure the acidity of gastric secretions
- Nursing interventions before the procedure
  - Withhold food and fluids after midnight
  - **Instruct the patient not to smoke for 8 to 12 hours before the test**
  - Withhold medications that can affect gastric secretions for 24 hours before the procedure
- Nursing interventions after the procedure
  - Obtain the patient's vital signs
  - Note reactions to gastric acid stimulant, if used

Ultrasonography

- Definition and purpose
  - Noninvasive procedure that uses echoes from sound waves
  - Visualization of body organs
- Nursing interventions before the procedure
  - Withhold food and fluids for 8 to 12 hours
  - Determine the patient's ability to lie still during the procedure

Cholangiography

- Invasive procedure using an injection of a radiopaque dye through a catheter
- Allows for examination of the biliary duct system
- Intervention: before the procedure, note the patient's allergies

Liver scan

- Invasive procedure using an I.V. injection of a radioisotope
- Provides an image of blood flow distribution in the liver
- Intervention: after the procedure, assess the patient for signs of delayed allergic reaction

Gastric analysis

- Aspiration of the contents of the stomach through an NG tube
- Measures the acidity of gastric secretions
- Intervention: instruct the patient not to smoke for 8 to 12 hours before the test

Ultrasonography

- Noninvasive procedure that uses echoes from sound waves
- Provides visualization of body organs
- Intervention: withhold food and fluids for 8 to 12 hours before the procedure

- Ask the patient not to smoke or chew gum for 8 to 12 hours before the test
- Administer enemas, as prescribed
- Remove abdominal dressings

Blood chemistry

Blood chemistry

- Laboratory test of a blood sample
- Analysis for potassium, sodium, calcium, glucose, BUN, and other substances
- Intervention: check the site for bleeding after the procedure

- Definition and purpose
  - Laboratory test of a blood sample
  - Analysis for potassium, sodium, calcium, phosphorus, glucose, bicarbonate, blood urea nitrogen (BUN), creatinine, protein, albumin, osmolality, amylase, lipase, alkaline phosphatase, ammonia, bilirubin, lactate dehydrogenase (LD), sulfobromophthalein test, aspartate aminotransferase (AST), serum alanine aminotransferase (ALT), hepatitis-associated antigens, carcinoembryonic antigen (CEA), and alpha-fetoprotein
- Nursing interventions
  - Withhold food and fluid, as directed, before the procedure
  - Check the site for bleeding after the procedure

Hematologic studies

Hematologic studies

- Blood test
- Analysis for RBCs, WBCs, platelets, PT, PTT, Hb, and HCT
- Intervention: note current drug therapy before the procedure

- Definition and purpose
  - Laboratory test of a blood sample
  - Analysis for red blood cells (RBCs), white blood cells (WBCs), platelets, prothrombin time (PT), partial thromboplastin time (PTT), hemoglobin (Hb), and hematocrit (HCT)
- Nursing interventions
  - Note current drug therapy before the procedure
  - Check the site for bleeding after the procedure

Liver biopsy

Liver biopsy

- Invasive procedure using a needle for the percutaneous removal of a small amount of liver tissue
- Interventions:
  - Before the procedure, assess baseline clotting studies and vital signs
  - After the procedure, observe the patient for signs of shock and pneumothorax; position on right lateral side for hemostasis

- Definition and purpose
  - Procedure using a needle for the percutaneous removal of a small amount of liver tissue
  - Histologic evaluation of liver tissue
- Nursing interventions before the procedure
  - Withhold food and fluids after midnight
  - Place obtained written informed consent in the patient's chart
  - **Assess baseline clotting studies and vital signs**
  - **Instruct patient to exhale and hold breath during insertion of the needle**
- Nursing interventions after the procedure
  - Check the insertion site for bleeding
  - Monitor the patient's vital signs
  - **Observe the patient for signs of shock and pneumothorax**
  - **Position the patient on the right lateral side for hemostasis**

Colonoscopy

- Definition and purpose
  - Procedure using a flexible, lighted scope
  - Direct visualization of large intestine; biopsies can be obtained

- Nursing interventions before the procedure
  - Provide clear liquid diet 48 hours before test, if indicated
  - Administer bowel preparation
  - Explain that the patient will feel cramping and the sensation of needing to have a bowel movement
  - Explain use of air to distend bowel lumen
- Nursing interventions after the procedure
  - **Monitor for gross bleeding**
  - Withhold food and fluids for 2 hours
  - Check for blood in the stool if polyps are removed

Endoscopic retrograde cholangiopancreatography (ERCP)

- Definition and purpose
  - Radiographic examination of the hepatobiliary tree and pancreatic ducts using contrast medium and a lighted scope
  - Used to evaluate the cause of obstructive jaundice
- Nursing interventions before the procedure
  - Withhold food and fluid after midnight
  - **Check for allergies to iodine or seafood**
  - Remove dentures
  - Explain that a local anesthetic will be used
- Nursing interventions after the procedure
  - **Check for signs of respiratory depression**
  - Check for signs of urine retention
  - Provide comfort measures for throat irritation
  - **Withhold food until gag reflex returns**

Percutaneous transhepatic cholangiography

- Definition and purpose
  - Fluoroscopic examination of the biliary ducts through the use of contrast medium
  - Used to evaluate cause of severe jaundice and diagnose obstruction
- Nursing interventions before the procedure
  - Inform the patient that the X-ray table will be tilted and rotated during the procedure
  - Explain that transient pain will be felt with the injection of the anesthetic
  - **Check for allergies to iodine or seafood**
  - **Check PT and PTT**
  - Withhold food and fluid after midnight
- Nursing interventions after the procedure
  - Instruct the patient to rest for at least 6 hours in right side-lying position
  - Check for bleeding at injection site
  - Monitor the patient's vital signs
  - Withhold food and fluids for 2 hours

Colonoscopy

- Invasive procedure
- Allows for direct visualization (and biopsy, if necessary) of the large intestine
- Intervention: after the procedure, monitor for gross bleeding

ERCP

- Radiographic examination of the hepatobiliary tree and pancreatic ducts using contrast medium and a lighted scope
- Used to evaluate the cause of obstructive jaundice
- Interventions:
  - Check for signs of respiratory depression
  - Withhold food until gag reflex returns

Percutaneous transhepatic cholangiography

- Fluoroscopic examination of the biliary ducts through the use of contrast medium
- Used to evaluate the cause of severe jaundice and diagnose obstruction
- Intervention: before the procedure, check for allergies; also check PT and PTT

Economic impact of GI disorders

- Disruption of employment
- Cost of special diet
- Cost of special diversion appli-ances
- Cost of medications

Social impact of GI disorders

- Changes in eating patterns and modes
- Changes in elimination patterns and modes
- Social withdrawal and isolation
- Changes in sexual function

Modifiable risk factors for GI disorders

- Low-fiber diet
- Smoking
- Inactivity
- Stress
- Contaminated water and food
- Anger, fear, or anxiety
- Culturally based reluctance to discuss personal hygiene and health habits

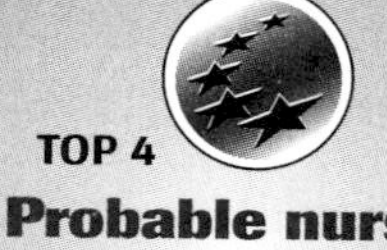

TOP 4

Probable nursing diagnoses for a GI disorder

1. Constipation
2. Diarrhea
3. Acute pain
4. Imbalanced nutrition: Less than body requirements

PSYCHOSOCIAL IMPACT OF GI DISORDERS

- **Developmental impact**
  - Changes in body image
  - Feeling of lack of control over body function
  - Fear of rejection
  - Embarrassment from changes in body function and structure
  - Decreased self-esteem
- **Economic impact**
  - Disruption of employment
  - Cost of special diet
  - Cost of special diversion appliances
  - Cost of medications
- **Occupational and recreational impact**
  - Change of occupation
  - Changes in leisure activity
  - Restrictions in physical activity
- **Social impact**
  - Changes in eating patterns and modes
  - Changes in elimination patterns and modes
  - Social withdrawal and isolation
  - Changes in sexual function

RISK FACTORS

- **Modifiable risk factors**
  - Diet: low-fiber
  - Smoking
  - Alcohol consumption
  - Inactivity
  - Stress
  - Contaminated water and food
  - Anger, fear, or anxiety
  - Culturally based reluctance to discuss personal hygiene and health habits
- **Nonmodifiable risk factors**
  - Family history of GI disorders
  - History of previous GI dysfunction

NURSING DIAGNOSES

- **Probable nursing diagnoses**
  - Constipation
  - Diarrhea
  - Acute pain
  - Imbalanced nutrition: Less than body requirements
  - Deficient fluid volume

Possible nursing diagnoses

- Disturbed body image
- Situational low self-esteem
- Impaired skin integrity
- Noncompliance (specify)
- Deficient knowledge (specify)
- Anxiety
- Sexual dysfunction
- Impaired swallowing
- Bowel incontinence
- Toileting self-care deficit

GALLBLADDER AND PANCREATIC SURGERIES

Description

- Cholecystostomy: surgical incision into the gallbladder to drain bile
- Choledochotomy: surgical incision into the common bile duct to remove stones
- Cholecystotomy: surgical incision into the gallbladder to remove gallstones
- Choledochostomy: surgical opening of the common bile duct to insert a T tube or catheter for drainage
- Cholecystectomy: surgical removal of the gallbladder
- Pancreatectomy: surgical removal of part or the entire pancreas
- Extracorporeal shock-wave lithotripsy (ESWL): use of shock waves to fragment gallstones into small pieces to either be removed by endoscopy or dissolved with solvents
- Laparoscopic cholecystectomy: removal of the gallbladder through a small incision in the abdomen and use of a fiber-optic endoscope

Gallbladder and pancreatic surgeries

- Cholecystostomy
- Choledochotomy
- Cholecystotomy
- Choledochostomy
- Cholecystectomy
- Pancreatectomy
- Extracorporeal shock-wave lithotripsy
- Laparoscopic cholecystectomy

Preoperative nursing interventions

- Complete patient and family preoperative teaching
  - Determine the patient's understanding of the procedure
  - Describe the operating room, postanesthesia care unit (PACU), and preoperative and postoperative routines
  - Demonstrate postoperative turning, coughing, deep breathing, splinting, and range-of-motion (ROM) exercises
  - Explain the postoperative need for drainage tubes, surgical dressings, oxygen therapy, I.V. therapy, and pain control
- Complete a preoperative checklist
- Administer preoperative medications, as prescribed
- Allay the patient's and his family's anxiety about surgery
- Document the patient's history and physical assessment database

Preoperative patient teaching

- Turning, coughing, and deep breathing
- Splinting of incision
- ROM exercises

Postoperative nursing interventions

- Check respiratory status and fluid balance
- Assess pain and administer postoperative analgesics, as prescribed
- Assess for return of peristalsis; give solid foods and liquids, as tolerated
- Administer I.V. fluids and transfusion therapy, as prescribed

Key nursing interventions after gallbladder and pancreatic surgeries

- Check respiratory status and fluid balance.
- Inspect the surgical dressing and change it, as directed.
- Reinforce turning, coughing, and deep breathing, and splinting of incision.
- Monitor and maintain position and patency of drainage tubes: NG, wound drainage, T tube.

Types of portosystemic shunts

- Portocaval shunt
- Splenorenal shunt
- Mesocaval shunt
- TIPS

Key nursing interventions before portosystemic shunt surgery

- Demonstrate postoperative turning, coughing, deep breathing, incentive spirometry, splinting, and ROM exercises.
- Administer vitamin K, as prescribed.
- Administer lactulose, as prescribed.
- Maintain patency of NG tube.
- Manage bleeding.

- Allay the patient's anxiety
- Inspect the surgical dressing and change it, as directed
- Reinforce turning, coughing, and deep breathing, and splinting of incision
- Keep the patient in semi-Fowler's position
- Provide incentive spirometry
- Maintain activity, as tolerated
- Monitor vital signs, intake and output (I/O), and laboratory studies
- Monitor and maintain position and patency of drainage tubes: NG, wound drainage, T tube
- Administer antibiotics, as prescribed
- Provide care for pancreatic surgery
  - **Perform blood glucose tests to monitor glucose**
  - **Monitor for signs of hyperglycemia**
- Individualize home care instructions
  - Avoid lifting for 6 weeks
  - Complete incision care daily
  - Continue care of the T tube
  - Adhere to a low-fat diet for 6 weeks

Surgical complications

- Pneumonia
- Atelectasis
- Peritonitis
- Hemorrhage

PORTOSYSTEMIC SHUNTS

Definition

- Portacaval shunt: surgical anastomosis of the portal vein to the inferior vena cava that diverts blood from the portal system and decreases pressure
- Splenorenal shunt: surgical anastomosis of the splenic vein to the left renal vein that diverts blood from the portal system and decreases pressure
- Mesocaval shunt: surgical anastomosis of the inferior vena cava to the side of the superior mesenteric vein that diverts blood from the portal system and decreases pressure
- Transjugular intrahepatic portosystemic shunt (TIPS): shunt between the portal and systemic venous circulation using the right internal jugular vein and placement of a stent

Preoperative nursing interventions

- Complete patient and family preoperative teaching
  - Determine the patient's understanding of the procedure
  - Describe the operating room, PACU, and preoperative and postoperative routines; demonstrate postoperative turning, coughing, deep breathing, incentive spirometry, splinting, and ROM exercises
  - Explain the postoperative need for drainage tubes, surgical dressings, oxygen therapy, I.V. therapy, and pain control

- Complete a preoperative checklist
- Administer preoperative medications, as prescribed
- Allay the patient's and his family's anxiety about surgery
- Document the patient's history and physical assessment database
- Administer antibiotics, as prescribed (neomycin sulfate)
- **Administer vitamin K, as prescribed**
- Administer I.V. and transfusion therapy, as prescribed
- Administer lactulose, as prescribed
- Maintain patency of NG tube
- Monitor central venous pressure (CVP)
- Manage bleeding
  - Administer vasopressin (Pitressin) or octreotide (Sandostatin)
  - Maintain Sengstaken-Blakemore tube
- Monitor laboratory values
- Provide fluids and electrolytes, as indicated
- Apply sequential compression devices

How to manage bleeding with portosystemic shunts

- Administer vasopressin or octreotide.
- Maintain Sengstaken-Blakemore tube.

Postoperative nursing interventions

- Assess cardiac, respiratory, and neurologic status and fluid balance
- Assess pain and administer postoperative analgesics, as prescribed
- Administer I.V. fluids, total parenteral nutrition (TPN), and transfusion therapy, as prescribed
- Allay the patient's anxiety
- Inspect the surgical dressing
- Reinforce turning, coughing, deep breathing, and incentive spirometry, and splinting of the incision
- Keep the patient in semi-Fowler's position
- Assess for return of peristalsis
- Provide suctioning, as needed
- Maintain activity: bed rest, active and passive ROM and isometric exercises
- Administer oxygen and maintain endotracheal tube to ventilator
- Monitor vital signs, I/O, CVP, laboratory studies, electrocardiogram (ECG), neurovital signs, and pulse oximetry
- Monitor and maintain position and patency of drainage tubes: NG, indwelling urinary catheter, wound drainage
- Allay the patient's anxiety verbally as well as with medication
- **Measure and record the patient's abdominal girth**
- **Monitor stool and NG tube drainage for occult blood**
- Monitor for hemorrhage
- Check for peripheral edema
- Provide skin, nares, and mouth care
- Reorient the patient frequently
- Administer antibiotics, as prescribed (neomycin sulfate)
- Administer vitamin K, as prescribed
- Elevate extremities
- Have the patient ambulate as soon as tolerated
- Use sequential compression devices while in bed
- Individualize home care instructions

Key nursing interventions after portosystemic shunt surgery

- Assess cardiac, respiratory, and neurologic status and fluid balance.
- Assess pain and administer postoperative analgesics, as prescribed.
- Assess for return of peristalsis.
- Monitor vital signs, I/O, CVP, laboratory studies, ECG, neurovital signs, and pulse oximetry.
- Measure and record the patient's abdominal girth.
- Monitor stool and NG tube drainage for occult blood.
- Monitor for hemorrhage.

- Adhere to activity limitations
- Complete incision care daily
- Avoid using alcohol
- Adhere indefinitely to a protein-restricted diet
- Avoid using over-the-counter (OTC) medications
- Observe for symptoms of encephalopathy

Home care instructions for a patient with a portosystemic shunt

- Avoid using alcohol.
- Adhere indefinitely to a protein-restricted diet.
- Observe for symptoms of encephalopathy.

Surgical complications

- Acute hepatic failure
- Chronic portosystemic encephalopathy
- Coagulopathy
- Shunt malfunction

GASTRIC SURGERY

Description

- Vagotomy: surgical ligation of the vagus nerve to decrease the secretion of gastric acid
- Antrectomy: surgical removal of the antrum of the stomach
- Pyloroplasty: surgical dilatation of the pyloric sphincter to increase the rate of gastric emptying
- Gastroduodenostomy (Billroth I): surgical removal of the lower portion of the stomach with anastomosis of the remaining portion of the stomach to the duodenum
- Gastrojejunostomy (Billroth II): surgical removal of the antrum and distal portion of the stomach and duodenum with anastomosis of the stomach to the jejunum
- Subtotal gastrectomy: surgical removal of 60% to 80% of the stomach
- Esophagojejunostomy (total gastrectomy): surgical removal of the entire stomach with a loop of the jejunum anastomosed to the esophagus

Types of gastric surgery

- Vagotomy
- Antrectomy
- Pyloroplasty
- Gastroduodenostomy
- Gastrojejunostomy
- Subtotal gastrectomy
- Esophagojejunostomy

Preoperative nursing interventions

- Complete patient and family preoperative teaching
  - Determine the patient's understanding of the procedure
  - Describe the operating room, PACU, and preoperative and postoperative routines
  - Demonstrate postoperative turning, coughing, deep breathing, splinting, and leg and ROM exercises
  - Explain the postoperative need for drainage tubes, surgical dressings, oxygen therapy, I.V. therapy, and pain control
- Complete a preoperative checklist
- Administer preoperative medications, as prescribed
- Allay the patient's and his family's anxiety about surgery
- Document the patient's history and physical assessment data
- Administer bowel preparation, as prescribed

Key nursing steps before gastric surgery

- Complete patient and family teaching.
- Administer preoperative medications, as prescribed.
- Administer bowel preparation, as prescribed.

Postoperative nursing interventions

- Assess respiratory status and fluid balance
- Assess pain and administer postoperative analgesics, as prescribed

- Administer I.V. fluids, NG tube feedings, and transfusion therapy, as prescribed
- Allay the patient's anxiety
- Inspect the surgical dressing and change it, as directed
- Reinforce turning, coughing, and deep breathing, and splinting of incision
- Keep the patient in semi-Fowler's position
- Assess for return of peristalsis
- Provide incentive spirometry
- Maintain activity, as tolerated
- Administer oxygen
- Monitor vital signs, I/O, laboratory studies, and pulse oximetry
- Monitor and maintain position and patency of drainage tubes: NG, indwelling urinary catheter, wound drainage
- Monitor NG tube drainage for overt bleeding
- **Irrigate NG tube gently; don't reposition it**
- Have the patient ambulate as soon as tolerated
- Administer anticoagulants, such as low-dose heparin or low-molecular-weight heparin, until patient is ambulatory
- Use sequential compression devices while in bed
- Weigh the patient daily
- Monitor gastric pH
- Individualize home care instructions
  - Identify ways to reduce stress
  - Increase food intake gradually
  - Eat six small meals a day
  - Limit fluids with meals

Surgical complications

- **Dumping syndrome after a partial gastrectomy**
- Hemorrhage
- Dehydration
- Infection
- Dehiscence

HEMORRHOIDECTOMY

Description

- Surgical removal of hemorrhoids by clamp, excision, or cautery

Preoperative nursing interventions

- Complete patient and family preoperative teaching
  - Determine the patient's understanding of the procedure
  - Describe the operating room, PACU, and preoperative and postoperative routines
  - Demonstrate postoperative turning, coughing, deep breathing, splinting, and ROM exercises
  - Explain the postoperative need for drainage tubes, surgical dressings, oxygen therapy, I.V. therapy, and pain control

Key nursing steps after gastric surgery

- Administer I.V. fluids, NG tube feedings, and transfusion therapy, as prescribed.
- Inspect the surgical dressing and change it, as directed.
- Assess for return of peristalsis.
- Monitor and maintain position and patency of drainage tubes: NG, indwelling urinary catheter, wound drainage.
- Administer anticoagulants, such as low-dose heparin or low-molecular-weight heparin, until patient is ambulatory.
- Use sequential compression devices while in bed.
- Irrigate NG tube gently; don't reposition it.

Hemorrhoidectomy defined

- Surgical removal of hemorrhoids
- Removed with clamp, excision, or cautery

Key nursing steps before hemorrhoidectomy

- Demonstrate postoperative turning, coughing, deep breathing, splinting, and ROM exercises.
- Explain postoperative needs.
- Administer bowel preparation, as prescribed.

Key nursing steps after hemorrhoidectomy

- Assess for return of peristalsis; give solid foods and liquids, as tolerated.
- Inspect the surgical dressing and remove anal packing, as directed.
- Administer analgesics, as prescribed.
- Provide sitz baths.
- Administer stool softeners, as prescribed.

Home precautions for a patient after hemorrhoidectomy

- Avoid heavy lifting and prolonged standing or sitting.
- Avoid constipation.
- Anticipate a small amount of bleeding with bowel movements.

Types of bowel surgery

- Abdominoperineal resection
- Colectomy
- Ileostomy
- Continent ileostomy
- Bowel resection
- Permanent colostomy
- Loop colostomy
- Double-barrel colostomy

- Complete a preoperative checklist
- Administer preoperative medications, as prescribed
- Allay the patient's and his family's anxiety about surgery
- Document the patient's history and physical assessment data
- Administer bowel preparation, as prescribed
  - Cleansing enemas
  - Laxatives

Postoperative nursing interventions

- Assess pain and administer postoperative analgesics, as prescribed
- Assess for return of peristalsis; give solid foods and liquids, as tolerated
- Administer I.V. fluids
- Allay the patient's anxiety
- Inspect the surgical dressing and remove anal packing, as directed
- Reinforce turning, coughing, and deep breathing
- Keep the patient prone or on his side
- Provide incentive spirometry
- Maintain activity, as tolerated
- Monitor vital signs, I/O, and laboratory studies
- Encourage the patient to discuss feelings of embarrassment and fear of defecation
- **Administer analgesics, as prescribed, before the first bowel movement**
- Provide sitz baths
- Provide a flotation pad when sitting
- Administer stool softeners, as prescribed
- Individualize home care instructions
  - Avoid heavy lifting and prolonged standing or sitting
  - Avoid constipation
  - Defecate when urge is felt
  - Provide perineal care daily
  - **Anticipate a small amount of bleeding with bowel movements postoperatively**
  - Avoid Valsalva's maneuver
  - Increase fluid intake

Surgical complications

- Rectal hemorrhage
- Urine retention

BOWEL SURGERY

Description

- Abdominoperineal resection: removal of distal sigmoid colon, rectum, and anus with the creation of a permanent colostomy (see *Reviewing types of ostomies*)
- Colectomy: surgical excision of the right colon (right hemicolectomy) or left colon (left hemicolectomy)

Reviewing types of ostomies

The type of ostomy appropriate for a patient depends on the patient's condition. Temporary ones, such as a double-barrel or loop colostomy, help treat perforated sigmoid diverticulitis and other conditions in which intestinal healing is expected. Permanent colostomy or ileostomy accompanies extensive abdominal surgery such as the removal of a malignant tumor.

DOUBLE-BARREL COLOSTOMY

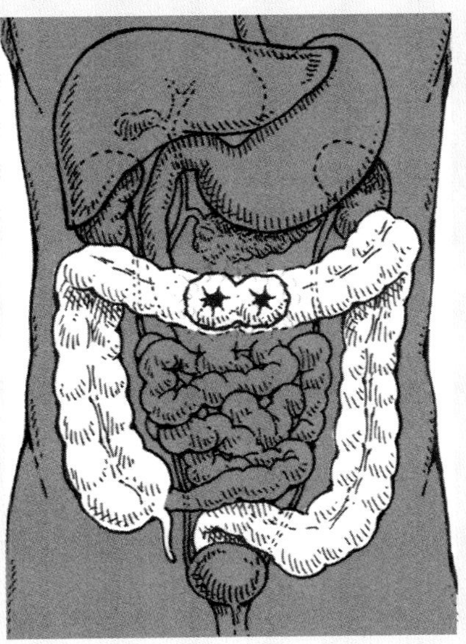

LOOP COLOSTOMY

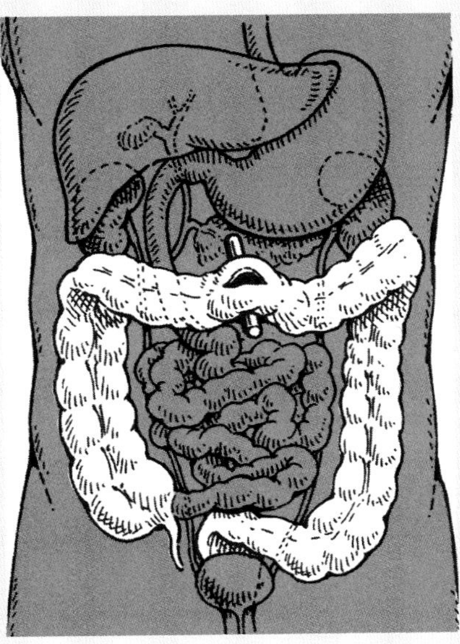

PERMANENT COLOSTOMY

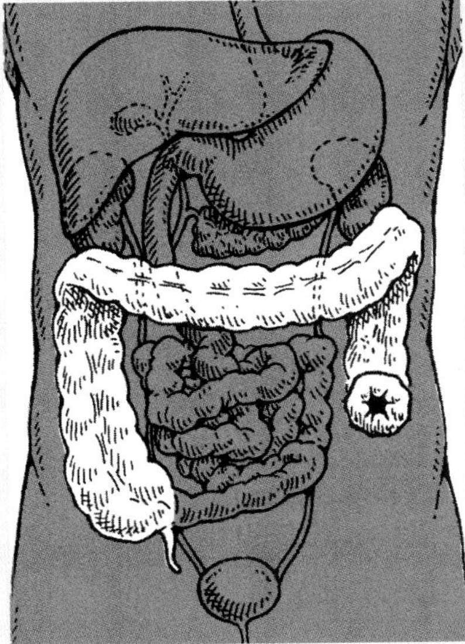

ILEOSTOMY

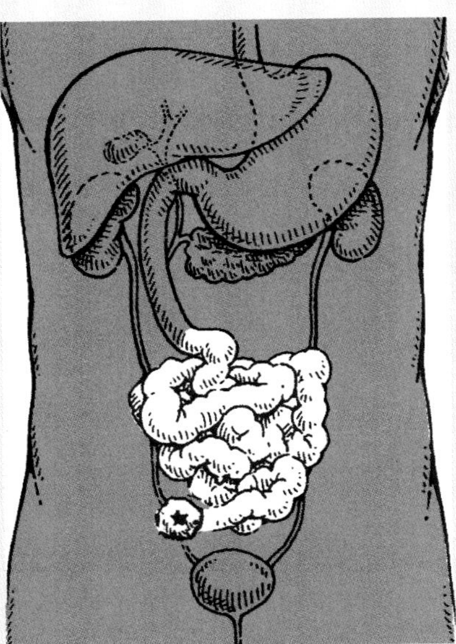

Types of ostomies

- Double-barrel colostomy: surgical opening of the colon to the abdominal surface to form two stomas to prevent passage of stool into the distal bowel
- Loop colostomy: creation of proximal and distal stomas from a loop of intestine that has been pulled through an abdominal incision and supported with a plastic or glass rod
- Permanent colostomy: surgical opening of the colon to the abdominal surface to form a single stoma after the distal portion of the bowel is removed
- Ileostomy: surgical opening of the ileum to the abdominal surface to form a stoma

- Ileostomy: surgical opening of the ileum to the abdominal surface to form a stoma
- Continent ileostomy: surgical creation of an intra-abdominal reservoir for stool
- Bowel resection: surgical excision of a portion of the bowel
- Permanent colostomy: surgical opening of the colon to the abdominal surface to form a single stoma after the distal portion of the bowel is removed
- Loop colostomy: creation of proximal and distal stomas from a loop of intestine that has been pulled through an abdominal incision and supported with a plastic or glass rod
- Double-barrel colostomy: surgical opening of the colon to the abdominal surface to form two stomas to prevent passage of stool into the distal bowel

Preoperative nursing interventions

- Complete patient and family preoperative teaching
  - Determine the patient's understanding of the procedure
  - Describe the operating room, PACU, and preoperative and postoperative routines
  - Demonstrate postoperative turning, coughing, deep breathing, splinting, and leg and ROM exercises
  - Explain the postoperative need for drainage tubes, gastrostomy feeding tube, surgical dressings, oxygen therapy, I.V. therapy, and pain control
- Complete a preoperative checklist
- Administer preoperative medications, as prescribed
- Allay the patient's and his family's anxiety about surgery
- Document the patient's history and physical assessment data
- Administer bowel preparation, as prescribed
  - Antibiotics
  - Cleansing enemas
- Arrange a preoperative visit with an enterostomal therapist
- Encourage the patient to express his feelings about changes in his body image

Key nursing steps before bowel surgery

- Administer bowel preparation, as prescribed.
- Encourage the patient to express his feelings about changes in his body image.
- Arrange a preoperative visit with an enterostomal therapist.

Postoperative nursing interventions

- Assess cardiac status and fluid balance
- Assess pain and administer postoperative analgesics, as prescribed
- Assess for return of peristalsis; give solid foods and liquids, as tolerated
- Administer I.V. fluids, TPN, and transfusion therapy, as prescribed
- Allay the patient's anxiety
- Inspect the surgical dressing and change it, as directed
- Reinforce turning, coughing, and deep breathing, and splinting of incision
- Keep the patient in semi-Fowler's position
- Provide incentive spirometry
- Maintain activity, as tolerated
- Apply antiembolism or pneumatic stockings
- Monitor vital signs, I/O, laboratory studies, and pulse oximetry

Key nursing steps after bowel surgery

- Assess for return of peristalsis; give solid foods and liquids, as tolerated.
- Monitor and maintain position and patency of drainage tubes: NG, indwelling urinary catheter, wound drainage.
- Monitor and record the color, consistency, and amount of the patient's stool.

- Monitor and maintain position and patency of drainage tubes: NG, indwelling urinary catheter, wound drainage
- Encourage the patient to express his feelings about changes in his body image
- Monitor and record the color, consistency, and amount of the patient's stool
- Provide routine colostomy care
  - Prevent skin breakdown by thoroughly cleaning the skin around the stoma
  - Check stoma
  - Control odor
  - Change ostomy bag, as needed
- **Increase fluid intake to 3 L/day**
- Individualize home care instructions
  - Recognize the signs and symptoms of intestinal obstruction
  - Complete incision care daily
  - Use ostomy bags
  - **Check the condition of the stoma daily and report bleeding and changes**
  - Report changes in consistency and color of stool
  - Perform colostomy care daily
  - Identify foods that cause flatus and irritability of the colon
  - Provide skin care around the stoma
  - Discuss concerns about sexual activities

Surgical complications

- Infection
- Hemorrhage
- Dehiscence
- Evisceration
- Paralytic ileus
- Prolapsed stoma
- Abscess

HIATAL HERNIA (ESOPHAGEAL HERNIA)

Definition

- Protrusion of the stomach through the diaphragm into the thoracic cavity

Causes

- Congenital weakness
- Obesity
- Pregnancy
- Trauma
- Increased abdominal pressure
- Aging

Pathophysiology

- The opening (hiatus) in the diaphragm where the esophagus enters the stomach becomes enlarged and weakened
- The upper portion of the stomach enters the lower thorax

Providing colostomy care after bowel surgery

- Prevent skin breakdown by thoroughly cleaning the skin around the stoma.
- Check stoma.
- Control odor.
- Change ostomy bag, as needed.

Hiatal hernia highlights

- Protrusion of the stomach through the diaphragm into the thoracic cavity
- Sliding of the stomach into the chest results in gastric acid reflux

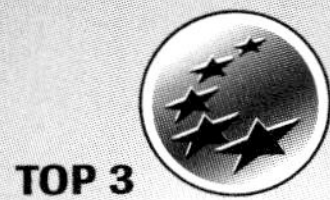

TOP 3

Causes of hiatal hernia

1. Congenital weakness
2. Obesity
3. Pregnancy

- Sliding of the esophagus and stomach into the chest results in gastric acid reflux

Chief assessment findings in hiatal hernia

- Dysphagia
- Regurgitation
- Sternal pain after eating

Key diagnostic test findings in hiatal hernia

- Esophagoscopy: incompetent cardiac sphincter
- Barium swallow: protrusion of the hernia
- Chest X-ray: protrusion of abdominal organs into thorax

Most common ways to manage hiatal hernia

- Bland diet with decreased intake of caffeine and spicy foods
- Anticholinergic
- H_2-receptor antagonists

Assessment findings

- Pyrosis
- Dysphagia
- Regurgitation
- Sternal pain after eating
- Vomiting
- Feeling of fullness
- Dyspnea
- Cough
- Tachycardia

Diagnostic test findings

- Esophagoscopy: incompetent cardiac sphincter
- Barium swallow: protrusion of the hernia
- Chest X-ray: protrusion of abdominal organs into thorax
- Gastric analysis: increased pH

Medical management

- Diet: bland diet with decreased intake of caffeine and spicy foods
- Oxygen therapy
- GI decompression: NG tube
- Position: semi-Fowler's
- Activity: as tolerated
- Monitoring: vital signs, and I/O
- Anticholinergic: propantheline (Pro-Banthine)
- Antacids: magnesium and aluminum hydroxide (Maalox), aluminum hydroxide gel (AlternaGEL)
- Histamine-2 (H_2) receptor antagonists: cimetidine (Tagamet), ranitidine (Zantac), famotidine (Pepcid), nizatidine (Axid)
- Weight loss

Nursing interventions

- Maintain the patient's diet
- Administer oxygen
- Assess respiratory status
- Maintain position, patency, and low suction of NG tube
- Keep the patient in semi-Fowler's position
- Monitor and record vital signs, I/O, and daily weight
- Administer medications, as prescribed
- Allay the patient's anxiety through verbalization and medication
- Avoid flexion at the waist when positioning the patient
- Individualize home care instructions (for more information about teaching, see *Patients with GI disorders*)
  - Eat small, frequent meals
  - Stop drinking carbonated beverages and alcohol
  - Stay upright for 2 hours after eating
  - Avoid wearing constrictive clothing

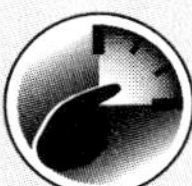

TIME-OUT FOR TEACHING

Patients with GI disorders

Be sure to include these topics in your teaching plan for patients with GI disorders.

- Smoking cessation
- Stool monitoring, including color, amount, and consistency
- Glucose level monitoring
- Signs of hyperglycemia
- Weight maintenance program
- Medication therapy, including the action, adverse effects, and scheduling of medications
- Dietary recommendations and restrictions
- Rest and activity patterns
- Signs and symptoms of GI bleeding
- Self-monitoring for infection

Key teaching topics for patients with GI disorders

- Glucose level monitoring
- Dietary recommendations and restrictions
- Medication therapy

 – Avoid lifting, bending, straining, and coughing

- **Complications**
  - Hemorrhage
  - Ulceration
  - Aspiration
  - Incarceration of stomach in chest
- **Surgical interventions**
  - Reduction of hiatal hernia
  - Fundoplication

Peptic ulcer defined

- Erosion of mucosal lining of the stomach
- Caused by an inflammatory reaction with tissue breakdown

PEPTIC ULCER

- **Definition**
  - Erosion of mucosal lining of the stomach
- **Causes**
  - Alcohol abuse
  - Stress
  - Drug-induced: salicylates, steroids, indomethacin, reserpine
  - Smoking
  - Gastritis
  - Zollinger-Ellison syndrome
  - Infection: *Helicobacter pylori*
- **Pathophysiology**
  - Increased emptying time of gastric acid from the gastric lumen into the small intestine causes an inflammatory reaction with tissue breakdown
  - Bile refluxes into the stomach if the pyloric valve is involved
  - Combination of hydrochloric acid and pepsin destroys gastric mucosa
  - Decreased resistance of gastric mucosa to action of hydrochloric acid
- **Assessment findings**
  - Left epigastric pain 1 to 2 hours after eating

Main causes of peptic ulcer

- Alcohol abuse
- Stress
- Drug-induced
- Smoking

- Weight loss
- Nausea and vomiting
- Hematemesis
- Melena
- Anorexia
- Relief from pain after administration of antacids

Key assessment findings in peptic ulcer

- Left epigastric pain 1 to 2 hours after eating
- Hematemesis
- Relief from pain after administration of antacids

Diagnostic test findings

- Hematology: decreased Hb, HCT, PT, and PTT
- Blood chemistry: increased sodium
- Gastric analysis: normal for gastric ulcer
- Upper GI: location of ulcer
- Barium swallow: ulceration of gastric mucosa
- Fecal occult blood: positive
- Serum gastrin: normal or increased

Key diagnostic test findings in peptic ulcer

- Upper GI: location of ulcer
- Barium swallow: ulceration of gastric mucosa

Medical management

- Diet: low-fiber in small, frequent feedings
- GI decompression: NG tube
- Position: semi-Fowler's
- Activity: bed rest
- Monitoring: vital signs, and I/O
- Laboratory studies: Hb and HCT
- Treatment: saline lavage by NG tube
- Transfusion therapy: packed RBCs
- Anticholinergics: propantheline (Pro-Banthine), dicyclomine (Bentyl)
- Antacids: magnesium and aluminum hydroxide (Maalox), aluminum hydroxide gel (AlternaGEL)
- H_2-receptor antagonists: cimetidine (Tagamet), ranitidine (Zantac), nizatidine (Axid), famotidine (Pepcid)
- Prostaglandin: misoprostol (Cytotec)
- Mucosal barrier fortifier: sucralfate (Carafate)
- Endoscopic laser
- Photocoagulation
- Hormone: vasopressin (Pitressin) for management of bleeding
- Antibiotic: if *H. pylori* present
- Sequential compression devices
- Gastric surgery, if hemorrhage present

Main medical treatment options for peptic ulcer

- H_2-receptor antagonists
- Prostaglandin
- Mucosal barrier fortifier
- Antibiotics
- Gastric surgery, if hemorrhage present

Nursing interventions

- Maintain the patient's diet with small, frequent feedings
- Assess respiratory, GI, and cardiovascular status
- Maintain position, patency, and low suction of NG tube if gastric decompression is ordered
- Keep the patient in semi-Fowler's position
- Monitor and record vital signs, I/O, laboratory studies, fecal occult blood, and gastric pH
- Administer medications, as prescribed
- Allay the patient's anxiety

- Provide nares and mouth care
- Minimize environmental stress
- Maintain a quiet environment
- **Irrigate the NG tube with normal saline to maintain patency; don't use water, which may interfere with fluid and electrolyte balance**
- Monitor the consistency, color, amount, and frequency of stools
- Apply sequential compression devices while in bed
- Individualize home care instructions
  - Identify ways to reduce stress
  - Follow dietary recommendations and restrictions; avoid caffeine, alcohol, and spicy and fried foods
  - Maintain a quiet environment

Complications
- Hemorrhage
- Perforation
- Chemical peritonitis
- Intestinal obstruction

Surgical interventions
- Billroth I
- Billroth II
- Vagotomy
- Pyloroplasty

GASTRIC CANCER

Definition
- Malignant stomach tumor that's primary or metastatic

Causes
- High intake of salty and smoked foods
- Low intake of vegetables and fruits
- Chronic gastritis
- Achlorhydria
- Pernicious anemia
- Gastric ulcer

Pathophysiology
- Unregulated cell growth and uncontrolled cell division result in the development of a neoplasm
- Tumor usually develops in the distal third of stomach and metastasizes to the abdominal organs, lungs, and bones
- Most common neoplasm is adenocarcinoma

Assessment findings
- Fatigue
- Weakness
- Syncope
- Shortness of breath

Key nursing interventions for a patient with a peptic ulcer

- Assess respiratory, GI, and cardiovascular status.
- Maintain position, patency, and low suction of NG tube if gastric decompression is ordered.
- Keep the patient in semi-Fowler's position.
- Irrigate the NG tube with normal saline to maintain patency.

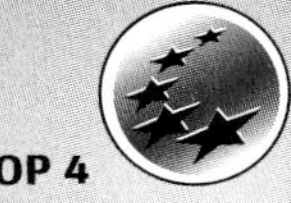

TOP 4

Things for the patient with peptic ulcers to avoid

1. Stress
2. Caffeine
3. Alcohol
4. Spicy and fried foods

Key facts about gastric cancer

- Malignant stomach tumor
- May be primary or metastatic
- Usually develops in the distal third of stomach
- Most common neoplasm is adenocarcinoma

Key signs and symptoms of gastric cancer

- Nausea and vomiting
- Weight loss
- Epigastric fullness and pain
- Melena
- Anorexia

Key test findings in gastric cancer

- Gastric analysis: positive cancer cells, achlorhydria
- Gastroscopy: biopsy positive for cancer cells

Most common treatments for gastric cancer

- Antineoplastics
- Vitamin supplements
- Gastric surgery

- Nausea and vomiting
- Weight loss
- Hematemesis
- Indigestion
- Epigastric fullness and pain
- Malaise
- Melena
- Regurgitation
- Anorexia

Diagnostic test findings

- Fecal occult blood: positive
- CEA: positive
- Hematology: decreased Hb and HCT; shortened or prolonged PT and PTT, depending on location of neoplasm
- Blood chemistry: increased AST, LD, and amylase
- Gastric analysis: positive cancer cells, achlorhydria
- GI series: gastric mass
- Gastroscopy: biopsy positive for cancer cells

Medical management

- Diet: high-protein, high-calorie, high-fat, and low-carbohydrate
- I.V. therapy: saline lock
- GI decompression: NG tube
- Position: semi-Fowler's
- Activity: as tolerated
- Monitoring: vital signs, and I/O
- Laboratory studies: Hb, HCT, and fecal occult blood
- Nutritional support: TPN
- Radiation therapy
- Antineoplastics: carmustine (BiCNU), 5-fluorouracil (Adrucil)
- Vitamin supplements: folic acid (Folvite), cyanocobalamin (vitamin B_{12})
- Analgesics: meperidine (Demerol), morphine (Roxanol)
- Antiemetic: prochlorperazine (Compazine)
- Gastric surgery

Nursing interventions

- Maintain the patient's diet
- Assess GI status
- Maintain position, patency, and low suction of NG tube
- Keep the patient in semi-Fowler's position
- Monitor and record vital signs, I/O, laboratory studies, and daily weight
- Administer TPN
- Administer medications, as prescribed
- Encourage the patient to express his feelings about a fear of dying
- Provide skin and mouth care
- Provide rest periods
- Monitor the consistency, amount, and frequency of stool
- Monitor the color of stool for blood

- Provide postchemotherapeutic and postradiation nursing care
  - Provide prophylactic skin and mouth care
  - Monitor dietary intake
  - Administer antiemetics and antidiarrheals, as prescribed
  - Monitor for bleeding, infection, and electrolyte imbalance
  - Provide rest periods
- Provide information about the American Cancer Society
- Individualize home care instructions
  - Avoid exposure to people with infections
  - Alternate rest periods with activity
  - Monitor self for infection by taking temperature frequently
  - Recognize the signs and symptoms of ulceration
  - Complete skin care daily

Complications
- Obstruction
- Ulceration
- Metastasis

Surgical interventions
- Subtotal gastrectomy
- Total gastrectomy
- Billroth I
- Billroth II

Key nursing interventions for a patient with gastric cancer

- Assess GI status.
- Maintain position, patency, and low suction of NG tube.
- Monitor the consistency, amount, and frequency of stool.
- Monitor the color of stool for blood.
- Provide postchemotherapeutic and postradiation nursing care.
- Provide information about the American Cancer Society.

ULCERATIVE COLITIS

Definition
- Inflammatory disorder of the large bowel

Causes
- Emotional stress
- Autoimmune disease
- Genetics
- Idiopathic cause
- Allergies
- Viral and bacterial infections

Pathophysiology
- Inflammatory edema of the mucous membrane of the colon and rectum leads to bleeding and shallow ulcerations
- Abscess formation causes bowel-wall shortening, thinning, fragility, hypermotility, and decreased absorption
- Mucosal ulcerations begin in the distal end of the colon and ascend the large intestine

Assessment findings
- Abdominal tenderness
- Weakness
- Debilitation

Ulcerative colitis defined

- Inflammatory disorder of the large bowel
- Leads to bleeding and shallow ulcerations

Causes of ulcerative colitis

- Emotional stress
- Autoimmune disease
- Genetics
- Idiopathic cause
- Allergies
- Viral and bacterial infections

- Anorexia
- Nausea and vomiting
- Dehydration
- **Bloody, purulent, mucoid, watery stools (15 to 20/day)**
- Elevated temperature
- Cachexia
- Weight loss
- Abdominal cramping
- Tenesmus
- **Hyperactive bowel sounds**
- Abdominal distention

Key assessment findings in ulcerative colitis

- Weight loss
- Abdominal cramping
- Bloody, purulent, mucoid, watery stools (15 to 20/day)
- Hyperactive bowel sounds

Diagnostic test findings

- Sigmoidoscopy: ulceration and hyperemia
- Barium enema: ulcerations
- Blood chemistry: decreased potassium; increased osmolality
- Hematology: decreased Hb and HCT
- Urine chemistry: increased urine specific gravity
- Stool specimen: positive for blood and mucus

Possible test findings in ulcerative colitis

- Sigmoidoscopy: ulceration and hyperemia
- Barium enema: ulcerations

Medical management

- Diet: two types
  - High-protein, high-calorie, low-residue; bland foods in small, frequent feedings with restricted intake of milk and gas-forming foods
  - No food and fluids
- I.V. therapy: hydration, electrolyte replacement, and saline lock
- GI decompression: NG tube
- Position: semi-Fowler's
- Activity: bed rest with bedside commode
- Monitoring: vital signs, I/O, daily weight, urine specific gravity, calorie count, and stools for occult blood
- Laboratory studies: potassium, Hb, HCT, and osmolality
- Nutritional support: TPN
- Treatments: indwelling urinary catheter, sitz baths
- Antibiotic: sulfasalazine (Azulfidine)
- Analgesic: meperidine (Demerol)
- Sedative: phenobarbital (Luminal)
- Anticholinergics: propantheline (Pro-Banthine), dicyclomine (Bentyl)
- Antacids: magnesium and aluminum hydroxide (Maalox), aluminum hydroxide gel (AlternaGEL)
- Corticosteroid: hydrocortisone (Solu-Cortef)
- Antiemetic: prochlorperazine (Compazine)
- Antidiarrheals: diphenoxylate (Lomotil), loperamide (Imodium)
- Transfusion therapy: packed RBCs
- Antianemics: ferrous sulfate (Feosol), ferrous gluconate (Fergon)
- Immunosuppressive agents: azathioprine (Imuran), cyclophosphamide (Cytoxan)
- Vitamins and minerals

Main medical options for ulcerative colitis

- I.V. therapy
- Nutritional support
- Antibiotics
- Anticholinergics
- Antiemetics
- Immunosuppressive agents
- Anti-inflammatory agents

- Tranquilizer: diazepam (Valium)
- Potassium supplements: potassium chloride (K-Lor), potassium gluconate (Kaon)
- Anti-inflammatory: olsalazine (Dipentum)

Nursing interventions

- Maintain the patient's diet; withhold food and fluids, as necessary
- Administer I.V. fluids
- Assess GI status and fluid balance
- Maintain position, patency, and low suction of NG tube
- Keep the patient in semi-Fowler's position
- Monitor and record vital signs, I/O, laboratory studies, daily weight, urine specific gravity, calorie count, and fecal occult blood
- Administer TPN and transfusion therapy
- Administer medications, as prescribed
- Allay the patient's anxiety
- Provide skin, mouth, nares, and perianal care
- Maintain bed rest with bedside commode
- Turn the patient every 2 hours
- Minimize environmental stress
- Provide rest periods
- Maintain a quiet environment
- Promote independence in activities of daily living (ADLs)
- Assess bowel sounds
- Administer sitz baths
- Monitor the number, amount, and character of stools
- Assess perineal excoriation
- Provide information about the United Ostomy Association and the National Foundation of Ileitis and Colitis
- Individualize home care instructions
  - Maintain a normal weight
  - Identify ways to reduce stress
  - Recognize the signs and symptoms of rectal hemorrhage and intestinal obstruction
  - Complete sitz baths and perianal care daily

Complications

- Anemia
- Malnutrition
- GI perforation
- Megacolon
- Dehydration
- GI obstruction
- Hypokalemia
- Massive rectal hemorrhage
- Amyloidosis

Surgical interventions

- Ileostomy

Key nursing interventions for a patient with ulcerative colitis

- Administer I.V. fluids.
- Assess GI status and fluid balance.
- Maintain position, patency, and low suction of NG tube.
- Administer TPN.
- Monitor the number, amount, and character of stools.
- Assess perineal excoriation.
- Provide information about the United Ostomy Association and the National Foundation of Ileitis and Colitis.

Home care checklist for a patient with ulcerative colitis

- Maintain normal weight.
- Identify ways to reduce stress.
- Recognize the signs and symptoms of rectal hemorrhage and intestinal obstruction.
- Complete sitz baths and perianal care daily.

- Colectomy

CROHN'S DISEASE (REGIONAL ENTERITIS)

Definition
- Chronic inflammatory disease typically of the small intestine, usually affecting the terminal ileum and sometimes affecting the large intestine (usually the ascending colon)
- Slowly progressive with exacerbations and remissions

Causes
- Unknown
- Emotional upsets
- Milk and milk products
- Fried foods

Pathophysiology
- Ulcerations of intestinal mucosa are accompanied by congestion, thickening of the small bowel, and fissure formations (see *Bowel changes in Crohn's disease)*
- Enlarged regional mesenteric lymph nodes accompany fibrosis and narrowing of intestinal wall

Assessment findings
- Pain in right lower quadrant
- Mesenteric lymphadenitis
- Abdominal cramps and spasms after meals
- Nausea
- Flatulence
- Weight loss
- Elevated temperature
- Chronic diarrhea with blood
- Borborygmus

Diagnostic test findings
- Abdominal X-ray: congested, thickened, fibrosed, and narrowed intestinal wall
- Proctosigmoidoscopy: ulceration
- Fecal occult blood: positive
- Fecal fat test: increased
- Upper GI: classic "string sign" at terminal ileum
- Barium enema: lesions in terminal ileum

Medical management
- Diet: two types
  - High-protein, high-calorie, low-residue, low-fat, low-fiber, high-carbohydrate; bland foods in small, frequent feedings with restricted intake of milk and gas-forming foods
  - No food and fluids
- I.V. therapy: saline lock
- Activity: as tolerated

Crohn's disease
- Chronic inflammatory disease typically of the small intestine
- Usually affects the terminal ileum
- Sometimes affects the large intestine, usually the ascending colon

Possible causes of Crohn's disease
- Emotional upsets
- Milk and milk products
- Fried foods

Key assessment findings in Crohn's disease
- Pain in right lower quadrant
- Abdominal cramps and spasms after meals
- Chronic diarrhea with blood

Key diagnostic test findings in Crohn's disease
- Abdominal X-ray: congested, thickened, fibrosed, and narrowed intestinal wall
- Upper GI: classic "string sign" at terminal ileum

Bowel changes in Crohn's disease

As Crohn's disease progresses, fibrosis thickens the bowel wall and narrows the lumen. Narrowing – or stenosis – can occur in any part of the intestine and cause varying degrees of intestinal obstruction. At first, the mucosa may appear normal, but as the disease progresses, it takes on a "cobblestone" appearance, as shown.

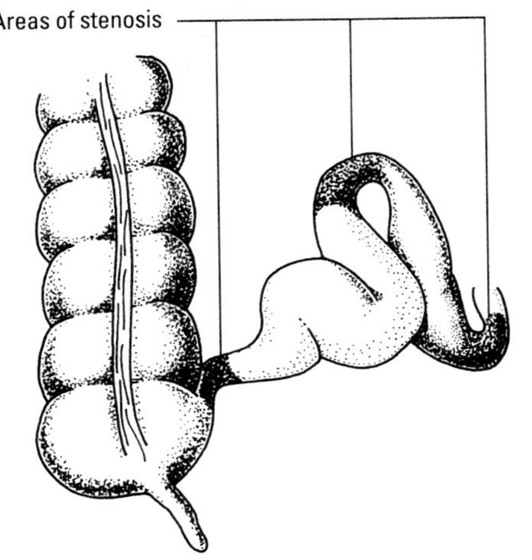

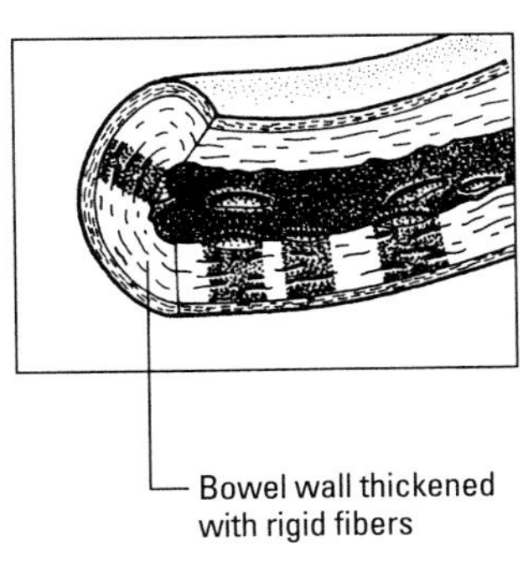

- Monitoring: vital signs, I/O, daily weight, stool for occult blood, and urine specific gravity
- Laboratory studies: potassium, Hb, HCT, and osmolality
- Nutritional support: TPN
- Antibiotic: sulfasalazine (Azulfidine)
- Analgesic: meperidine (Demerol)
- Anticholinergics: propantheline (Pro-Banthine), dicyclomine (Bentyl)
- Antacids: magnesium and aluminum hydroxide (Maalox), aluminum hydroxide gel (AlternaGEL)
- Corticosteroid: prednisone (Deltasone)
- Antiemetic: prochlorperazine (Compazine)
- Antidiarrheal: diphenoxylate (Lomotil)
- Antianemics: ferrous sulfate (Feosol), ferrous gluconate (Fergon)
- Vitamins and minerals
- Potassium supplements: potassium chloride (K-Lor), potassium gluconate (Kaon)
- Anti-inflammatory: olsalazine (Dipentum)
- Antibacterial: metronidazole (Flagyl)
- Immunosuppressants: mercaptopurine (Purinethol), azathioprine (Imuran)

Nursing interventions

- Maintain the patient's diet; withhold food and fluids, as necessary
- Assess GI status and fluid balance

Bowel changes in Crohn's disease

- Thickening of the bowel wall and narrowing of the lumen can cause varying degrees of intestinal obstruction
- "Cobblestone" appearance of the intestinal mucosa

Common ways to treat Crohn's disease

- Antibiotics
- Anticholinergics
- Corticosteroids
- Antidiarrheals
- Anti-inflammatory agents
- Immunosuppressants

Key nursing steps in the care of a patient with Crohn's disease

- Assess GI status and fluid balance.
- Minimize stress and encourage expression of feelings.
- Monitor the number, amount, and character of stools.
- Assess abdominal distention.

Diverticulum defined

- Outpouching of intestinal mucosa through the muscular wall of the intestine
- Multiple diverticula is called *diverticulosis*
- Inflammation of diverticula is called *diverticulitis*

Causes of diverticulosis and diverticulitis

- Stress
- Congenital weakening of the intestinal wall
- Low intake of roughage and fiber
- Straining at defecation
- Chronic constipation

- Monitor and record vital signs, I/O, laboratory studies, daily weight, urine specific gravity, and fecal occult blood
- Administer TPN
- Administer medications, as prescribed
- Allay the patient's anxiety
- Provide skin and perianal care
- Minimize the patient's stress and encourage expression of his feelings
- Maintain a quiet environment
- Promote independence in ADLs
- **Monitor the number, amount, and character of stools**
- **Assess abdominal distention**
- Individualize home care instructions
  - Avoid laxatives and aspirin
  - Complete perianal care daily
  - Identify ways to reduce stress
  - **Recognize the signs and symptoms of rectal hemorrhage and intestinal obstruction**

Complications

- Intestinal obstruction
- Intestinal fistulas
- Intestinal perforation
- Hemorrhage
- Malnutrition
- Anemia

Surgical interventions

- Bowel resection with anastomosis
- Gastrojejunostomy with vagotomy
- Ileoanal reservoir
- Colectomy with ileostomy

DIVERTICULOSIS AND DIVERTICULITIS

Definition

- Diverticulum: outpouching of intestinal mucosa through the muscular wall of the intestine
- Diverticulosis: multiple diverticula
- Diverticulitis: inflammation of diverticula

Causes

- Stress
- Congenital weakening of the intestinal wall
- Low intake of roughage and fiber
- Straining at defecation
- Chronic constipation

Pathophysiology

- Muscle tone is weakened in the intestinal wall, resulting in a saclike outpouching (diverticulum)

- Inflammation (diverticulitis) is caused by bacteria and fecal material trapped in the diverticula
- Intestinal wall thickens and narrows
- Common site is sigmoid colon

Assessment findings

- Left lower quadrant pain
- Constipation and diarrhea
- Bloody stools
- Elevated temperature
- Rectal bleeding
- Change in bowel habits
- Flatulence
- Nausea

Diagnostic test findings

- Sigmoidoscopy: diverticula, thickened wall
- Barium enema (contraindicated in acute diverticulitis): inflammation, narrow lumen of the bowel, diverticula
- Hematology: increased WBCs and erythrocyte sedimentation rate (ESR)

Medical management

- Diet: high-fiber, high-residue; avoid foods with seeds
- I.V. therapy: hydration, saline lock
- GI decompression: NG tube
- Position: semi-Fowler's
- Activity: bed rest, active ROM and isometric exercises
- Monitoring: vital signs and I/O
- Laboratory studies: Hb, HCT, and WBCs
- Nutritional support: TPN
- Antibiotics: gentamicin (Garamycin), tobramycin (Nebcin), clindamycin (Cleocin)
- Anticholinergic: propantheline (Pro-Banthine)
- Stool softener: docusate (Colace)

Nursing interventions

- Maintain the patient's diet
- Assess abdominal distention
- Maintain position, patency, and low suction of NG tube
- Keep the patient in semi-Fowler's position
- Monitor and record vital signs, I/O, and laboratory studies
- Administer TPN
- Administer medications, as prescribed
- Allay the patient's anxiety through verbalization and medication
- Provide nares and mouth care
- Provide rest periods
- Administer cleansing enemas
- Monitor stool for occult blood
- Assess bowel sounds
- Individualize home care instructions

Key signs and symptoms of diverticulosis and diverticulitis

- Left lower quadrant pain
- Bloody stools
- Change in bowel habits
- Flatulence
- Nausea

Key steps in the medical management of diverticulosis and diverticulitis

- High-fiber, high-residue diet; avoid foods with seeds
- Antibiotics
- Anticholinergics
- Stool softeners

Key nursing steps for a patient with diverticulosis and diverticulitis

- Assess abdominal distention.
- Monitor stool for occult blood.
- Assess bowel sounds.

– Identify ways to decrease constipation
– Follow dietary recommendations and restrictions; avoid corn, nuts, and fruits and vegetables with seeds
– Monitor stools for bleeding

- **Complications**
  - Bowel perforation
  - Peritonitis
  - Abscess
  - Fistula
  - Hemorrhage
- **Surgical intervention**
  - Bowel resection

INTESTINAL OBSTRUCTION

- **Definition**
  - Blockage of intestinal lumen
- **Causes**
  - Adhesions
  - Hernias
  - Tumors
  - Fecal impaction
  - Mesenteric thrombosis
  - Paralytic ileus
  - Diverticulitis
  - Inflammation (Crohn's disease)
  - Volvulus
- **Pathophysiology**
  - Gas, fluid, and digested substances accumulate proximal to the obstruction
  - Fluids and gases cause bowel distention
  - Peristalsis increases proximal to the obstruction
  - Water and electrolytes are secreted into the blocked bowel
  - Bowel inflammation increases and absorption by bowel mucosa is inhibited
  - Fluid loss results in dehydration
- **Assessment findings**
  - Cramping pain
  - Nausea
  - Abdominal distention
  - Vomiting fecal material
  - Constipation
  - Singultus
  - Elevated temperature
  - Diminished or absent bowel sounds
  - Weight loss

Intestinal obstruction highlights

- Blockage of the intestinal lumen
- Fluid and gases cause bowel distention
- Fluid loss results in dehydration

Key causes of intestinal obstruction

- Adhesions
- Hernias
- Tumors
- Fecal impaction

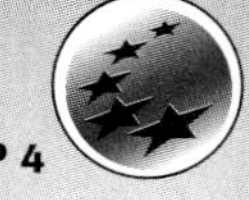

TOP 4

Assessment findings in intestinal obstruction

1. Cramping pain
2. Abdominal distention
3. Vomiting fecal material
4. Diminished or absent bowel sounds

Diagnostic test findings

- Blood chemistry: decreased sodium, potassium
- Hematology: increased WBCs
- Barium enema: stops at obstruction
- Abdominal X-rays: increased amount of gas in bowel

Medical management

- Diet: withhold food and fluids
- I.V. therapy: hydration, electrolyte replacement, saline lock
- GI decompression: NG tube, Miller-Abbott tube, Cantor tube
- Position: semi-Fowler's
- Activity: bed rest
- Monitoring: vital signs, and I/O
- Laboratory studies: sodium, potassium, and WBCs
- Treatments: indwelling urinary catheter, NG tube irrigation
- Antibiotic: gentamicin (Garamycin)
- Analgesic: meperidine (Demerol)
- Anticoagulation: low-molecular-weight heparin
- Sequential compression devices

Nursing interventions

- Withhold food and fluids
- Administer I.V. fluids
- Assess bowel sounds
- Measure and record the patient's abdominal girth
- Monitor and record the frequency, color, and amount of stools
- Maintain position, patency, and low suction of NG or Miller-Abbott tube
- Keep the patient in semi-Fowler's position
- Use sequential compression devices or administer low-molecular-weight heparin while on bed rest
- Have the patient ambulate as soon as possible
- Encourage incentive spirometry
- Monitor and record vital signs, I/O, and laboratory studies
- Administer medications, as prescribed
- Allay the patient's anxiety through verbalization and medication
- Provide nares and mouth care
- Provide information about the American Ostomy Association
- Individualize home care instructions
  - Avoid constipating foods
  - Monitor the frequency and color of stools
  - Recognize the signs and symptoms of diverticulitis

Complications

- Peritonitis
- Strangulation of bowel
- Infection
- Sepsis
- Bowel necrosis

Key test findings in an intestinal obstruction

- Barium enema: stops at obstruction
- Abdominal X-rays: increased amount of gas in bowel

Key ways to treat intestinal obstruction with GI decompression

- NG tube
- Miller-Abbott tube
- Cantor tube

Key nursing interventions for a patient with an intestinal obstruction

- Administer I.V. fluids.
- Assess bowel sounds.
- Measure and record the patient's abdominal girth.
- Maintain position, patency, and low suction of NG or Miller-Abbott tube.
- Have the patient ambulate as soon as possible.

- **Surgical interventions**
  - Bowel resection
  - Colostomy

PERITONITIS

Peritonitis defined
- Inflammation of the peritoneal cavity
- May be localized or generalized

Most common causes of peritonitis
- Bacterial infection
- Pancreatitis
- Blunt or penetrating trauma
- Inflammation of colon or kidneys
- Volvulus

Key assessment findings in peritonitis
- Constant, diffuse, and intense abdominal pain
- Rebound tenderness
- Elevated temperature
- Abdominal rigidity and distention
- Weak, rapid pulse
- Decreased or absent bowel sounds

- **Definition**
  - Localized or generalized inflammation of peritoneal cavity
- **Causes**
  - Bacterial infection
  - Pancreatitis
  - Blunt or penetrating trauma
  - Inflammation of colon or kidneys
  - Volvulus
  - Intestinal ischemia
  - Intestinal obstruction
  - Peptic ulceration
  - Biliary tract disease
  - Neoplasms
  - Nephrosis
  - Cirrhosis
  - Intestinal perforation
- **Pathophysiology**
  - Peritoneal irritants cause inflammatory edema, vascular congestion, and hypermotility of the bowel
  - Movement of extracellular fluid into the peritoneal cavity leads to hypovolemia and decreased urine output
- **Assessment findings**
  - Constant, diffuse, and intense abdominal pain
  - **Rebound tenderness**
  - Malaise
  - Nausea
  - Elevated temperature
  - **Abdominal rigidity and distention**
  - Anorexia
  - Decreased urine output
  - Shallow respirations
  - Weak, rapid pulse
  - Decreased peristalsis
  - Decreased or absent bowel sounds
  - Abdominal resonance and tympany on percussion
- **Diagnostic test findings**
  - Hematology: increased WBCs and HCT
  - Peritoneal aspiration: positive for blood, pus, bile, bacteria, or amylase
  - Abdominal X-ray: free air in abdomen under diaphragm

Medical management

- Diet: withhold food and fluids
- I.V. therapy: hydration, electrolyte replacement, saline lock
- GI decompression: NG tube
- Position: semi-Fowler's
- Activity: bed rest
- Monitoring: vital signs, I/O, CVP, and urine specific gravity
- Laboratory studies: Hb, HCT, potassium, sodium, calcium, osmolality, and WBCs
- Nutritional support: TPN
- Treatments: indwelling urinary catheter, incentive spirometry, SCDs
- Antibiotics: gentamicin (Garamycin), clindamycin (Cleocin), cephalothin (Keflin), ampicillin or sulbactam (Unasyn)
- Analgesic: meperidine (Demerol)
- Anticoagulant: low-molecular-weight heparin

Nursing interventions

- Withhold food and fluids
- Administer I.V. fluids
- Provide turning, coughing, and deep breathing, and incentive spirometry
- Assess respiratory status and fluid balance
- Maintain position, patency, and low suction of NG tube
- Keep the patient in semi-Fowler's position
- Apply sequential compression devices while on bed rest
- Monitor and record vital signs, I/O, laboratory studies, CVP, daily weight, and urine specific gravity
- Administer TPN
- Administer medications, as prescribed
- Allay the patient's anxiety
- Provide nares and mouth care
- Turn the patient every 2 hours
- Maintain bed rest
- Assess pain and administer analgesics, as necessary
- Assess bowel sounds
- Measure and record the patient's abdominal girth
- Avoid giving the patient laxatives
- **Don't apply heat to the patient's abdomen**
- Individualize home care instructions
  - Recognize the signs and symptoms of infection
  - Monitor temperature daily
  - Recognize the signs and symptoms of GI obstruction

Complications

- Adhesions
- Abscesses
- Obstruction
- Septic shock
- Paralytic ileus

Key treatment options for a patient with peritonitis

- Diet: withhold food and fluids
- I.V. therapy: hydration, electrolyte replacement, saline lock
- GI decompression: NG tube
- Antibiotics

Key nursing interventions for a patient with peritonitis

- Withhold food and fluids.
- Maintain position, patency, and low suction of NG tube.
- Monitor and record vital signs, I/O, laboratory studies, CVP, daily weight, and urine specific gravity.
- Assess bowel sounds.
- Don't apply heat to the patient's abdomen.

Home care checklist for a patient with peritonitis

- Recognize the signs and symptoms of infection.
- Monitor temperature daily.
- Recognize the signs and symptoms of GI obstruction.

- **Surgical interventions**
  - Exploratory laparotomy
  - Bowel resection
  - Incision and drainage of abscess
  - Closure of perforation

Hemorrhoids highlights

- Congested and dilated vessels of the rectum and anus
- May be internal or external

HEMORRHOIDS

- **Definition**
  - Congested and dilated internal or external vessels of the rectum and anus
- **Causes**
  - Chronic constipation
  - Prolonged sitting or standing
  - Straining at defecation
  - Pregnancy
  - Heavy lifting
  - Portal hypertension
  - Heredity
  - Obesity
  - Anal infection

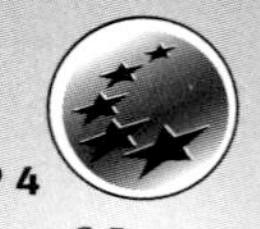

TOP 4

Causes of hemorrhoids

1. Chronic constipation
2. Prolonged sitting or standing
3. Straining at defecation
4. Pregnancy

- **Pathophysiology**
  - Increased abdominal pressure impairs blood flow through the hemorrhoidal venous plexus
  - Decreased blood flow causes dilation and congestion of the vessels of the rectum and anus
- **Assessment findings**
  - Anal pain with defecation, sitting, or walking
  - Anal pruritus
  - Protrusion of hemorrhoids
  - Rectal bleeding
  - Rectal mucus discharge
  - Bleeding during defecation
  - Sensation of incomplete fecal evacuation

Key assessment findings for hemorrhoids

- Anal pain with defecation, sitting, or walking
- Anal pruritus
- Rectal bleeding

- **Diagnostic test findings**
  - Digital examination: hemorrhoids
  - Barium enema: hemorrhoids
  - Proctoscopy: internal hemorrhoids
  - Hematology: decreased Hb and HCT
- **Medical management**
  - Diet: high-fiber, low-roughage with increased fluid intake
  - Position: side-lying or prone
  - Activity: as tolerated
  - Monitoring: vital signs, frequency of stools
  - Laboratory studies: Hb and HCT
  - Treatments: witch hazel compresses, sitz baths

- Corticosteroid: hydrocortisone (Hydrocortisone Cream)
- Analgesic: acetaminophen (Tylenol)
- Antipruritic: diphenhydramine (Benadryl)
- Stool softener: docusate (Colace)
- Anesthetic: lidocaine (Xylocaine)
- Laxative: magnesium hydroxide (milk of magnesia)
- Cryodestruction

Nursing interventions

- Maintain the patient's diet with increased fluids
- Assess bowel elimination and rectal bleeding
- Keep the patient on his side or prone while in bed
- Encourage ambulation
- Monitor and record vital signs, I/O, and laboratory studies
- Administer medications, as prescribed
- Allay the patient's anxiety through verbalization and medication
- Provide perineal care
- Administer sitz baths and witch hazel compresses for comfort
- Provide privacy and time for defecation
- Individualize home care instructions
  - Use sitz baths and witch hazel compresses for comfort
  - Defecate when urge is felt
  - Avoid constipation
  - Complete perineal care daily
  - Avoid prolonged sitting or standing
  - Avoid heavy lifting
  - Recognize the signs and symptoms of rectal bleeding

Complications

- Megacolon
- Diverticulitis
- Hemorrhage

Surgical interventions

- Hemorrhoidectomy
- Barron rubber-band ligation

COLORECTAL CANCER

Definition

- Malignant tumor of the colon or rectum that's primary or metastatic

Causes

- Diverticulosis
- Chronic ulcerative colitis
- Familial polyposis
- Aging
- Low-fiber, high-carbohydrate diet
- Chronic constipation

Key steps in managing hemorrhoids

- High-fiber, low-roughage diet with increased fluid intake
- Side-lying or prone position
- Treatments: witch hazel compresses, sitz baths
- Corticosteroid
- Laxative

Key nursing interventions for a patient with hemorrhoids

- Maintain the patient's diet with increased fluids.
- Assess bowel elimination and rectal bleeding.
- Keep the patient on his side or prone while in bed.
- Administer sitz baths and witch hazel compresses.

Key facts about colorectal cancer

- Malignant tumor of the colon or rectum
- May be primary or metastatic
- Key causes include diverticulosis, chronic ulcerative colitis, and familial polyposis

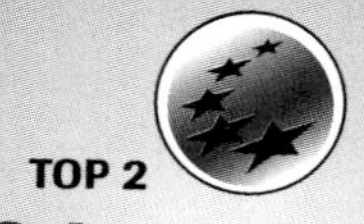
TOP 2

Colorectal cancer signs and symptoms

1. Rectal bleeding
2. Change in bowel habits

Key tests to diagnose colorectal cancer

- Fecal occult blood: positive
- Sigmoidoscopy: identification and location of mass

Key ways to manage colorectal cancer

- Radiation therapy
- Antineoplastics

Pathophysiology

- Unregulated cell growth and uncontrolled cell division result in the development of a neoplasm
- Metastasis commonly occurs in the liver
- Adenocarcinomas occur in the colon, rectum, jejunum, and duodenum
- Adenocarcinomas infiltrate and cause obstruction, ulcerations, and hemorrhage

Assessment findings

- Abdominal cramps
- Abdominal distention
- Diarrhea and constipation
- Weakness
- Pallor
- Weight loss
- Anorexia
- Change in shape of stool
- **Rectal bleeding**
- **Change in bowel habits**
- Fecal oozing
- Palpable mass
- Melena
- Vomiting

Diagnostic test findings

- Fecal occult blood: positive
- Hematology: decreased Hb and HCT; decreased PT and PTT, and International Normalized Ratio (INR)
- Sigmoidoscopy: identification and location of mass
- Barium enema: location of mass
- Biopsy: cytology positive for cancer cells
- CEA: positive
- GI series: location of mass

Medical management

- Diet: high-fiber, low-fat, low-refined carbohydrate
- I.V. therapy: saline lock
- Position: semi-Fowler's
- Activity: as tolerated
- Use sequential compression devices while on bed rest
- Monitoring: vital signs and I/O
- Laboratory studies: Hb and HCT
- Nutritional support: TPN
- Radiation therapy
- Antineoplastics: doxorubicin (Adriamycin), 5-fluorouracil (Adrucil)
- Immunomodulator: levamisole (Ergamisol)
- Folic acid derivative: leucovorin (citrovorum factor)
- Antiemetics: prochlorperazine (Compazine), ondansetron (Zofran)
- Anticoagulant: low-molecular-weight heparin

Nursing interventions

- Maintain the patient's diet
- Keep the patient in semi-Fowler's position
- Apply sequential compression devices while in bed
- Monitor and record vital signs, I/O, laboratory studies, and daily weight
- Administer TPN
- Administer medications, as prescribed
- Encourage the patient to express his feelings about changes in his body image and a fear of dying
- Provide skin and mouth care
- Provide rest periods
- Monitor and record the color, consistency, amount, and frequency of stools
- Assess for signs and symptoms of intestinal obstruction and rectal bleeding
- Provide postchemotherapeutic and postradiation nursing care
  - Provide prophylactic skin and mouth care
  - Monitor dietary intake
  - Administer antiemetics and antidiarrheals, as prescribed
  - Monitor for bleeding, infection, and electrolyte imbalance
  - Provide rest periods
- Provide information about the United Ostomy Association and the American Cancer Society
- Individualize home care instructions
  - Monitor changes in bowel elimination
  - Monitor self for infection
  - Alternate rest periods with activity

Complications

- Anemia
- Hemorrhage
- Intestinal obstruction

Surgical interventions

- Abdominoperineal resection
- Colostomy

CHOLECYSTITIS

Definition

- Acute or chronic inflammation of the gallbladder; most commonly associated with cholelithiasis

Causes

- Cholelithiasis: cholesterol, bile pigment, calcium stones
- Obesity
- Infection of the gallbladder
- Estrogen therapy

Key nursing interventions for a patient with colorectal cancer

- Encourage the patient to express his feelings about changes in his body image and a fear of dying.
- Provide postchemotherapeutic and postradiation nursing care.
- Provide information about the United Ostomy Association and the American Cancer Society.

Cholecystitis defined

- Inflammation of the gallbladder
- May be acute or chronic
- Commonly associated with cholelithiasis

Causes of cholecystitis

- Cholelithiasis
- Obesity
- Infection of the gallbladder
- Estrogen therapy

Key signs and symptoms of cholecystitis

- Indigestion or chest pain after eating fatty or fried foods
- Episodic colicky pain in epigastric area, which radiates to back and shoulder
- Jaundice
- Flatulence

Key test findings for cholecystitis

- Cholangiogram: stones in biliary tree
- Blood chemistry: increased alkaline phosphatase, bilirubin, direct bilirubin transaminase, amylase, lipase, AST, and LD

Key treatment options for a patient with cholecystitis

- Low-fat diet
- Vitamins

Pathophysiology

- Inflamed gallbladder can't contract in response to fatty foods entering the duodenum because of obstruction by calculi or edema
- Inability to constrict causes pain
- Accumulated bile is absorbed into the blood

Assessment findings

- Indigestion or chest pain after eating fatty or fried foods
- **Episodic colicky pain in epigastric area, which radiates to back and shoulder**
- **Jaundice**
- Nausea and vomiting
- Elevated temperature
- Flatulence
- Belching
- Clay-colored stools
- Dark amber urine
- Pruritus
- Ecchymosis
- Steatorrhea

Diagnostic test findings

- Cholangiogram: stones in biliary tree
- Gallbladder series: stones in biliary tree
- Ultrasound: bile duct distention and calculi
- Liver scan: obstruction of biliary tree
- Blood chemistry: increased alkaline phosphatase, bilirubin, direct bilirubin transaminase, amylase, lipase, AST, and LD
- Hematology: increased WBCs

Medical management

- Diet: two types
  - Low-fat, high-carbohydrate, high-protein, high-fiber, low-calorie meals in small, frequent feedings with restricted intake of gas-forming foods
  - No food and fluids, as directed
- I.V. therapy: hydration, electrolyte replacement, saline lock
- GI decompression: NG tube, Miller-Abbott tube
- Position: semi-Fowler's
- Activity: bed rest
- Monitoring: vital signs, I/O, and urine specific gravity
- Laboratory studies: amylase, lipase, bilirubin, alkaline phosphatase, and WBCs
- Treatments: incentive spirometry, tepid baths without soap
- Antilithic: chenodiol (Chenix)
- Antibiotic: cephalothin (Keflin)
- Analgesic: meperidine (Demerol)
- Anticholinergics: propantheline (Pro-Banthine), dicyclomine (Bentyl)
- Antiemetic: prochlorperazine (Compazine)
- Antipruritic: diphenhydramine (Benadryl)

- Vitamins: phytonadione (AquaMEPHYTON), cyanocobalamin (vitamin B_{12})
- ESWL
- Endoscopic sphincterotomy

Nursing interventions

- Maintain the patient's diet; withhold food and fluids
- Administer I.V. fluids
- Provide turning, coughing, deep breathing, and incentive spirometry
- Assess pain and administer analgesics, as indicated
- Maintain position, patency, and low suction of NG tube
- Keep the patient in semi-Fowler's position
- Monitor and record vital signs, I/O, laboratory studies, and urine specific gravity
- Administer medications, as prescribed
- Allay the patient's anxiety
- Provide skin, nares, and mouth care
- Have the patient ambulate, as tolerated
- Maintain a quiet environment
- Administer tepid baths without soap
- Prevent scratching if pruritus occurs
- Individualize home care instructions
  - Complete skin care daily
  - Recognize the signs and symptoms of renal colic

Complications

- Hemorrhage
- Cirrhosis
- Intestinal perforation
- Peritonitis
- Pancreatitis

Surgical interventions

- Cholecystectomy
- Choledochostomy
- Cholecystostomy
- Laparoscopic laser cholecystectomy

PANCREATITIS

Definition

- Acute or chronic inflammation of the pancreas with varying degrees of pancreatic edema, fat necrosis, and hemorrhage

Causes

- Biliary tract disease
- Alcoholism
- Hyperparathyroidism
- Hyperlipidemia
- Blunt trauma to pancreas or abdomen

Key nursing interventions for a patient with cholecystitis

- Withhold food and fluids.
- Assess pain and administer analgesics, as indicated.
- Maintain position, patency, and low suction of NG tube.

Pancreatitis defined

- Inflammation of the pancreas with varying degrees of pancreatic edema, fat necrosis, and hemorrhage
- May be acute or chronic

Common causes of pancreatitis

- Biliary tract disease
- Alcoholism
- Hyperparathyroidism
- Hyperlipidemia

Key assessment findings in pancreatitis

- Nausea and vomiting
- Tachycardia
- Abrupt onset of pain in epigastric area that radiates to the shoulder, substernal area, back, and flank
- Aching, burning, stabbing, pressing pain
- Abdominal tenderness and distention

Key test findings in pancreatitis

- Blood chemistry: increased amylase, lipase, LD, glucose, AST, and lipids; decreased calcium and potassium
- Turner's sign: positive
- Ultrasonography: cysts, bile duct inflammation and dilation
- Cullen's sign: positive

- Bacterial or viral infection
- Duodenal ulcer
- Medication induced: steroids, thiazide diuretics, hormonal contraceptives

Pathophysiology

- Acute: pancreatic enzymes are activated in the pancreas rather than the duodenum, resulting in tissue damage and autodigestion of the pancreas
- Chronic: chronic inflammation results in fibrosis and calcification of the pancreas, obstruction of the ducts, and destruction of the secreting acinar cells

Assessment findings

- Nausea and vomiting
- Tachycardia
- **Abrupt onset of pain in epigastric area that radiates to the shoulder, substernal area, back, and flank**
- **Aching, burning, stabbing, pressing pain**
- Abdominal tenderness and distention
- Elevated temperature
- Steatorrhea
- Weight loss
- Jaundice
- Hypotension
- Pain upon eating
- Dyspnea
- Decreased or absent bowel sounds
- Positioning knee-chest, fetal, or leaning forward for comfort

Diagnostic test findings

- Computed tomography (CT) scan: enlarged pancreas
- Blood chemistry: increased amylase, lipase, LD, glucose, AST, and lipids; decreased calcium and potassium
- Hematology: increased WBCs and RBCs
- Turner's sign (a bruiselike discoloration of the skin of the flanks): positive
- Ultrasonography: cysts, bile duct inflammation and dilation
- Cullen's sign (irregular, bluish hemorrhagic patches on the skin around the umbilicus): positive
- Urine chemistry: increased amylase
- Fecal fat: positive
- Arteriography: fibrous tissue and calcification of pancreas
- Glucose tolerance test: increased
- ERCP: biliary obstruction

Medical management

- Diet: low-fat, low-protein, high-carbohydrate in small, frequent feedings with restricted intake of caffeine, alcohol, and gas-forming foods
- I.V. therapy: hydration, electrolyte replacement, saline lock
- GI decompression: NG tube
- Position: semi-Fowler's
- Activity: bed rest

- Monitoring: vital signs, I/O, CVP, urine specific gravity, and urine glucose and ketones
- Laboratory studies: glucose, potassium, amylase, lipase, calcium, and lipids
- Nutritional support: TPN
- Transfusion therapy: packed RBCs
- Antibiotic: cephalothin (Keflin)
- Analgesic: morphine
- Anticholinergics: propantheline (Pro-Banthine), dicyclomine (Bentyl)
- Antacids: magnesium and aluminum hydroxide (Maalox), aluminum hydroxide gel (AlternaGEL)
- Corticosteroid: hydrocortisone (Solu-Cortef)
- Antiemetic: prochlorperazine (Compazine)
- Histamine antagonists: cimetidine (Tagamet), ranitidine (Zantac)
- Vitamins and minerals
- Tranquilizers: lorazepam (Ativan), alprazolam (Xanax)
- Digestants: pancrelipase (Viokase, Cotazym)
- Potassium supplements: potassium chloride (K-Lor), potassium gluconate (Kaon)
- Peritoneal lavage
- Dialysis
- Calcium supplements: calcium gluconate (Kalcinate), calcium carbonate (Os-Cal)
- Antidiabetic agent: insulin
- Mucosal barrier fortifier: sucralfate (Carafate)

Nursing interventions

- Maintain the patient's diet; withhold food and fluids, as necessary
- Administer I.V. fluids
- Assess fluid balance
- Assess GI, cardiac, and respiratory status
- Maintain position, patency, and low suction of NG tube
- Keep the patient in semi-Fowler's position
- Monitor and record vital signs, I/O, laboratory studies, CVP, daily weight, urine specific gravity, blood glucose levels, and urine glucose and ketones
- Administer TPN
- Administer medications, as prescribed
- Encourage incentive spirometry
- Allay the patient's anxiety through verbalization and medication
- Provide skin, nares, and mouth care
- Have the patient ambulate, as tolerated
- Provide a quiet, restful environment
- Monitor urine and stool for color, character, and amount
- Individualize home care instructions
  - Monitor glucose levels with blood glucose monitoring machine
  - Monitor stool for steatorrhea
  - Monitor self for infection
  - Recognize the signs and symptoms of increased blood glucose

Key ways to manage pancreatitis

- I.V. therapy: hydration, electrolyte replacement, saline lock
- Bed rest
- Transfusion therapy
- Analgesics
- Corticosteroids
- Potassium supplements
- Antidiabetic agents

Key nursing interventions for a patient with pancreatitis

- Assess fluid balance.
- Assess GI, cardiac, and respiratory status.
- Monitor and record vital signs, I/O, laboratory studies, CVP, daily weight, urine specific gravity, blood glucose levels, and urine glucose and ketones.

– Adhere to activity limitations
– Alternate rest periods with activity

Complications

- Ileus
- Hypovolemic shock
- Diabetes mellitus
- Infection
- Jaundice
- Pancreatic fistula
- Pancreatic abscess
- Hypocalcemia
- Septic shock

Key complications of pancreatitis

- Ileus
- Hypovolemic shock
- Diabetes mellitus
- Infection

Surgical intervention

- Pancreatectomy

HEPATIC CIRRHOSIS

Definition

- Chronic, progressive disease characterized by inflammation, fibrosis, and degeneration of liver parenchymal cells
- Three types of hepatic cirrhosis
  - Laënnec's (micronodular)
  - Postnecrotic (macronodular)
  - Biliary

Hepatic cirrhosis highlights

- Chronic, progressive disease
- Characterized by inflammation, fibrosis, and degeneration of liver parenchymal cells
- Three types: Laënnec's, postnecrotic, and biliary

Causes

- Alcohol use or abuse
- Malnutrition
- Viral hepatitis
- Cholecystitis
- Obstructions from neoplasms, strictures, or gallstones

Pathophysiology

- Inflammation causes liver parenchymal cell destruction, with subsequent fibrosis
- Fibrotic changes cause obstruction of hepatic blood flow and normal liver function
- Obstruction causes portal hypertension
- Decreased liver function results in changes in body chemistry
  - Decreased absorption and utilization of fat-soluble vitamins (A, D, E, and K)
  - Increased secretion of aldosterone
  - Ineffective detoxification of protein wastes
  - Prolonged clotting times

Changes in body chemistry with decreased liver function

- Decreased absorption and utilization of fat-soluble vitamins (A, D, E, and K)
- Increased secretion of aldosterone
- Ineffective detoxification of protein wastes
- Prolonged clotting times

Assessment findings

- Nausea and vomiting
- Weakness and fatigue

- Anorexia and weight loss
- Jaundice
- Ecchymosis
- Palmar erythema
- Indigestion
- Pruritus
- Irregular bowel habits
- Pain in the right upper quadrant
- Peripheral edema
- Petechiae
- Epistaxis
- Hematemesis
- Telangiectasis
- Gynecomastia and impotence
- Amenorrhea
- Hemorrhoids
- Hepatomegaly
- Melena
- Esophageal varices

Diagnostic test findings

- Blood chemistry: increased AST, ALT, LD, alkaline phosphatase, ammonia, bilirubin, and sulfobromophthalein test; decreased albumin and total protein
- Hematology: decreased Hb, HCT, and WBCs; increased PT, PTT, and INR
- Liver scan: fibrotic liver, increased uptake
- Liver biopsy: destruction of parenchymal cells
- Esophagoscopy: esophageal varices
- Arterial blood gas (ABG) analysis: metabolic acidosis, respiratory acidosis, respiratory alkalosis
- Urine chemistry: proteinuria
- CT scan: ascites

Medical management

- Diet: high-calorie, high-carbohydrate, low-fat, low-sodium in small, frequent feedings with restricted intake of alcohol and fluids
- I.V. therapy: hydration, electrolyte replacement, saline lock
- Oxygen therapy
- GI decompression: NG tube
- Position: semi-Fowler's
- Activity: bed rest
- Monitoring: vital signs, I/O, neurovital signs, ECG, hemodynamic variables, and stools for occult blood
- Laboratory studies: AST, ALT, LD, PT, amylase, lipase, Hb, HCT, bilirubin, albumin, WBCs, and ABG analysis
- Nutritional support: TPN, NG tube feedings
- Treatments: indwelling urinary catheter; incentive spirometry; tepid bath; cool, moist compresses

Key signs and symptoms of hepatic cirrhosis

- Nausea and vomiting
- Anorexia
- Jaundice
- Pain in the right upper quadrant

Key test findings in hepatic cirrhosis

- Blood chemistry: increased AST, ALT, LD, alkaline phosphatase, ammonia, bilirubin, and sulfobromophthalein test; decreased albumin and total protein
- Liver biopsy: destruction of parenchymal cells
- CT scan: ascites

Key treatment options for hepatic cirrhosis

- GI decompression: NG tube
- Transfusion therapy: platelets, packed RBCs, FFP
- Hemostatic
- Diuretics
- Ammonia detoxicant
- Vitamins
- Abdominal paracentesis
- Balloon tamponade of varices: Sengstaken-Blakemore tube

Key nursing interventions for a patient with hepatic cirrhosis

- Assess respiratory status, GI bleeding, and fluid balance.
- Assess for bleeding.
- Monitor and record vital signs, I/O, laboratory studies, hemodynamic variables, daily weight, urine specific gravity, fecal occult blood, and neurovital signs.
- Prevent scratching and administer antipruritic medication, as needed.
- Use small-gauge needles to decrease risk of bleeding.
- Apply prolonged pressure after venipuncture.
- Observe for signs of behavioral or personality changes.
- Monitor ammonia levels.
- Provide information on Alcoholics Anonymous or make a referral to a treatment program.

- Precautions: standard
- Transfusion therapy: platelets, packed RBCs, fresh frozen plasma (FFP)
- Antibiotic: neomycin (Neobiotic)
- Hemostatic: vasopressin (Pitressin)
- Diuretics: spironolactone (Aldactone), furosemide (Lasix)
- Sedative: phenobarbital (Luminal)
- Stool softener: docusate (Colace)
- Ammonia detoxicant: lactulose (Cephulac)
- Vitamins: phytonadione (AquaMEPHYTON), cyanocobalamin (vitamin B_{12})
- Antacids: magnesium and aluminum hydroxide (Maalox), aluminum hydroxide gel (AlternaGEL)
- Analgesic: oxycodone (Tylox)
- Enzyme replacement: pancrelipase (Viokase)
- Endoscopy sclerotherapy: ethanolamine (Ethamolin)
- Abdominal paracentesis
- Balloon tamponade of varices: Sengstaken-Blakemore tube

Nursing interventions

- Maintain the patient's diet; withhold food and fluids, as necessary
- Administer I.V. fluids
- Administer oxygen
- Provide turning, coughing, deep breathing, and incentive spirometry
- Assess respiratory status, GI bleeding, and fluid balance
- Assess for bleeding
- Maintain position, patency, and low suction of NG tube
- Keep the patient in semi-Fowler's position
- Monitor and record vital signs, I/O, laboratory studies, hemodynamic variables, daily weight, urine specific gravity, fecal occult blood, and neurovital signs
- Observe for signs of behavioral or personality changes
- Monitor ammonia levels
- Measure and record the patient's abdominal girth
- Monitor for infection
- Administer TPN
- Administer medications, as prescribed
- Allay the patient's anxiety through verbalization and medication
- Provide skin, nares, and mouth care
- Maintain standard precautions
- Maintain bed rest
- Maintain a quiet environment
- Administer tepid baths without soap; apply cool, moist compresses
- Prevent scratching and administer antipruritic medication, as needed
- Use small-gauge needles to decrease risk of bleeding; avoid I.M. injections where possible
- Apply prolonged pressure after venipuncture
- Monitor stool for color, consistency, and amount
- Provide information on Alcoholics Anonymous (AA) or make a referral to a treatment program

- Individualize home care instructions
  - Avoid using OTC medications
  - Avoid drinking alcohol
  - Avoid exposure to people with infections
  - Know the action, adverse effects, and scheduling of medications
  - Complete skin care daily
  - Avoid straining while defecating, vigorously blowing nose, coughing, and using a hard toothbrush
  - Eat the same amounts of green vegetables daily
  - Keep appointments for blood work

Complications

- Ascites
- Esophageal varices
- Hemorrhoids
- Hemorrhage
- Estrogen and androgen imbalance
- Portal hypertension
- Hepatic coma
- Pancytopenia

Surgical interventions

- Portacaval shunt
- LeVeen peritoneovenous shunt
- TIPS

Home care instructions for a patient with hepatic cirrhosis

- Avoid using OTC medications.
- Avoid drinking alcohol.
- Avoid exposure to people with infections.
- Know the action, adverse effects, and scheduling of medications.
- Complete skin care daily.
- Avoid straining while defecating, vigorously blowing nose, coughing, and using a hard toothbrush.
- Eat the same amounts of green vegetables daily.
- Keep appointments for blood work.

HEPATITIS

Definition

- Inflammation of the liver
- Five types of hepatitis (see *Viral hepatitis from A to E,* pages 242 and 243)
  - Hepatitis A
  - Hepatitis B
  - Hepatitis C
  - Hepatitis D
  - Hepatitis E

Causes, transmission

- Hepatitis A: Contaminated food (usually by preparers with poor hand washing), milk, water, feces (food-borne most common)
- Hepatitis B: Parenteral, sexual, oral, transmitted through contact with any infected body fluid
- Hepatitis C: Blood or serum (blood transfusions, exposure to contaminated blood), transmitted through contact with any infected body fluid
- Hepatitis D: Similar to type B virus (HBV); can only become active in presence of HBV
- Hepatitis E: Fecal (usually from contact with sewage-contaminated water), oral route

Key characteristics of hepatitis

- Inflammation of liver tissue causes inflammation of hepatic cells, hypertrophy, and proliferation of Kupffer's cells and bile stasis
- Five types: hepatitis A, hepatitis B, hepatitis C, hepatitis D, and hepatitis E

Incubation period for the types of hepatitis

- Hepatitis A: 15 to 45 days
- Hepatitis B: 30 to 180 days
- Hepatitis C: 15 to 160 days
- Hepatitis D: 14 to 64 days
- Hepatitis E: 14 to 60 days

Key preicteric symptoms of hepatitis

- Fatigue
- Weight loss
- Right upper quadrant pain
- Pruritus

Viral hepatitis from A to E

This chart compares the features of each (characterized) type of viral hepatitis. Other types are emerging.

FEATURE	HEPATITIS A	HEPATITIS B
Incubation	15 to 45 days	30 to 180 days
Onset	Acute	Insidious
Age group most affected	Children, young adults	Any age
Transmission	Fecal-oral, sexual (especially oral-anal contact), nonpercutaneous (sexual, maternal-neonatal), percutaneous (rare)	Blood-borne; parenteral route, sexual, maternal-neonatal; virus is shed in all body fluids
Severity	Mild	Often severe
Prognosis	Generally good	Worsens with age and debility
Progression to chronicity	None	Occasional

Pathophysiology

- Inflammation of liver tissue causes inflammation of hepatic cells, hypertrophy, and proliferation of Kupffer's cells and bile stasis
- Type A virus (HAV) is transmitted by fecal or oral route and causes hepatitis A
- HBV is transmitted by blood and body fluids and causes hepatitis B

Assessment findings

- Preicteric
  - Anorexia
  - Nausea and vomiting
  - Fatigue
  - Constipation and diarrhea
  - Weight loss
  - Right upper quadrant pain
  - Hepatomegaly
  - Splenomegaly
  - Malaise
  - Elevated temperature
  - Pharyngitis

HEPATITIS C	HEPATITIS D	HEPATITIS E
15 to 160 days	14 to 64 days	14 to 60 days
Insidious	Acute and chronic	Acute
More common in adults	Any age	Ages 20 to 40
Blood-borne; parenteral route	Parenteral route; most people infected with hepatitis D are also infected with hepatitis B	Primarily fecal-oral
Moderate	Can be severe and lead to fulminant hepatitis	Highly virulent with common progression to fulminant hepatitis and hepatic failure, especially in pregnant patients
Moderate	Fair, worsens in chronic cases; can lead to chronic hepatitis D and chronic liver disease	Good unless pregnant
10% to 50% of cases	Occasional	None

  - Nasal discharge
  - Headache
  - Pruritus
- Icteric
  - Fatigue
  - Weight loss
  - **Clay-colored stools**
  - **Dark urine**
  - Hepatomegaly
  - Jaundice
  - Splenomegaly
  - Pruritus
- Posticteric
  - Fatigue
  - Decreasing hepatomegaly
  - Decreasing jaundice
  - Improved appetite

Severity of the types of hepatitis

- Hepatitis A: mild
- Hepatitis B: often severe
- Hepatitis C: moderate
- Hepatitis D: fair; worsens in chronic cases
- Hepatitis E: good, unless pregnant

Key icteric symptoms of hepatitis

- Fatigue
- Weight loss
- Clay-colored stools
- Dark urine

Key posticteric symptoms of hepatitis

- Fatigue
- Decreasing hepatomegaly
- Decreasing jaundice

Diagnostic test findings

- Blood chemistry: increased ALT, AST, alkaline phosphatase, LD, bilirubin, ESR, positive anti-HAV (IgM) or positive hepatitis B surface antigen (HB_sAg)
- Hematology: increased PT
- Sulfobromophthalein: increased
- Urine chemistry: increased urobilinogen
- Stool: HAV

Blood chemistry findings

- Increased ALT, AST, alkaline phosphatase, LD, bilirubin, ESR
- Positive anti-HAV (IgM) or positive HB_sAg

Medical management

- Diet: high-calorie, moderate-protein, high-carbohydrate, and low-fat
- Activity: bed rest
- Monitoring: vital signs and I/O
- Laboratory studies: ALT, AST, LD, bilirubin, PT, and PTT
- Precautions: standard
- Antiemetic: prochlorperazine (Compazine)
- Vitamins and minerals: vitamin K (AquaMEPHYTON), vitamin C and B-complex

Key medical therapies for hepatitis

- Vitamins and minerals
- High-calorie, moderate protein, high-carbohydrate, low-fat diet

Nursing interventions

- Maintain the patient's diet
- Monitor and record vital signs, I/O, and laboratory studies
- Administer medications, as prescribed
- Allay the patient's anxiety
- Maintain standard precautions
- Provide rest periods
- Encourage small, frequent meals
- Avoid skin irritation
- Prevent complications of bleeding
- Individualize home care instructions
  - Administer gamma globulin to individuals exposed to hepatitis
  - Avoid exposure to people with infections
  - Avoid alcohol
  - Maintain good personal hygiene
  - Refrain from donating blood
  - Increase fluid intake to 3 L/day
  - Abstain from sexual intercourse until serum liver studies are within normal limits

Key nursing interventions for a patient with hepatitis

- Provide rest periods.
- Encourage small, frequent meals.
- Avoid skin irritation.
- Prevent complications of bleeding.

Complications

- Pancreatitis
- Aplastic anemia
- Glomerulonephritis
- Vasculitis
- Cirrhosis

Surgical interventions

- None

ESOPHAGEAL VARICES

Definition
- Dilation of esophageal veins in the lower part of the esophagus

Causes
- Portal hypertension
- Increased intra-abdominal pressure
- Alcohol abuse
- Cirrhosis

Pathophysiology
- Venous drainage from the liver into the portal vein is decreased
- Drainage obstruction results in portal hypertension
- Return of venous blood from the intestinal tract and spleen to the right atrium via the collateral circulation is obstructed
- The increased pressure dilates the esophageal veins, which then protrude into the esophageal lumen

Assessment findings
- Anorexia
- Nausea and vomiting
- Hematemesis
- Fatigue and weakness
- Splenomegaly
- Ascites
- Peripheral edema
- Melena
- Dysphagia
- Pallor

Diagnostic test findings
- Hematology: increased PT; decreased RBCs, Hb, and HCT
- Blood chemistry: increased BUN, LD, and AST; decreased albumin
- Barium swallow: narrowed and irregular esophagus
- Esophagoscopy: varices

Medical management
- Diet: soft; withhold food and fluids with active bleeding
- I.V. therapy: hydration, saline lock
- Oxygen therapy
- GI decompression: NG tube
- Position: semi-Fowler's
- Activity: bed rest
- Monitoring: vital signs and I/O
- Laboratory studies: Hb, HCT, PT, and PTT
- Treatments: indwelling urinary catheter
- Transfusion therapy: packed RBCs and FFP
- Esophageal balloon tamponade: Sengstaken-Blakemore or Minnesota tube

Esophageal varices defined
- Dilation of esophageal veins in the lower part of the esophagus
- After the esophageal veins dilate, they protrude into the esophageal lumen

Key assessment findings in esophageal varices
- Hematemesis
- Melena

Key test findings in esophageal varices
- Hematology: increased PT; decreased RBCs, Hb, and HCT
- Blood chemistry: increased BUN, LD, and AST; decreased albumin

Key treatment options for a patient with esophageal varices

- Food and fluid restrictions with active bleeding
- I.V. therapy: hydration
- Transfusion therapy: packed RBCs and FFP
- Esophageal balloon tamponade: Sengstaken-Blakemore or Minnesota tube
- Endoscopy sclerotherapy
- Hormones
- Vitamins
- Iced saline lavage by NG tube

Key nursing interventions for a patient with esophageal varices

- Maintain position, patency, and low suction of NG tube and Sengstaken-Blakemore tube.
- Check for signs of bleeding.
- Avoid activities that increase intra-abdominal pressure.
- Assess level of consciousness and impending encephalopathy.

Key home care instructions for a patient with esophageal varices

- Monitor stools for occult blood.
- Avoid lifting and straining.
- Avoid using alcohol.

- Paracentesis
- Endoscopy sclerotherapy: ethanolamine (Ethamolin)
- Diuretic: furosemide (Lasix)
- Hormone: I.V. vasopressin (Pitressin) with nitroglycerin therapy or octreotide (Sandostatin)
- Antacids: magnesium and aluminum hydroxide (Maalox), aluminum hydroxide gel (AlternaGEL)
- Histamine antagonists: cimetidine (Tagamet), ranitidine (Zantac)
- Vitamins: vitamin K (AquaMEPHYTON)
- Iced saline lavage by NG tube
- Stool softener: docusate (Colace)
- Mucosal barrier fortifier: sucralfate (Carafate)

Nursing interventions

- Withhold food and fluids
- Administer I.V. fluids
- Administer oxygen
- Assess cardiovascular and respiratory status
- Maintain position, patency, and low suction of NG tube and Sengstaken-Blakemore tube
  - Maintain emergency measures for gastric balloon rupture
  - Have suction, scissors to cut tube available
- Keep the patient in semi-Fowler's position
- Monitor and record vital signs, I/O, laboratory studies, CVP, and daily weight
- Administer medications, as prescribed
- Allay the patient's anxiety
- Provide nares and mouth care
- Minimize environmental stress
- Check for signs of bleeding
- Avoid activities that increase intra-abdominal pressure
- Monitor and record amount, color, frequency, and consistency of stools
- Assess level of consciousness and impending encephalopathy
- Provide information about AA or refer to a treatment program
- Individualize home care instructions
  - Monitor stools for occult blood
  - Avoid lifting and straining
  - Avoid using alcohol

Complications

- Hemorrhage
- Shock
- Metabolic imbalance

Surgical interventions

- Ligation of varices
- Portacaval shunt
- Splenorenal shunt
- Mesocaval shunt
- TIPS

GASTROESOPHAGEAL REFLUX DISEASE (GERD)

Definition
- Backflow of gastric or duodenal contents into the esophagus and past the lower esophageal sphincter (LES)

Causes
- Impaired LES functioning
- Increased intra-abdominal pressure — for example, obesity, pregnancy, constricting waistline, and bending over
- Hiatal hernia
- Alcohol ingestion
- Smoking
- Gastric distention such as from large meals or ascites
- Prolonged NG intubation
- Ingestion of peppermint or spearmint
- Medications, such as morphine, calcium channel blockers, anticholinergics, and nitrates

Pathophysiology
- Reflux occurs when LES pressure is deficient or when pressure within the stomach exceeds LES pressure (see *How heartburn occurs,* page 248)
- Acidic contents cause injury and inflammation to esophageal mucosa

Assessment findings
- Dyspepsia (pyrosis or heartburn) in epigastric region, may radiate to jaw or arms, occurs after meals
- Pain worsens with lying down or bending over
- Hypersalivation (water brash)
- Regurgitation of warm, sour, or bitter fluid in throat

Diagnostic test findings
- Esophageal acidity tests: reveals reflux
- Endoscopy: allows visualization and confirmation of pathologic changes in the mucosa
- Barium swallow: identifies hiatal hernia as the cause
- Esophageal manometry: evaluates LES pressure

Medical management
- Diet: small, frequent meals; avoid meals before bedtime
- Fluids: increase fluid intake
- Position: upright during and after meals; sleep with head of bed elevated
- Antacids: magnesium and aluminum hydroxide (Maalox), aluminum hydroxide gel (AlternaGEL)
- H_2-antagonists: cimetidine (Tagamet), ranitidine (Zantac), famotidine (Pepcid), nizatidine (Axid)
- Proton pump inhibitors: omeprazole (Prilosec), lansoprazole (Prevacid)
- Cholinergic agents: bethanechol (Urecholine)
- Smoking cessation

Key characteristics of GERD
- Backflow of gastric or duodenal contents into the esophagus and past the LES
- Acidic contents cause injury and inflammation to esophageal mucosa

Key causes of GERD
- Impaired LES functioning
- Increased intra-abdominal pressure
- Hiatal hernia
- Alcohol ingestion

Common assessment findings in GERD
- Dyspepsia (pyrosis or heartburn) in epigastric region, may radiate to jaw or arms, occurs after meals
- Pain worsens with lying down or bending over
- Regurgitation of warm, sour, or bitter fluid in throat

Key ways to manage GERD
- Fluids: increase fluid intake
- Position: upright during and after meals; sleep with head of bed elevated
- Antacids
- H_2-antagonists
- Proton pump inhibitors
- Cholinergic agents

What happens in heartburn

- Hormonal fluctuations, mechanical stress, and the effects of certain foods and drugs can lower LES pressure.
- When LES pressure falls and intra-abdominal or intragastric pressure rises, the normally contracted LES relaxes inappropriately and allows reflux of gastric acid or bile secretions in the lower esophagus.
- The reflux irritates and inflames the esophageal mucosa, causing pyrosis.

Nursing interventions for a patient with GERD

- Maintain an upright position during and after meals.
- Provide information on alcohol and smoking cessation.
- Individualize home care instructions such as instructing the patient to eat small, frequent meals.

How heartburn occurs

Hormonal fluctuations, mechanical stress, and the effects of certain foods and drugs can decrease lower esophageal sphincter (LES) pressure. When LES pressure falls and intra-abdominal or intragastric pressure rises, the normally contracted LES relaxes inappropriately and allows reflux of gastric acid or bile secretions into the lower esophagus. There, the reflux irritates and inflames the esophageal mucosa, causing pyrosis.

Persistent inflammation can cause LES pressure to decrease even more and may trigger a recurrent cycle of reflux and pyrosis.

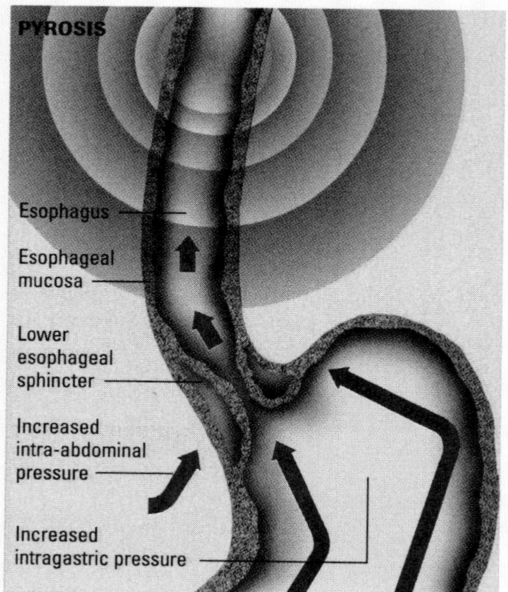

Nursing interventions

- Maintain patient's diet with small frequent feedings
- Maintain an upright position during and after meals
- Monitor and record vital signs, I/O, and laboratory studies
- Monitor respiratory status
- Provide information on alcohol and smoking cessation
- Encourage increased fluid intake
- Administer medications, as prescribed
- Individualize home care instructions
  - Eat small, frequent meals
  - Maintain prescribed position during and after meals and during sleep
  - Recognize signs and symptoms of reflux
  - Follow alcohol and smoking cessation
  - Identify ways to avoid increasing intra-abdominal pressure

Complications

- Barrett's epithelium
- Esophagitis with possible ulceration
- Esophageal stricture
- Bleeding
- Aspiration pneumonia
- Tracheoesophageal fistula

- **Surgical interventions**
  - Belsey Mark IV operation (invaginates the esophagus into the stomach)
  - Hill or Nissen procedures (creates a gastric wraparound with or without fixation)
  - Vagotomy
  - Pyloroplasty

APPENDICITIS

- **Definition**
  - Inflammation of the appendix
- **Causes**
  - Mucosal ulceration
  - Fecal mass
  - Stricture
  - Barium ingestion
  - Viral infection
  - Parasitic infection
- **Pathophysiology**
  - Lumen of the appendix becomes obstructed and inflammation occurs
  - Mucosa continues to secrete fluid and pressure in lumen of appendix increases
  - Blood flow is restricted and infection occurs
  - Gangrene from hypoxia or perforation may occur
- **Assessment findings**
  - Generalized abdominal pain that becomes localized in right lower abdomen
  - Anorexia
  - Nausea
  - Vomiting
  - Abdominal rigidity (boardlike)
  - Rebound tenderness
  - Low-grade fever (late sign)
  - Sudden cessation of pain (indicates rupture)
- **Diagnostic test findings**
  - Hematology: elevated WBCs
  - Ultrasound: inflammation of the appendix
  - CT scan: enlarged appendix
- **Medical management**
  - Diet: nothing by mouth
  - I.V. therapy: fluid and electrolyte replacement, saline lock
  - GI decompression: NG tube
  - Position: Fowler's
  - Activity: bed rest
  - Monitoring: vital signs, I/O, and laboratory values
  - Antibiotics

Appendicitis defined

- Inflammation of the appendix
- Blood flow is restricted and infection occurs

Most common causes of appendicitis

- Mucosal ulceration
- Fecal mass
- Stricture

Key assessment findings in appendicitis

- Abdominal rigidity
- Rebound tenderness
- Generalized abdominal pain that becomes localized in right lower abdomen
- Anorexia

- Analgesics: meperidine (Demerol), morphine

Key medical options for appendicitis

- GI decompression: NG tube
- Antibiotics
- Analgesics

Nursing interventions

- Withhold food and fluids
- Administer I.V. fluids
- Assess GI status and fluid balance
- Maintain position, patency, and low suction of NG tube
- Keep the patient in Fowler's position
- Monitor and record vital signs, I/O, and laboratory studies
- Administer medications, as prescribed
- Allay the patient's anxiety verbally and with medications
- Maintain bed rest
- **Never administer cathartics or enemas because they may rupture the appendix**
- **Never apply heat to the right lower abdomen; this may cause the appendix to rupture**
- Individualize home care instructions
  - Follow activity restrictions
  - Recognize signs and symptoms of infection

Key nursing interventions for a patient with appendicitis

- Withhold food and fluids.
- Never administer cathartics or enemas because they may rupture the appendix.
- Never apply heat to the right lower abdomen (may cause the appendix to rupture).

Complications

- Peritonitis
- Infection
- Intra-abdominal abscess
- Intestinal obstruction
- Fecal fistula
- Death

Surgical intervention

- Appendectomy

GASTROENTERITIS

Definition

- Inflammation of the digestive tract

Gastroenteritis highlights

- Inflammation of the digestive tract
- Common causes include amoebae, bacteria, and drug reactions

Causes

- Amoebae, especially *Entamoeba histolytica*
- Bacteria (responsible for acute food poisoning): *Staphylococcus aureus, Salmonella, Shigella, Clostridium botulinum, Escherichia coli, C. perfringens*
- Drug reactions (especially antibiotics)
- Enzyme deficiencies
- Food allergens
- Ingestion of toxins: plants or toadstools
- Parasites: *Ascaris, Enterobius, Trichinella spiralis*
- Viruses (may be responsible for traveler's diarrhea): adenovirus, echovirus, or coxsackievirus

Pathophysiology

- Infecting organism may attack the intestinal mucosa through the release of an enterotoxin
- The organism may attach to the mucosal epithelium, destroying the intestinal villi
- The organism may overwork the absorptive capacity of the small bowel
- The result is hypermotility of the GI tract, leading to altered secretions of fluids and electrolytes

Assessment findings

- **Watery, frequent diarrhea**
- Vomiting
- Increased or hyperactive bowel sounds
- Nausea
- Abdominal tenderness
- Malaise
- Signs and symptoms of dehydration, if prolonged

Diagnostic test findings

- Stool culture: identifies the organism
- Blood culture: identifies the organism

Medical management

- Diet: advance diet from clear liquid to soft foods, as tolerated
- Nutritional support
- I.V. therapy: fluid and electrolyte replacement, saline lock
- Activity: as tolerated, bed rest with acute episodes
- Monitoring: vital signs, I/O, and laboratory tests
- Antibiotics
- Bismuth-containing compounds: bismuth subsalicylate (Pepto Bismol)
- Antiemetics: prochlorperazine (Compazine), trimethobenzamide (Tigan)

Nursing interventions

- Maintain the patient's diet: advance diet as tolerated
- Assess GI status and fluid balance
- Monitor and record vital signs, I/O, daily weight, and laboratory studies
- Administer medications, as ordered
- Allay the patient's anxiety
- Provide skin and perianal care using moisture-barrier products
- Provide warm compresses or sitz baths for anal irritation
- Maintain bed rest with acute episodes
- **Report infection to local health department, depending on the type of gastroenteritis**
- Individualize home care instructions
  - Use proper hand-washing technique
  - Take warm sitz baths
  - Recognize signs and symptoms of gastroenteritis

Complications

- Dehydration

Key signs of gastroenteritis

- Watery, frequent diarrhea
- Vomiting
- Nausea
- Abdominal tenderness

Key treatment options for gastroenteritis

- I.V. therapy: fluid and electrolyte replacement
- Bismuth-containing compounds
- Antiemetics

Key nursing interventions for a patient with gastroenteritis

- Assess GI status and fluid balance.
- Provide skin and perianal care using moisture-barrier products.
- Provide warm compresses or sitz baths for anal irritation.

- Sepsis
- Death

Surgical interventions
- None

Key facts about IBS
- Functional GI disorder
- Characterized by chronic diarrhea, abdominal pain, and bloating

Common symptoms of IBS
- Diarrhea, constipation, or both
- Mucus with stool passage
- Abdominal pain or cramps
- Abdominal distention

Key ways to manage IBS
- Avoidance of food irritants
- Antidiarrheals
- Antispasmodics
- Stress management and behavior modification

IRRITABLE BOWEL SYNDROME (IBS)

Definition
- A functional GI disorder characterized by chronic diarrhea, constipation, abdominal pain, and bloating

Causes
- Stress
- Ingestion of irritants
- Lactose intolerance
- Hormonal changes

Pathophysiology
- Impaired motor function of the GI tract, results in changes in normal bowel elimination patterns
- Follows pattern of remissions and exacerbations

Assessment findings
- Diarrhea, constipation, or both
- Abdominal pain or cramps relieved by defecation
- Abdominal distention
- Mucus with stool passage
- Flatus
- Pasty, pencil-like stools

Diagnostic test findings
- Barium enema: may reveal colonic spasm
- Sigmoidoscopy or colonoscopy: normal bowel mucosa, spastic contractions
- Stool culture: to rule out ova, parasites, and bacteria
- Lactose intolerance testing: to rule out lactose intolerance
- Rectal biopsy: to rule out malignancy

Medical management
- Diet: avoid food irritants
- I.V. therapy: saline lock
- Activity: as tolerated
- Monitoring: vital signs, I/O, and laboratory values
- Antidiarrheal: diphenoxylate with atropine (Lomotil), loperamide (Imodium)
- Antispasmodic: propantheline (Pro-Banthine), hyoscyamine (Levbid), dicyclomine (Bentyl)
- Bulk-forming laxatives for constipation
- Calcium channel blockers
- Stress management and behavior modification

Nursing interventions
- Identify dietary habit and food irritants

- Assess GI status and fluid balance
- Monitor and record vital signs, I/O, and laboratory values
- Administer medications, as prescribed
- Teach stress-management techniques
- Allay the patient's anxiety through verbalization and medications
- Provide skin and perianal care
- Monitor the number, amount, and character of stools
- Individualize home care instructions
  - Take medications, as directed
  - Exercise regularly
  - Practice stress-management techniques
  - Avoid food irritants

Complications

- Malnutrition
- Dehydration
- Malabsorption

Surgical interventions

- None

Key nursing steps in caring for a patient with IBS

- Identify dietary habit and food irritants.
- Assess GI status and fluid balance.
- Teach stress-management techniques.

CHOLELITHIASIS

Definition

- Stones or calculi (gallstones) in the gallbladder (see *Common sites of calculi formation,* page 254)

Causes

- Pregnancy
- Hormonal contraceptives
- Diabetes
- Celiac disease
- Cirrhosis of the liver
- Pancreatitis

Pathophysiology

- Results from changes in bile components
- Stones are made up of cholesterol and calcium bilirubinate or a mixture of cholesterol and bilirubin pigment
- Stones arise during periods of sluggishness in the gallbladder

Assessment findings

- Attacks commonly follow meals rich in fats or at night, suddenly awakening the patient
- Acute abdominal pain in the right upper quadrant; may radiate to back, between the shoulders
- Recurring fat intolerance
- Biliary colic
- Belching
- Flatulence

Cholelithiasis defined

- Stones or calculi in the gallbladder
- Results from changes in bile components
- Stones arise during periods of sluggishness in the gallbladder

Key signs and symptoms of cholelithiasis

- Attacks commonly follow meals rich in fats or at night, suddenly awakening the patient
- Acute abdominal pain in the right upper quadrant; may radiate to back, between the shoulders
- Flatulence
- Nausea
- Vomiting

Sites of calculi formation

- Liver
- Small bile duct
- Hepatic duct
- Cystic duct
- Pancreas
- Common bile duct
- Pancreatic ducts
- Greater duodenal papilla
- Gallbladder
- Duodenum

Key test findings in cholelithiasis

- Laboratory tests: elevated total bilirubin, urine bilirubin, amylase, lipase, AST, LD, and alkaline phosphatase
- Cholangiogram: reveals stones in the biliary tree

Common sites of calculi formation

The illustration below shows sites where calculi typically collect. Stones vary in size; small stones may travel.

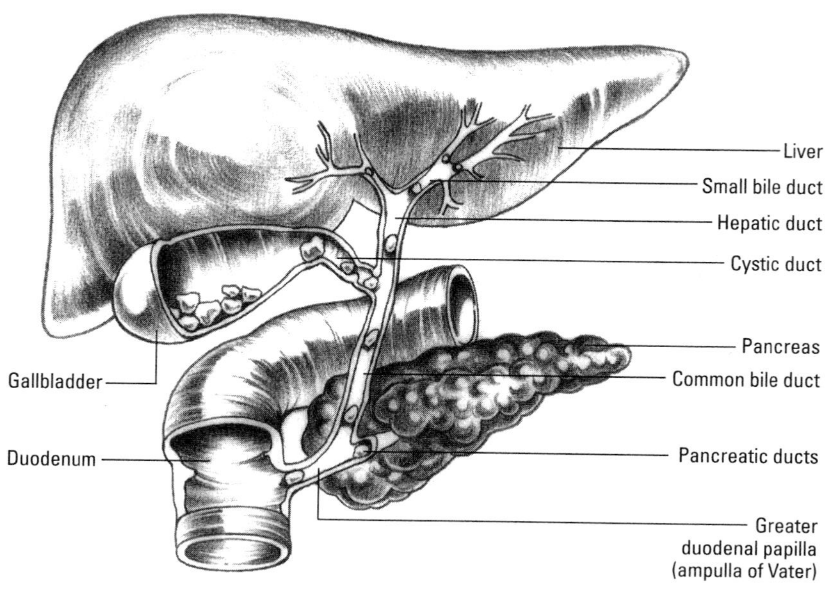

- Indigestion
- Diaphoresis
- Nausea
- Vomiting
- Chills
- Low-grade fever
- Jaundice
- Clay-colored stools

Diagnostic test findings

- Echography and X-rays: detect gallstones
- Ultrasound: reflects gallstones
- Gallbladder nuclear scan: detects obstruction of the cystic duct
- Flat plate of the abdomen: identifies calcified, but not cholesterol, stones
- Oral cholecystography: shows stones in the gallbladder and biliary duct obstruction
- Laboratory tests: reveal elevated total bilirubin, urine bilirubin, amylase, lipase, AST, LD, and alkaline phosphatase
- Cholangiogram: reveals stones in the biliary tree

Medical management

- Diet: nothing by mouth during an acute attack

- I.V. therapy: fluid replacement, saline lock
- Activity: as tolerated
- Monitoring: vital signs, I/O, and laboratory values
- Treatments: NG tube
- Solubilizing agent: ursodiol (Actigall), chenodiol (Chenix)
- Antibiotic: cephalothin (Keflin)
- Analgesic: meperidine (Demerol), morphine
- ESWL

Nursing interventions

- Maintain the patient's diet; withhold food and fluids, as necessary
- Assess GI status
- Monitor and record vital signs, I/O, and laboratory studies
- Assess for pain and medicate, as indicated
- Maintain position, patency, and suction of NG tube
- Administer medications, as ordered
- Provide preoperative and postoperative care
- Individualize home care instructions
  - Report signs and symptoms of infection
  - Provide care of T tube
  - Adhere to low-fat diet for 6 weeks after surgery
  - Avoid lifting for 6 weeks

Complications

- Medical
  - Cholangitis
  - Cholecystitis
  - Choledocholithiasis
  - Gallstone ileus
- Surgical
  - Pneumonia
  - Atelectasis
  - Peritonitis
  - Hemorrhage

Possible surgical interventions

- Laparoscopic cholecystectomy
- Choledochotomy
- Cholecystotomy

Main treatment options for a patient with cholelithiasis

- I.V. therapy: fluid replacement
- Solubilizing agents
- Analgesics
- ESWL

Key nursing interventions for a patient with cholelithiasis

- Assess GI status.
- Assess for pain and medicate, as indicated.
- Maintain position, patency, and suction of NG tube.
- Provide preoperative and postoperative care.

NCLEX CHECKS

It's never too soon to begin your NCLEX preparation. Now that you've reviewed this chapter, carefully read each of the following questions and choose the best answer. Then compare your responses to the correct answers.

1. The nurse is providing discharge teaching for a patient with gastroesophageal reflux disease (GERD). Which statement by the patient indicates that he understands the instructions?

- ☐ A. "I will lie down after meals."
- ☐ B. "I will restrict fluids."
- ☐ C. "I will sleep with the head of the bed elevated."
- ☐ D. "I will no longer use a pillow."

2. Which finding in a patient with appendicitis alerts the nurse to a ruptured appendix?

- ☐ A. Pain in the right lower abdomen
- ☐ B. Sudden cessation of abdominal pain
- ☐ C. Rebound tenderness
- ☐ D. Abdominal "boardlike" rigidity

3. While preparing a patient for an endoscopy, the nurse should implement which of the following? (Select all that apply.)

- ☐ A. Administer a preparation to clean the GI tract, such as Golytely or Fleets Phospha-Soda.
- ☐ B. Tell the patient he shouldn't eat or drink for 6 to 12 hours before the procedure.
- ☐ C. Tell the patient he must be on a clear liquid diet for 24 hours before the procedure.
- ☐ D. Inform the patient that he'll receive a sedative before the procedure.
- ☐ E. Tell the patient that he may eat and drink immediately after the procedure.

4. A nurse is evaluating the effectiveness of dietary instructions in a patient with diverticulitis. Regular consumption of which food would indicate that the patient hasn't understood the instructions?

- ☐ A. Fiber
- ☐ B. Bananas
- ☐ C. Milk products
- ☐ D. Cucumbers

5. A patient with a history of peptic ulcer disease develops a fever of 101° F (38.3° C). Which accompanying sign most strongly indicates the patient has peritonitis?

- ☐ A. Leukopenia
- ☐ B. Hyperactive bowel sounds
- ☐ C. Abdominal rigidity
- ☐ D. Polyuria

6. The nurse is planning care for a female patient with acute hepatitis A. What's the primary mode of transmission for hepatitis A?

- ☐ A. Fecal contamination and oral ingestion
- ☐ B. Exposure to contaminated blood
- ☐ C. Sexual activity with an infected partner
- ☐ D. Sharing a contaminated needle or syringe

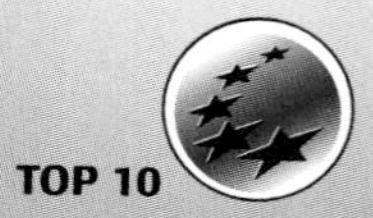

TOP 10

Items to study for your next test on the GI system

1. Organs of the GI system
2. Nursing interventions after a barium enema
3. The purpose of a colonoscopy
4. Types of ostomies performed in bowel surgery
5. Colostomy care
6. The differences between ulcerative colitis and Crohn's disease
7. Peritonitis and appendicitis assessment findings
8. Key signs of colorectal cancer
9. The five types of viral hepatitis
10. Mealtime tips for patients with GERD

ANSWERS AND RATIONALES

1. CORRECT ANSWER: C
The patient with GERD should sleep with the head of the bed elevated to reduce intra-abdominal pressure. The head of the bed should remain elevated during and after meals to reduce reflux. Fluid intake should be increased to wash gastric contents out of the esophagus. Lying flat in bed increases intra-abdominal pressure and the risk of reflux.

2. CORRECT ANSWER: B
Sudden cessation of abdominal pain indicates perforation or infarction of the appendix. Pain in the right lower abdomen, rebound tenderness, and abdominal "boardlike" rigidity are all signs and symptoms of appendicitis.

3. CORRECT ANSWER: B, D
The patient shouldn't eat or drink for 6 to 12 hours before the procedure to ensure that his upper GI tract is clear for viewing. The patient will receive a sedative before the endoscope is inserted that will help him relax, but allow him to remain conscious. GI tract cleaning and a clear liquid diet are interventions for a patient having a lower GI tract procedure such as colonoscopy. Food and fluids must be withheld until the gag reflex returns.

4. CORRECT ANSWER: D
In diverticulitis, vegetables with seeds are prohibited in the diet because the seeds can lodge in diverticula and cause flare-ups of diverticulitis. Fiber and residue are recommended in the diet. Bananas and milk products aren't contraindicated.

5. CORRECT ANSWER: C
Abdominal rigidity is a classic sign of peritonitis. The patient would typically have leukocytosis, hypoactive bowel sounds, and decreased urine output.

6. CORRECT ANSWER: A
Hepatitis A is predominantly transmitted by the ingestion of fecally contaminated food. Transmission is more likely to occur with poor hygiene, crowded conditions, and poor sanitation. Hepatitis B and C may be transmitted through exposure to contaminated blood and blood products. Sexual activity with an infected partner and sharing contaminated needles or syringes may transmit hepatitis B.

6

Endocrine system

LEARNING OBJECTIVES

After studying this chapter, you should be able to:

- Describe the psychosocial impact of endocrine disorders.
- Differentiate between modifiable and nonmodifiable risk factors in the development of an endocrine disorder.
- List three probable and three possible nursing diagnoses for a patient with an endocrine disorder.
- Identify the nursing interventions for a patient with an endocrine disorder.
- Identify three teaching topics for a patient with an endocrine disorder.

CHAPTER OVERVIEW

Caring for the patient with an endocrine disorder requires a sound understanding of endocrine anatomy and physiology and fluid and electrolyte balance. A thorough assessment is essential to planning and implementing appropriate patient care. The assessment includes a complete history, a physical examination, diagnostic testing, identification of modifiable and nonmodifiable risk factors, and information related to the psychosocial impact of the disorder on the patient.

Nursing diagnoses focus primarily on altered nutrition, fluid volume excess or deficit, and body image disturbance. Nursing interventions are designed to assess patient hydration and nutritional status, teach the patient and his family about long-term use of medications, and assist the patient in adjusting to changes in body image and the effects of chronic illness. Patient teaching—a crucial nursing activity—involves providing information about medical follow-up, medication regimens, signs and symptoms of possible complications, and reducing modifiable risk factors through adherence to dietary and medication recommendations and restrictions.

ANATOMY AND PHYSIOLOGY REVIEW

Hypothalamus

- Controls temperature, respiration, and blood pressure
- Affects the emotional states of fear, anxiety, anger, rage, pleasure, and pain
- Produces hypothalamic-stimulating hormones, which affect the inhibition and release of pituitary hormones

Pituitary gland

- Considered the"master gland"
- Composed of anterior and posterior lobes
  - Posterior lobe (neurohypophysis) secretes vasopressin (antidiuretic hormone [ADH]) and oxytocin
  - Anterior lobe (adenohypophysis) secretes follicle-stimulating hormone (FSH), luteinizing hormone (LH), prolactin, corticotropin, thyroid-stimulating hormone (TSH), and growth hormone (GH)
- Affects all hormonal activity; factors altering pituitary gland function affect all hormonal activity

Thyroid gland

- Accelerates cellular reactions, including basal metabolic rate and growth
- Controlled by secretion of TSH
- Produces thyroxine (T_4), tri-iodothyronine (T_3), and thyrocalcitonin

Parathyroid glands

- Secrete parathyroid hormone (parathormone [PTH]), which regulates calcium and phosphorus metabolism
- Require active form of vitamin D for PTH function

Adrenal glands

- Adrenal cortex secretes three major hormones
  - Glucocorticoids (cortisol)
  - Mineralocorticoids (aldosterone)
  - Sex hormones (androgens, estrogens, and progesterone)
- Adrenal medulla secretes two hormones
  - Norepinephrine
  - Epinephrine

Pancreas

- Accessory gland of digestion
  - Exocrine function: secretion of digestive enzymes
    - Amylase
    - Lipase
    - Trypsin

What the hypothalamus controls

- Temperature
- Respiration
- Blood pressure

Pituitary gland

- Considered the "master gland"
- Affects all hormone activity

Thyroid gland's role

- Accelerates cellular reactions
- Produces T_4, T_3, and thyrocalcitonin

Parathyroid glands

- Secrete PTH
- Require active form of vitamin D

Adrenal glands

- Adrenal cortex: secretes hormones such as glucocorticoids
- Adrenal medulla: secretes hormones such as norepinephrine

- Endocrine function: secretion of hormones from islets of Langerhans
  - Insulin
  - Glucagon
  - Somatostatin
- Main pancreatic duct joins the common bile duct and empties into the duodenum at the ampulla of Vater

Roles of the pancreas

- Aids in digestion
- Secretes digestive enzymes
- Secretes hormones such as insulin

ASSESSMENT FINDINGS

History

- Changes in weight; hair quality and distribution; body proportions, muscle mass, and fat distribution (see *Assessing endocrine dysfunction: Some common signs and symptoms*)
- Fatigue and weakness
- Change in mood or behavior
- Anorexia
- Constipation, diarrhea, urinary frequency
- Change in menses and libido
- History of infections
- Intolerance of heat or cold

Key assessment findings

- Changes in weight; hair quality and distribution; body proportions, muscle mass, and fat distribution
- Change in mood or behavior
- Changes in menses and libido
- Intolerance of heat or cold

Physical examination

- Vital sign changes
- Skin color and temperature changes
- Change in skin texture
- Change in level of consciousness (LOC)
- Pattern and character of respirations
- Change in urinary patterns
- Change in thirst
- Abnormalities of nails
- Change in visual acuity

Key physical examination findings

- Skin color and temperature changes
- Change in skin texture
- Change in LOC
- Change in urinary patterns
- Change in thirst

DIAGNOSTIC TESTS AND PROCEDURES

Hematologic studies

- Definition and purpose
  - Laboratory test of a blood sample
  - Analysis for white blood cells (WBCs), red blood cells (RBCs), erythrocyte sedimentation rate, platelets, prothrombin time, partial thromboplastin time, hemoglobin (Hb), and hematocrit (HCT)
- Nursing interventions
  - **Note current drug therapy that might alter test results**
  - Check the venipuncture site for bleeding after the procedure

Characteristics of hematologic studies

- Laboratory test of blood
- Analyzes blood cells
- Intervention: note current drug therapy that might alter test results

Blood chemistry

- Definition and purpose
  - Laboratory test of a blood sample

Assessing endocrine dysfunction: Some common signs and symptoms

SIGN OR SYMPTOM	POSSIBLE CAUSES
Abdominal pain	Diabetic ketoacidosis (DKA), myxedema, addisonian crisis, thyroid storm
Anemia	Hypothyroidism, panhypopituitarism, adrenal insufficiency, Cushing's disease, hyperparathyroidism
Anorexia	Hyperparathyroidism, Addison's disease, DKA, hypothyroidism
Body temperature changes	*Increase:* Thyrotoxicosis, thyroid storm, primary hypothalamic disease (after pituitary surgery) *Decrease:* Addison's disease, hypoglycemia, myxedema coma, DKA
Hypertension	Primary aldosteronism, pheochromocytoma, Cushing's syndrome
Libido changes, sexual dysfunction	Thyroid or adrenocortical hypofunction or hyperfunction, diabetes mellitus, hypopituitarism, gonadal failure
Skin changes	*Hyperpigmentation:* Addison's disease (after bilateral adrenalectomy for Cushing's syndrome), corticotropin-secreting pituitary tumor *Hirsutism:* Cushing's syndrome; adrenal hyperplasia, adrenal tumor, acromegaly *Coarse, dry skin:* Myxedema, hypoparathyroidism, acromegaly *Excessive sweating:* Thyrotoxicosis, acromegaly, pheochromocytoma, hypoglycemia
Tachycardia	Hyperthyroidism, pheochromocytoma, hypoglycemia, DKA
Weakness, fatigue	Addison's disease, Cushing's syndrome, hypothyroidism, hyperparathyroidism, hyperglycemia or hypoglycemia, pheochromocytoma
Weight gain	Cushing's syndrome, hypothyroidism, pituitary tumor
Weight loss	Hyperthyroidism, pheochromocytoma, Addison's disease, hyperparathyroidism, diabetes mellitus, diabetes insipidus

- – Analysis for potassium, sodium, calcium, phosphorus, ketones, glucose, osmolality, chloride, blood urea nitrogen (BUN), creatinine, T_3, T_4, protein-bound iodine, cortisol
- Nursing interventions
  - Withhold food and fluids, as directed, before the procedure
  - Check for recent studies using radiopaque dyes that may alter test results
  - Note pregnancy
  - List current medications that contain iodine
  - Check the venipuncture site for bleeding after the procedure

Fasting serum glucose and 2-hour postprandial glucose test

- Definition and purpose

Common signs and symptoms of endocrine dysfunction

- Abdominal pain
- Anemia
- Anorexia
- Body temperature changes
- Hypertension
- Libido changes, sexual dysfunction
- Skin changes
- Tachycardia
- Weakness, fatigue
- Weight gain
- Weight loss

What blood chemistry analyzes

- Potassium
- Sodium
- Calcium
- Phosphorus
- Ketones
- Glucose
- Osmolality
- Chloride
- BUN
- Creatinine
- T_3
- T_4
- Protein-bound iodine
- Cortisol

- Laboratory test of a blood sample
- Analysis to measure the body's use and disposal of glucose
- Nursing interventions
  - Withhold food and fluids for 12 hours before fasting sample is drawn
  - Withhold insulin until the test is completed
  - Administer ordered amount of glucose orally, and request the laboratory to draw blood 2 hours later
  - Assess the patient for hypoglycemia or hyperglycemia

Fasting serum glucose and 2-hour postprandial glucose test

- Laboratory test of blood sample
- Measures the body's use and disposal of glucose
- Intervention: assess the patient for hypoglycemia or hyperglycemia

Glucose tolerance test (GTT)

- Definition and purpose
  - Laboratory test of blood and urine
  - Analysis to measure absorption of carbohydrates
- Nursing interventions
  - List any medications that might interfere with the test
  - Note pregnancy, trauma, or infectious disease
  - Provide the patient with a high-carbohydrate diet 2 days before the test; then have the patient fast for 12 hours before the test
  - Instruct the patient to avoid smoking, caffeine, alcohol, and exercise for 12 hours before the procedure
  - Withhold all medications after midnight
  - Obtain fasting serum glucose and urine specimen
  - Administer test load oral glucose, and record time
  - Request laboratory collection of serum glucose and urine specimens at 30, 60, 120, and 180 minutes
  - Refrigerate samples
  - Assess the patient for hyperglycemia or hypoglycemia

Glucose tolerance test

- Laboratory test of blood and urine
- Measures absorption of carbohydrates
- Intervention: list any medications that might interfere with the test

Adrenocorticotropic hormone stimulation test

- Definition and purpose
  - Laboratory test of a blood sample
  - Analysis for cortisol
- Nursing interventions
  - List any medications that might interfere with the test
  - Monitor 24-hour I.V. infusion of corticotropin after baseline serum sample is drawn
  - Check the venipuncture site for bleeding

Adrenocorticotropic hormone stimulation test

- Laboratory test of a blood sample
- Analyzes cortisol
- Intervention: monitor 24-hour I.V. infusion of corticotropin after sample is drawn

Dexamethasone suppression test

- Definition and purpose
  - Laboratory test of urine samples
  - Analysis of serum cortisol and urinary 17-hydroxycorticosteroids (17-OHCS) after administration of dexamethasone
- Nursing interventions
  - Administer dexamethasone and an antacid, as prescribed
  - Obtain single urine and 24-hour urine samples, as directed
  - List any medications that might interfere with the test

Dexamethasone suppression test

- Laboratory test of urine
- Analyzes serum cortisol and 17-OHCS after dexamethasone administration
- Intervention: obtain single urine and 24-hour urine samples, as directed

24-hour urine test for 17-ketosteroids (17-KS) and 17-OHCS

- Definition and purpose
  - Laboratory test of urine samples
  - Quantitative laboratory analysis of urine collected over 24 hours to determine hormone precursors
- Nursing interventions
  - Withhold all medications for 48 hours before the test
  - Instruct the patient to void and note the time (collection of urine starts with the next voiding)
  - Place urine container on ice
  - Measure each voided urine
  - Instruct the patient to void at the end of the 24-hour period
  - List any medications that might interfere with the test

Urine vanillylmandelic acid (VMA) test

- Definition and purpose
  - Laboratory test of urine samples
  - Quantitative analysis of urine collected over 24 hours to determine the end products of catecholamine metabolism (epinephrine and norepinephrine)
- Nursing interventions
  - List any medications, previous tests, and medical conditions that might interfere with the test
  - **Restrict foods that contain vanilla, coffee, tea, citrus fruits, bananas, nuts, and chocolate for 3 days before 24-hour urine collection**
  - Instruct the patient to void and note the time (collection of urine starts with the next voiding)
  - Place urine container on ice
  - Measure each voided urine
  - Instruct the patient to void at the end of the 24-hour period

Basal metabolic rate test

- Definition and purpose
  - Noninvasive test
  - Indirect measurement of oxygen consumed by the body during a given time
- Nursing interventions
  - List medications taken before the procedure
  - Note environmental and emotional stressors

Visual acuity and field testing

- Definition and purpose
  - Noninvasive test
  - Measurement of central and peripheral vision
- Nursing interventions
  - Ask the patient to wear or bring corrective lenses for the test
  - Determine the patient's hearing and ability to follow directions

24-hour urine test

- Laboratory test of urine samples
- Analyzes urine collected over 24 hours
- Intervention: withhold all medications for 48 hours before the test

VMA test

- Laboratory test of urine
- Analyzes urine collected over 24 hours to determine end products of epinephrine and norepinephrine metabolism
- Intervention: restrict foods that contain vanilla, coffee, tea, citrus fruits, bananas, nuts, and chocolate before 24-hour urine collection

Basal metabolic rate test

- Noninvasive test
- Indirect measurement of oxygen consumed by the body during a given time
- Intervention: list medications taken before the procedure

Visual acuity and field testing

- Noninvasive test
- Measures central and peripheral vision
- Intervention: ask the patient to bring corrective lenses for the test

Computed tomography

- Noninvasive scan
- Visualizes the sella turcica and abdomen
- Intervention: note the patient's allergies before the procedure

Ultrasonography

- Noninvasive procedure
- Uses echoes from sound waves to visualize the thyroid, pelvis, and abdomen
- Intervention: withhold food and fluids 8 to 12 hours before the procedure

Closed percutaneous thyroid biopsy

- Involves aspiration of thyroid tissue
- Histologic evaluation
- Intervention: assess the patient for esophageal or tracheal puncture

Thyroid uptake test

- Uses oral or I.V. radioactive iodine
- Measures the amount of radioactive iodine taken up by the thyroid gland
- Intervention: advise the patient not to eat iodine-rich foods for 24 hours before the test

Computed tomography (CT)

- Definition and purpose
  - Noninvasive scan that may use I.V. injection of contrast dye
  - Visualization of the sella turcica and abdomen
- Nursing interventions
  - Explain the procedure
  - Note the patient's allergies to iodine, seafood, and radiopaque dyes
  - Allay the patient's anxiety
  - Inform the patient about possible throat irritation and flushing of the face

Ultrasonography

- Definition and purpose
  - Noninvasive procedure using echoes from sound waves
  - Visualization of the thyroid, pelvis, and abdomen
- Nursing interventions
  - Withhold food and fluids 8 to 12 hours before the test
  - Determine the patient's ability to lie still
  - Ask the patient not to smoke or chew gum for 8 to 12 hours before the test
  - Administer an enema before the procedure, as directed
  - Remove abdominal dressing before the procedure

Closed percutaneous thyroid biopsy

- Definition and purpose
  - Procedure involving a percutaneous, sterile aspiration of a small amount of thyroid tissue
  - Histologic evaluation
- Nursing interventions before the procedure
  - Withhold food and fluids after midnight
  - Place obtained written informed consent in the patient's chart
- Nursing interventions after the procedure
  - Maintain bed rest for 24 hours
  - Monitor vital signs
  - Check the biopsy site for bleeding
  - Assess the patient for esophageal or tracheal puncture

Thyroid uptake (radioactive iodine uptake [RAIU])

- Definition and purpose
  - Procedure using oral or I.V. radioactive iodine
  - Measurement of the amount of radioactive iodine taken up by the thyroid gland in 24 hours
- Nursing interventions before the procedure
  - Advise the patient not to eat iodine-rich foods, such as iodized salt or shellfish, for 24 hours before the test
  - Discontinue all thyroid and cough medications 7 to 10 days before the test
  - Schedule a thyroid scan before tests using iodine-based dyes

Thyroid scan

- Definition and purpose
  - Procedure using an oral or I.V. radioactive isotope
  - Visual imaging of radioactivity distribution in the thyroid gland
- Nursing interventions before the procedure
  - Advise the patient not to eat iodine-rich foods, such as iodized salt or shellfish, for 24 hours before the test
  - Discontinue all thyroid and cough medications 7 to 10 days before the test
  - Schedule the scan before other tests using iodine-based dyes or radioactive iodine

Arteriography

- Definition and purpose
  - Procedure using an injection of a radiopaque dye through a catheter
  - Fluoroscopic examination of the arterial blood supply to the parathyroid, adrenal, or pancreatic glands
- Nursing interventions before the procedure
  - Place obtained written informed consent in the patient's chart
  - **Note the patient's allergies to iodine, seafood, and radiopaque dyes**
  - Inform the patient about possible throat irritation and flushing of the face after the dye injection
  - Withhold food and fluids after midnight
- Nursing interventions after the procedure
  - Monitor vital signs
  - Check the insertion site for bleeding

Sulkowitch's test

- Definition and purpose
  - Laboratory test of urine
  - Analysis to measure the amount of calcium being excreted
- Nursing interventions
  - If hypercalcemia is indicated, collect a single urine sample before a meal
  - If hypocalcemia is indicated, collect a single urine sample after a meal

PSYCHOSOCIAL IMPACT OF ENDOCRINE DISORDERS

Developmental impact

- Decreased self-esteem
- Changes in body image
- Embarrassment from the changes in body function and structure, such as changes in secondary sex characteristics and sexual functioning

Economic impact

- Disruption of employment
- Cost of vocational retraining

Thyroid scan

- Uses an oral or I.V. radioactive isotope
- Provides visual imaging of radioactivity distribution in the thyroid gland
- Intervention: advise the patient not to eat iodine-rich foods for 24 hours before the procedure

Arteriography

- Uses an injection of radiopaque dye through a catheter
- Examines the arterial blood supply
- Intervention: note the patient's allergies before the procedure

Sulkowitch's test

- Laboratory test of urine
- Measures the amount of calcium being excreted
- Intervention: collect a urine sample before or after a meal, depending on what disorder is indicated

- Cost of medications
- Cost of special diet
- Cost of hospitalizations and follow-up care

Economic impact of endocrine disorders

- Disruption of employment
- Cost of vocational retraining
- Cost of medications
- Cost of special diet
- Cost of hospitalizations and follow-up care

Occupational and recreational impact

- Physical activity restrictions
- Adjustment to change in occupation

Social impact

- Social withdrawal and isolation
- Changes in eating patterns
- Changes in role performance
- Changes in sexual function

RISK FACTORS

Modifiable risk factors

- Medication
- Stress
- Diet
- Obesity

Modifiable risk factors

- Medication
- Stress
- Diet
- Obesity

Nonmodifiable risk factors

- Family history of endocrine illness
- History of trauma
- Aging

NURSING DIAGNOSES

Probable nursing diagnoses

- Excess fluid volume
- Risk for imbalanced fluid volume
- Risk for imbalanced nutrition: More than body requirements
- Disturbed body image
- Impaired urinary elimination
- Imbalanced nutrition: Less than body requirements

Probable nursing diagnoses

- Excess fluid volume
- Risk for imbalanced fluid volume
- Risk for imbalanced nutrition: More than body requirements
- Disturbed body image
- Impaired urinary elimination
- Imbalanced nutrition: Less than body requirements

Possible nursing diagnoses

- Risk for injury
- Social isolation
- Deficient knowledge
- Noncompliance
- Disturbed sensory perception: visual
- Disturbed sensory perception: tactile
- Risk for impaired skin integrity
- Disturbed thought processes

ADRENALECTOMY

Description

- Surgical removal of one or both adrenal glands

Preoperative nursing interventions

- Complete patient and family preoperative teaching
  - Determine the patient's understanding of the procedure
  - Describe the operating room, postanesthesia care unit (PACU), and preoperative and postoperative routines
  - Demonstrate postoperative turning, coughing, deep breathing, splinting, and range-of-motion (ROM) exercises
  - Explain the postoperative need for drainage tubes, surgical dressings, oxygen therapy, I.V. therapy, and pain control
- Complete a preoperative checklist
- Administer preoperative medications, as prescribed
- Allay the patient's and his family's anxiety about surgery
- Document the patient's history and physical assessment data
- Administer steroids, as prescribed
- Administer vasopressors, as prescribed

Postoperative nursing interventions

- Assess cardiac, respiratory, and neurologic status
  - Monitor fluid intake and output (I/O) and serum electrolyte levels
  - **Keep in mind that adrenalectomy disturbs mineralocorticoid and glucocorticoid secretion, resulting in altered fluid and electrolyte balance**
- Assess pain and administer postoperative analgesics, as prescribed
- Assess for return of peristalsis; provide solid foods and liquids, as tolerated
- Administer I.V. fluids
- Allay the patient's anxiety
- Inspect the surgical dressing and change, as directed
- Reinforce turning, coughing, and deep breathing, and splinting of incision
- Keep the patient in semi-Fowler's position
- Provide incentive spirometry
- Maintain activity, as tolerated
- Monitor vital signs, I/O, central venous pressure (CVP), laboratory studies, electrocardiogram (ECG), neurovital signs, daily weight, specific gravity, urine for glucose and ketones, and pulse oximetry
- Monitor and maintain position and patency of drainage tubes: nasogastric, indwelling urinary catheter, and wound drainage
- Encourage the patient to express his feelings about changes in his body image and the need for lifelong medication replacement
- Administer antacids, as prescribed
- Maintain a quiet environment
- Administer hormone replacements, as prescribed
- Administer vasopressors, as prescribed
- Individualize home care instructions

Adrenalectomy defined

- Surgical removal of one or both adrenal glands

Key nursing interventions before adrenalectomy

- Administer steroids, as prescribed.
- Administer vasopressors, as prescribed.

Key nursing interventions after adrenalectomy

- Assess cardiac, respiratory, and neurologic status.
- Monitor fluid I/O and serum electrolyte levels.
- Monitor vital signs, I/O, CVP, laboratory studies, ECG, neurovital signs, daily weight, specific gravity, urine for glucose and ketones, and pulse oximetry.
- Administer hormone replacements and vasopressors.

Key home care instructions for a patient after adrenalectomy

- Recognize the signs and symptoms of infection, hypovolemia, and hypoglycemia.
- Comply with lifelong hormone replacement.
- Monitor blood pressure daily.

Hypophysectomy defined

- Surgical removal of part or all of the pituitary gland

Key nursing interventions before hypophysectomy

- Administer steroids, as prescribed.
- Administer antibiotics, as prescribed.

    - Recognize the signs and symptoms of infection, hypovolemia, and hypoglycemia
    - **Avoid exposure to people with infections**
    - Complete incision care daily, as directed
    - Comply with lifelong hormone replacement
    - Monitor blood pressure daily
    - Explore methods to reduce insomnia
    - Avoid extreme temperatures

Surgical complications
- Shock
- Hypoglycemia
- Hemorrhage
- Peptic ulcers
- Adrenal crisis
- Pneumothorax
- Acute renal failure
- Infection

HYPOPHYSECTOMY

Description
- Surgical removal of part or all of the pituitary gland

Preoperative nursing interventions
- Complete patient and family preoperative teaching
    - Determine the patient's understanding of the procedure
    - Describe the operating room, PACU, and preoperative and postoperative routines
    - Demonstrate postoperative turning, coughing, deep breathing, splinting, and ROM exercises
    - Explain the postoperative need for drainage tubes, surgical dressings, oxygen therapy, I.V. therapy, and pain control
- Complete a preoperative checklist
- Administer preoperative medications, as prescribed
- Allay the patient's and his family's anxiety about surgery
- Document the patient's history and physical assessment data
- Administer steroids, as prescribed
- Administer antibiotics, as prescribed

Postoperative nursing interventions
- Assess cardiac, respiratory, and neurologic status and fluid balance
- Assess pain and administer postoperative analgesics, as prescribed
- Assess for return of peristalsis: provide solid foods and liquids, as tolerated
- Administer I.V. fluids
- Allay the patient's anxiety
- Inspect the surgical dressing or nasal drip pad and change, as directed
- Test nasal drainage for glucose
- Reinforce turning, coughing, and deep breathing

- Keep the patient in semi-Fowler's position
- Provide incentive spirometry
- Maintain activity, as tolerated
- Monitor vital signs, I/O, CVP, laboratory studies, neurovital signs, daily weight, specific gravity, urine glucose and ketones, and pulse oximetry
- Monitor and maintain the position and patency of the indwelling urinary catheter
- Institute seizure precautions
- Encourage the patient to express his feelings about changes in his body image and a fear of dying
- Administer antibiotics, as prescribed
- Administer hormone replacements, as prescribed
- Observe the patient for signs of increased intracranial pressure (ICP)
- Check for rhinorrhea
- Provide mouth and eye care
- Avoid brushing the patient's teeth
- Administer stool softeners, as prescribed
- Individualize home care instructions
  - Recognize the signs and symptoms of infection, seizure activity, and hormone deficiencies
  - Avoid coughing, blowing nose, lifting, straining while defecating, and sneezing
  - Comply with lifelong hormone replacement

Surgical complications

- Diabetes insipidus
- Increased ICP
- Hemorrhage
- Adrenal crisis
- Thyroid storm
- Meningitis
- Diplopia

Key interventions after hypophysectomy

- Assess cardiac, respiratory, and neurologic status and fluid balance.
- Inspect the surgical dressing or nasal drip pad and change, as directed.
- Test nasal drainage for glucose.
- Monitor vital signs, I/O, CVP, laboratory studies, neurovital signs, daily weight, specific gravity, urine glucose and ketones, and pulse oximetry.
- Institute seizure precautions.
- Administer antibiotics.
- Administer hormone replacements.
- Check for rhinorrhea.
- Avoid brushing the patient's teeth.

THYROID AND PARATHYROID SURGERIES

Description

- Thyroidectomy: surgical removal of part or all of the thyroid gland
- Parathyroidectomy: surgical removal of one or more parathyroid glands

Preoperative nursing interventions

- Complete patient and family preoperative teaching
  - Determine the patient's understanding of the procedure
  - Describe the operating room, PACU, and preoperative and postoperative routines
  - Demonstrate postoperative turning, coughing, deep breathing, splinting, and ROM exercises
  - Explain the postoperative need for drainage tubes, surgical dressings, oxygen therapy, I.V. therapy, and pain control

Thyroidectomy

- Surgical removal of part or all of the thyroid gland

Parathyroidectomy

- Surgical removal of one or more parathyroid glands

Key nursing interventions before thyroidectomy

- Administer iodine preparations.
- Administer antithyroid medications.

Key nursing interventions after thyroidectomy

- Assess respiratory status.
- Monitor vital signs, I/O, CVP, laboratory studies (especially calcium and phosphorous), urine glucose and ketones, and pulse oximetry.
- Provide specific parathyroidectomy care.

Key home care instructions for a patient after thyroid or parathyroid surgery

- Recognize the signs and symptoms of infection, seizure activity, and hypothyroidism.
- Alternate periods of talking with voice rest.
- Complete ROM exercises of the neck daily.

- Complete a preoperative checklist
- Administer preoperative medications, as prescribed
- Allay the patient's and his family's anxiety about surgery
- Document the patient's history and physical assessment data
- Administer iodine preparations and antithyroid medications, as prescribed

Postoperative nursing interventions

- Assess respiratory status (see *Caring for the thyroidectomy patient*)
- Assess pain and administer postoperative analgesics, as prescribed
- Assess for return of peristalsis: provide solid foods and liquids, as tolerated
- Administer I.V. fluids
- Allay the patient's anxiety
- **Inspect the surgical dressing for bleeding, especially at the back of the neck, and change the dressing, as directed**
- Reinforce turning, coughing, and deep breathing, and splinting of incision
- Keep the patient in semi-Fowler's position, with neutral alignment and support to his neck
- Provide incentive spirometry
- Maintain activity, as tolerated
- Provide humidified cold steam nebulizer
- Monitor vital signs, I/O, CVP, laboratory studies (especially calcium and phosphorous), urine glucose and ketones, and pulse oximetry
- Monitor and maintain position and patency of wound drainage tubes
- **Maintain seizure precautions**
- Encourage the patient to express his feelings about a fear of choking or the loss of his voice
- **Assess for tetany**
- **Assess for hoarseness and aphasia**
- **Assess for thyroid storm**
- **Have calcium gluconate and tracheostomy tray available**
- Discourage talking
- Provide specific parathyroidectomy care
  - Provide a high-calcium diet with vitamin D
  - Administer calcium and vitamin D supplements, as prescribed
- Individualize home care instructions
  - Recognize the signs and symptoms of infection, seizure activity, and hypothyroidism
  - Alternate periods of talking with voice rest
  - Complete incision care daily, as directed
  - Complete ROM exercises of the neck daily

Surgical complications

- Hypocalcemia
- Laryngeal nerve damage
- Hypothyroidism
- Respiratory distress

Caring for the thyroidectomy patient

Keep these crucial points in mind when caring for the patient who has undergone thyroidectomy:

- Keep the patient in semi-Fowler's position to promote venous return from the head and neck and to decrease oozing into the incision.
- Watch for signs of respiratory distress (tracheal collapse, tracheal mucus accumulation, and laryngeal edema).
- Note that vocal cord paralysis can cause respiratory obstruction with sudden stridor and restlessness.
- Keep a tracheotomy tray at the patient's bedside for 24 hours after surgery and be prepared to assist with emergency tracheotomy if necessary.
- Assess for signs of hemorrhage.
- Assess for hypocalcemia (tingling and numbness of the extremities, muscle twitching, cramps, laryngeal spasm, and positive Chvostek's and Trousseau's signs), which may occur when parathyroid glands are damaged.
- Keep calcium gluconate available for emergency I.V. administration.
- Be alert for signs of thyroid storm (tachycardia, hyperkinesis, fever, vomiting, and hypertension).

- Hemorrhage
- Arrhythmias

HYPERTHYROIDISM

Definition

- Increased synthesis of thyroid hormone from overactivity (Graves' disease) or change in thyroid gland (toxic nodular goiter)

Causes

- Autoimmune disease
- Genetic
- Psychological or physiologic stress
- Thyroid adenomas
- Pituitary tumors
- Infection

Pathophysiology

- Thyroid-stimulating antibodies have a slow, sustained, stimulating effect on thyroid metabolism
- Accelerated metabolism causes increased synthesis of thyroid hormone and signs and symptoms of sympathetic nervous system stimulation

Assessment findings

- Anxiety
- Flushed, smooth skin
- Heat intolerance
- Mood swings

Key nursing interventions after thyroidectomy

- Keep the patient in semi-Fowler's position.
- Watch for respiratory distress.
- Prepare for possible emergency tracheotomy.
- Assess for hemorrhage.
- Assess for hypocalcemia.
- Have calcium gluconate available.
- Watch for thyroid storm.

Hyperthyroidism defined

- Increased synthesis of thyroid hormone from overactivity or change in thyroid gland

Key symptoms of hyperthyroidism

- Heat intolerance
- Diaphoresis
- Tachycardia
- Palpitations
- Exophthalmos
- Bruit or thrill over thyroid

- Diaphoresis
- Tachycardia
- Palpitations
- Dyspnea
- Weakness
- Increased hunger
- Increased systolic blood pressure
- Tachypnea
- Fine hand tremors
- Exophthalmos
- Weight loss
- Diarrhea
- Hyperhidrosis
- Bruit or thrill over thyroid

Diagnostic test findings for hyperthyroidism

- Blood chemistry: increased T_3, T_4, protein-bound iodine, ^{131}I, decreased TSH, cholesterol
- ECG: atrial fibrillation

Diagnostic test findings

- Thyroid scan: nodules
- Blood chemistry: increased T_3, T_4, protein-bound iodine, radioactive iodine (^{131}I); decreased TSH, cholesterol
- ECG: atrial fibrillation
- RAIU: increased

Key steps in the management of hyperthyroidism

- I.V. therapy
- Radiation therapy
- Antihyperthyroids
- Iodine preparations
- Beta-adrenergic blocking agents
- Glucocorticoids

Medical management

- Diet: high-protein, high-carbohydrate, high-calorie; restrict stimulants, such as coffee and caffeine
- I.V. therapy: saline lock
- Activity: bed rest
- Monitoring: vital signs and I/O
- Laboratory studies: T_3, T_4
- Sedative: lorazepam (Ativan)
- Radiation therapy
- Antihyperthyroids: methimazole (Tapazole), propylthiouracil (Propyl-Thyracil)
- Iodine preparations: potassium iodide, radioactive iodine
- Beta-adrenergic blocking agents: propranolol (Inderal)
- Vitamins: thiamine (vitamin B_1), ascorbic acid (vitamin C)
- Cardiac glycoside: digoxin (Lanoxin)
- Glucocorticoids: prednisone (Deltasone); I.V. hydrocortisone (Solu-Cortef) for thyroid storm
- I.V. glucose

Key nursing interventions for a patient with hyperthyroidism

- Maintain the patient's diet.
- Avoid stimulants.
- Assess fluid balance.

Nursing interventions

- Maintain the patient's diet
- Avoid stimulants, such as drugs and foods that contain caffeine
- Administer I.V. fluids
- Assess fluid balance
- Assess cardiovascular status
- Monitor and record vital signs, I/O, and laboratory studies
- Administer medications, as prescribed

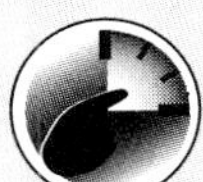

TIME-OUT FOR TEACHING

Patients with endocrine disorders

Be sure to include the following topics in your teaching plan when caring for patients with endocrine disorders.

- Follow-up appointments
- Optimal body weight maintenance
- Medication therapy including the action, adverse effects, and scheduling of medications
- Dietary recommendations and restrictions
- Fluid intake recommendations and restrictions
- Rest and activity patterns, including any limitations or restrictions
- Community agencies and resources for supportive services
- Ways to reduce stress
- Medical identification jewelry
- Safe, quiet environment

- Weigh the patient daily
- Provide rest periods
- Provide a quiet, cool environment
- Provide eye care
- Allay the patient's anxiety
- Encourage the patient to express his feelings about changes in his body image
- Provide postradiation nursing care
  - Provide prophylactic skin, mouth, and perineal care
  - Monitor dietary intake
  - Provide rest periods
- Individualize home care instructions (for teaching tips, see *Patients with endocrine disorders*)
  - Stop smoking
  - Recognize the signs and symptoms of thyroid storm
  - Adhere to activity limitations
  - Avoid exposure to people with infections
  - Monitor self for infection

Complications

- **Thyroid storm (thyroid crisis): tachycardia, delirium, agitation, coma, death, hyperpyrexia, dehydration, arrhythmias, diarrhea** (see *Understanding thyroid storm,* page 274)
- Arrhythmias
- Diabetes mellitus

Surgical intervention

- Subtotal thyroidectomy when euthyroid state is established

Key teaching topics for a patient with an endocrine disorder

- Medication therapy
- Fluid intake recommendations and restrictions
- Ways to reduce stress

Key postradiation care for hyperthyroidism

- Provide prophylactic skin, mouth, and perineal care.
- Monitor dietary intake.
- Provide rest period.

Key home care instructions for a patient with hyperthyroidism

- Recognize the signs and symptoms of thyroid storm.
- Avoid exposure to people with infections.

Facts about thyroid storm

- Overproduction of T_3 and T_4 hormones cause an increase in systemic adrenergic activity that results in severe hypermetabolism
- Leads to cardiac, GI, and sympathetic nervous system decompensation
- Initial symptoms include tachycardia, vomiting, and stupor
- Onset is usually abrupt

Understanding thyroid storm

Thyrotoxic crisis – also known as thyroid storm – usually occurs in patients with preexisting, though often unrecognized, thyrotoxicosis. Left untreated, it's usually fatal.

PATHOPHYSIOLOGY

The thyroid gland secretes the thyroid hormones triiodothyronine (T_3) and thyroxine (T_4). When T_3 and T_4 are overproduced, systemic adrenergic activity increases. The result is epinephrine overproduction and severe hypermetabolism, leading rapidly to cardiac, GI, and sympathetic nervous system decompensation.

ASSESSMENT FINDINGS

Initially, the patient may have marked tachycardia, vomiting, and stupor. If left untreated, he may experience vascular collapse, hypotension, coma, and death. Other findings may include a combination of irritability and restlessness; visual disturbances such as diplopia; tremor and weakness; angina; shortness of breath; cough; and swollen extremities. Palpation may disclose warm, moist, flushed skin, and a high fever that begins insidiously and rises rapidly to a lethal level.

PRECIPITATING FACTORS

Onset is usually abrupt and evoked by a stressful event, such as trauma, surgery, or infection. Other less common precipitating factors include:

- insulin-induced ketoacidosis
- hypoglycemia or diabetic ketoacidosis
- stroke
- myocardial infarction
- pulmonary embolism
- sudden discontinuation of antithyroid drug therapy
- initiation of radioactive iodine therapy
- preeclampsia
- subtotal thyroidectomy with accompanying excessive intake of synthetic thyroid hormone.

Hypothyroidism defined

- Underactive state of thyroid gland
- Results in absence or decreased secretion of thyroid hormone

Pathophysiology of hypothyroidism

- Thyroid gland fails to secrete enough thyroid hormone
- Hyposecretion of thyroid hormone causes decreased metabolism

HYPOTHYROIDISM

Definition

- Underactive state of thyroid gland, resulting in absence or decreased secretion of thyroid hormone

Causes

- Autoimmune disease: Hashimoto's thyroiditis
- Thyroidectomy
- Overuse of antithyroid drugs
- Malfunction of pituitary gland
- Use of radioactive iodine

Pathophysiology

- Thyroid gland fails to secrete a satisfactory quantity of thyroid hormone
- Hyposecretion of thyroid hormone results in overall decrease in metabolism

Assessment findings

- Fatigue
- Weight gain
- Dry, flaky, "doughy" skin

- Edema
- Cold intolerance
- Coarse hair
- Alopecia
- Thick tongue, swollen lips
- Mental sluggishness
- Menstrual disorders
- Constipation
- Hypersensitivity to narcotics, barbiturates, and anesthetics
- Anorexia
- Decreased diaphoresis
- Hypothermia

Diagnostic test findings

- Blood chemistry: decreased T_3, T_4, protein-bound iodine, sodium; increased TSH, cholesterol
- RAIU: decreased
- ECG: sinus bradycardia

Medical management

- Diet: high-fiber, high-protein, low-calorie with increased fluid intake
- Activity: as tolerated
- Monitoring: vital signs and I/O
- Laboratory studies: T_3, T_4, and sodium
- Stool softener: docusate (Colace)
- Thyroid hormone replacements: levothyroxine (Synthroid), liothyronine (Cytomel), thyroglobulin (Proloid), liotrix (Thyrolar)

Nursing interventions

- Maintain the patient's diet
- Encourage fluids
- Monitor and record vital signs, I/O, and laboratory studies
- Administer medications, as prescribed
- Encourage the patient to express his feelings of depression
- Encourage physical activity and mental stimulation
- Provide a warm environment
- **Avoid sedation: administer one-third to one-half the normal dose of sedatives or narcotics**
- Check for constipation and edema
- Prevent skin breakdown
- Provide frequent rest periods
- Individualize home care instructions
  - Exercise regularly
  - Recognize the signs and symptoms of myxedema coma (see *Understanding myxedema coma,* page 276)
  - Monitor self for constipation
  - Use additional protection in cold weather
  - Limit activity in cold weather
  - Avoid using sedatives

Common signs and symptoms of hypothyroidism

- Fatigue
- Weight gain
- Dry, flaky, "doughy" skin
- Cold intolerance
- Mental sluggishness
- Menstrual disorders
- Hypothermia

Types of thyroid hormone replacements to manage hypothyroidism

- Levothyroxine
- Liothyronine
- Thyroglobulin
- Liotrix

Key nursing interventions for a patient with hypothyroidism

- Encourage fluids.
- Check for constipation and edema.
- Encourage physical activity and mental stimulation.

Facts about patients in myxedema coma

- Have significantly depressed respirations
- Have decreased cardiac output and worsening of cerebral hypoxia
- Become stuporous and hypothermic
- Need life-saving interventions

Understanding myxedema coma

Myxedema coma is a medical emergency that commonly has a fatal outcome. Progression is usually gradual but when stress – such as infection, exposure to cold, or trauma – aggravates severe or prolonged hypothyroidism, coma may develop abruptly. Other precipitating factors are thyroid medication withdrawal and the use of sedatives, narcotics, or anesthetics.

WHAT HAPPENS

Patients in myxedema coma have significantly depressed respirations, so their partial pressure of carbon dioxide in arterial blood may rise. Decreased cardiac output and worsening cerebral hypoxia may also occur. The patient becomes stuporous and hypothermic. Vital signs reflect bradycardia and hypotension. Lifesaving interventions are necessary.

– Complete skin care daily

Complications

- Coronary artery disease (CAD)
- Heart failure
- Acute organic psychosis
- Angina
- Myocardial infarction (MI)
- Myxedema coma: hypoventilation, hypothermia, respiratory acidosis, syncope, bradycardia, hypotension, seizures, and cerebral hypoxia

Complications of hypothyroidism

- CAD
- Heart failure
- Acute organic psychosis
- Angina
- MI
- Myxedema coma

Surgical interventions

- None

THYROID CANCER

Characteristics of thyroid cancer

- Malignant, primary tumor of the thyroid
- Doesn't affect thyroid hormone secretion
- Types of thyroid carcinomas: papillary, follicular, anaplastic, and medullary

Definition

- Malignant, primary tumor of the thyroid that doesn't affect thyroid hormone secretion

Causes

- Chronic overstimulation of the pituitary gland
- Chronic overstimulation of the thymus gland
- Neck radiation

Pathophysiology

- Unregulated cell growth and uncontrolled cell division result in the development of a neoplasm
- Papillary carcinoma: well-differentiated columnar cells form a solitary nodule in the thyroid gland that spreads to the cervical lymph nodes
- Follicular carcinoma: encapsulated, well-differentiated cells that invade blood vessels and lymphatics
- Anaplastic carcinoma: either squamous, spindle, or small round cells

- Medullary carcinoma: solid, differentiated tumor arising from calcitonin-producing C cells

Assessment findings

- Enlarged thyroid gland
- Painless, firm, irregular, and enlarged thyroid nodule or mass
- Palpable cervical lymph nodes
- Dysphagia
- Hoarseness
- Dyspnea

Diagnostic test findings

- RAIU: "cold" or nonfunctioning nodule
- Ultrasound: thyroid nodules
- Thyroid biopsy: cytology positive for cancer cells
- Thyroid function tests: normal
- Blood chemistry: increased calcitonin, serotonin, and prostaglandins

Medical management

- Diet: high-protein, high-carbohydrate, high-calorie with supplemental feedings
- I.V. therapy: saline lock
- Activity: as tolerated
- Monitoring: vital signs and I/O
- Laboratory studies: calcitonin, serotonin
- Radiation therapy
- Chemotherapy: chlorambucil (Leukeran), doxorubicin (Adriamycin), vincristine (Oncovin)
- Thyroid hormone replacements: levothyroxine (Synthroid), liothyronine (Cytomel), thyroglobulin (Proloid)
- Pulse oximetry
- Antiemetics: prochlorperazine (Compazine), ondansetron (Zofran)

Nursing interventions

- Maintain the patient's diet
- Assess respiratory status
- Assess ability to swallow
- Monitor and record vital signs, I/O, and laboratory studies
- Administer medications, as prescribed
- Encourage the patient to express feelings about fear of dying
- Provide postchemotherapeutic and postradiation nursing care
  - Provide prophylactic skin, mouth, and perineal care
  - Monitor dietary intake
  - Administer antiemetics and antidiarrheals, as prescribed
  - Monitor for bleeding, infection, and electrolyte imbalance
  - Provide rest periods
- Individualize home care instructions
  - Provide information about the American Cancer Society

Most common signs and symptoms of thyroid cancer

- Enlarged thyroid gland
- Painless, firm, irregular, and enlarged thyroid nodule or mass

Key test findings for thyroid cancer

- RAIU: "cold" or nonfunctioning nodule
- Thyroid biopsy: cytology positive for cancer cells
- Blood chemistry: increased calcitonin, serotonin, and prostaglandins

Key management options for thyroid cancer

- Radiation therapy
- Chemotherapy
- Thyroid hormone replacements

Key nursing interventions for thyroid cancer

- Assess respiratory status.
- Assess ability to swallow.
- Provide postchemotherapeutic and postradiation nursing care.

– Recognize the signs and symptoms of respiratory distress and difficulty swallowing

Complications

- Laryngotracheal obstruction
- Respiratory distress
- Esophageal obstruction

Surgical interventions

- Thyroidectomy
- Modified neck dissection

SIMPLE GOITER

Simple goiter defined

- An enlarged thyroid gland caused when low levels of thyroid hormone stimulate increased secretion of TSH
- Key symptoms include dysphagia and enlarged thyroid gland

Definition

- Enlarged thyroid gland

Causes

- Decreased iodine intake
- Intake of goitrogenic foods: soybeans, peanuts, peaches, strawberries
- Use of goitrogenic drugs: iodine, lithium, propylthiouracil
- Genetic defects

Pathophysiology

- Low levels of thyroid hormone stimulate increased secretion of TSH by the pituitary gland
- TSH stimulation causes the thyroid to increase in size to compensate for the low levels of thyroid hormone

Assessment findings

- Dysphagia
- Enlarged thyroid gland
- Dyspnea

Diagnostic test findings for a simple goiter

- Blood chemistry: normal or decreased T_4
- RAIU: normal or increased
- TSH: increased

Diagnostic test findings

- Blood chemistry: normal or decreased T_4
- RAIU: normal or increased
- TSH: increased

Treating a simple goiter with thyroid hormone replacements

- Levothyroxine
- Liothyronine
- Thyroglobulin

Medical management

- Diet: avoid goitrogenic foods; use iodized salt
- Activity: as tolerated
- Monitoring: vital signs and I/O
- Laboratory studies: T_4
- Thyroid hormone replacements: levothyroxine (Synthroid), liothyronine (Cytomel), thyroglobulin (Proloid)
- Avoid goitrogenic drugs, such as sulfonamides, salicylates, and lithium

Nursing interventions

- Maintain the patient's diet
- Assess respiratory status

- Monitor and record vital signs, I/O, and laboratory studies
- Administer medications, as prescribed
- Encourage the patient to express his feelings about changes in his body image
- Assess the patient's ability to swallow
- Individualize home care instructions regarding the signs and symptoms of respiratory distress and difficulty swallowing

Complications
- Respiratory distress
- Laryngotracheal obstruction

Surgical intervention
- Subtotal thyroidectomy

Key nursing interventions for a patient with a simple goiter

- Maintain the patient's diet.
- Assess the patient's ability to swallow.
- Provide individualized home care instructions.

HYPERPARATHYROIDISM

Definition
- Overactivity of one or more parathyroid glands, resulting in increased PTH secretion

Causes
- Chronic renal failure
- Bone disease
- Benign adenomas
- Hypertrophy of parathyroid gland
- Malignant tumors of parathyroid gland
- Vitamin D deficiency
- Malabsorption

Pathophysiology
- Excessive secretion of PTH leads to bone demineralization and hypocalcemia
- Hypercalcemia increases the risk of renal calculi

Assessment findings
- Renal colic
- Renal calculi
- Arrhythmias
- Constipation
- Bowel obstruction
- Anorexia
- Weight loss
- Nausea and vomiting
- Depression
- Mental dullness
- Fatigue
- Osteoporosis
- Muscle weakness
- Mood swings

Facts about hyperparathyroidism

- Overactivity of one or more parathyroid glands, resulting in increased PTH secretion
- Hypercalcemia, which increases the risk of renal calculi
- Excessive PTH secretion, which leads to demineralization and hypocalcemia

Key assessment findings in hyperparathyroidism

- Renal calculi
- Anorexia
- Nausea and vomiting
- Muscle weakness
- Mood swings
- Deep bone pain

- Deep bone pain
- Hematuria
- Paresthesia
- Thick nails
- Pathologic fractures

Key diagnostic test findings in hyperparathyroidism

- Urine chemistry: decreased phosphorus; increased calcium
- X-ray: osteoporosis

Diagnostic test findings

- ECG: shortened QT interval
- Urine chemistry: decreased phosphorus; increased calcium
- Blood chemistry: increased calcium, BUN, creatinine, chloride, alkaline phosphatase; decreased phosphorus
- X-ray: osteoporosis

Medical management

- Diet: low-calcium, high-fiber, high-phosphorus in small frequent feedings; increase fluid intake to 3,000 ml/day
- I.V. therapy: saline lock
- Activity: as tolerated
- Monitoring: vital signs and I/O
- Laboratory studies: calcium, phosphorus, BUN, creatinine, potassium, and sodium
- Radiation therapy
- Treatments: strain urine, bed cradle
- Analgesic: oxycodone (Vicodin)
- Diuretics: furosemide (Lasix), ethacrynic acid (Edecrin)
- Antacid: aluminum hydroxide gel (AlternaGEL)
- Estrogen: estrogen (Premarin)
- Antineoplastic: plicamycin (Mithracin)
- Phosphate salts: K-Phos, Neutra-Phos
- Dialysis using calcium-free dialysate
- I.V. saline

Medical treatment options for hyperparathyroidism

- Radiation therapy
- Diuretics
- Antineoplastics
- Phosphate salts
- I.V. saline

Nursing interventions

- Maintain the patient's diet
- Encourage fluids with acidifying solutions: cranberry juice
- Administer I.V. fluids
- Assess urinary status
- Monitor and record vital signs, I/O, and laboratory studies
- Administer medications, as prescribed
- Encourage the patient to express his feelings about chronic illness
- Encourage the patient to walk
- Prevent falls
- Strain urine
- Assess bone and flank pain
- Move the patient carefully to prevent pathologic fractures
- Limit strenuous activity
- Assess the patient for constipation
- Provide postradiation nursing care
  - Provide skin and mouth care

Key nursing interventions for a patient with hypoparathyroidism

- Encourage fluids with acidifying solutions.
- Administer I.V. fluids.
- Strain urine.
- Assess bone and flank pain.
- Move the patient carefully to prevent pathologic fractures.

  - Monitor dietary intake
  - Provide rest periods
- Individualize home care instructions
  - Recognize the signs and symptoms of renal calculi
  - Strain urine
  - Prevent falls
  - Prevent constipation

Complications
- Peptic ulcer
- Psychosis
- Arrhythmias
- Renal failure
- Pathologic fractures

Surgical intervention
- Parathyroidectomy

HYPOPARATHYROIDISM

Definition
- Decrease in PTH secretion

Causes
- Thyroidectomy
- Autoimmune disease
- Parathyroidectomy
- Radiation
- Use of radioactive iodine
- Parathyroid tumor

Pathophysiology
- Decreased PTH decreases stimulation to osteoclasts, resulting in decreased release of calcium and phosphorus from bone (see *What happens in acute hypoparathyroidism,* page 282)
- Decreased circulating PTH reduces GI absorption of calcium and increases absorption of phosphorus
- Decreased blood calcium causes a rise in serum phosphates and decreased phosphate excretion by the kidney

Assessment findings
- Lethargy
- Calcification of ocular lens
- Muscle and abdominal spasms
- **Trousseau's sign: positive**
- **Chvostek's sign: positive**
- Tingling in fingers
- Arrhythmias
- Seizures
- Vision disturbances: diplopia, photophobia, blurring

Key home care instructions for a patient with hyperparathyroidism

- Recognize the signs and symptoms of renal calculi.
- Strain urine.
- Prevent falls.
- Prevent constipation.

Hypoparathyroidism highlights

- A decrease in PTH secretion
- Causes decreased stimulation to osteoclasts
- Reduces GI absorption of calcium
- Increases absorption of phosphorus
- Raises serum phosphates and decreases phosphate excretion

Key assessment findings in hypoparathyroidism

- Tingling in fingers
- Increased deep tendon reflexes

Causes of hypoparathyroidism

- Injury to the glands
- Accidental removal of the parathyroid glands
- Autoimmune disease
- Tumor
- Tuberculosis
- Sarcoidosis
- Hemochromatosis
- Severe magnesium deficiency

Results of acute hypoparathyroidism

- Seizures
- Tetany
- Laryngospasm
- CNS abnormalities

Key test findings in hypoparathyroidism

- Blood chemistry: decreased PTH, calcium; increased phosphorus
- Urine chemistry: decreased calcium

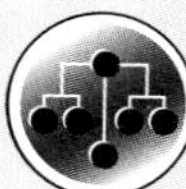

GO WITH THE FLOW

What happens in acute hypoparathyroidism

Causes of acute hypoparathyroidism include injury to the glands, accidental removal of the parathyroid glands during thyroidectomy or other neck surgery, autoimmune disease, tumor, tuberculosis, sarcoidosis, hemochromatosis, and severe magnesium deficiency associated with alcoholism and intestinal malabsorption. These disorders and conditions cause a cascade of effects that result in severe hypocalcemia and hyperphosphatemia, which can lead to seizures, tetany, laryngospasm, and central nervous system (CNS) abnormalities, as shown in the flow chart below.

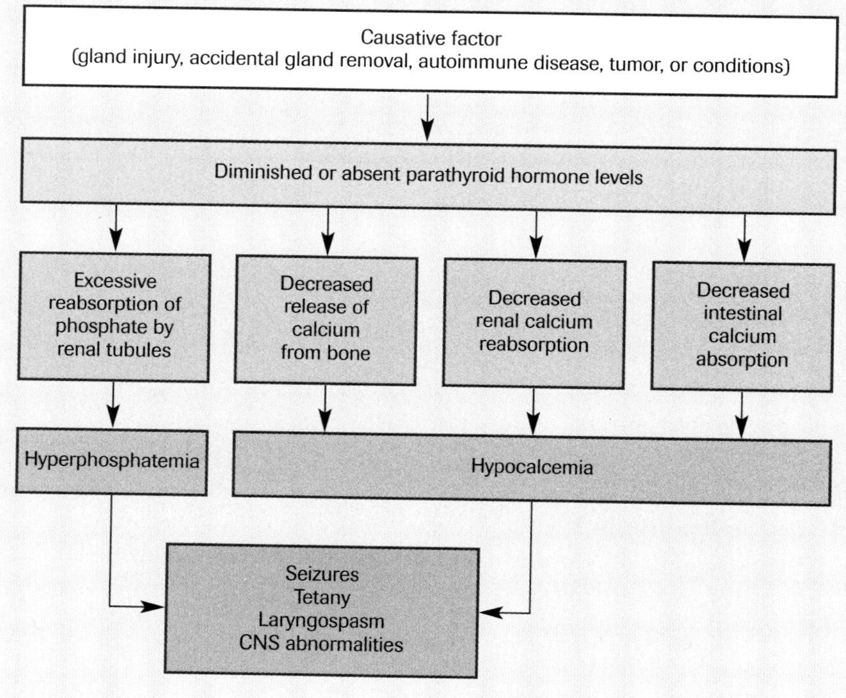

- Dyspnea
- Laryngeal stridor
- Personality changes
- Brittle nails
- Alopecia
- Deep tendon reflexes: increased

Diagnostic test findings

- Blood chemistry: decreased PTH, calcium; increased phosphorus
- Urine chemistry: decreased calcium
- X-ray: calcification of basal ganglia; increased bone density
- ECG: prolonged QT interval

- Sulkowitch's test: decreased

Medical management

- Diet: high-calcium, low-phosphorus, low-sodium with spinach restriction
- Activity: as tolerated
- I.V. therapy: saline lock
- Monitoring: vital signs and I/O
- Laboratory studies: PTH, calcium, and phosphorus
- Precautions: seizure
- Antacid: aluminum hydroxide gel (AlternaGEL)
- Sedative: zolpidem (Ambien)
- Anticonvulsants: phenytoin (Dilantin), magnesium sulfate (Epsom salt)
- Vitamins: ergocalciferol (vitamin D), dihydrotachysterol (Hytakerol)
- Oral calcium salts: calcium gluconate (Kalcinate), calcium carbonate (Os-Cal)
- Diuretic: furosemide (Lasix)
- Hormone replacement: parathyroid extract (PTH)
- I.V. calcium salts: calcium chloride or calcium gluconate

Nursing interventions

- Maintain the patient's diet
- Assess neurologic status
- **Maintain seizure precautions**
- Monitor and record vital signs, I/O, and laboratory studies
- Administer medications, as prescribed
- Allay the patient's anxiety
- Keep tracheostomy tray and I.V. calcium gluconate available
- Maintain a calm environment
- Individualize home care instruction
  - Recognize the signs and symptoms of seizure activity
  - Follow dietary recommendations

Complications

- Heart failure
- Mental retardation
- Blindness

Surgical interventions

- None

CUSHING'S SYNDROME (HYPERCORTISOLISM)

Definition

- Hyperactivity of the adrenal cortex that results in excessive secretion of glucocorticoids, particularly cortisol
- Possible increase in mineralocorticoids and sex hormones

Causes

- Hyperplasia of the adrenal glands
- Hypothalamic stimulation of the pituitary gland

Medications to help manage hypoparathyroidism

- Sedatives
- Anticonvulsants
- Vitamins
- Oral calcium salts
- I.V. calcium salts

Key nursing interventions for a patient with hyperparathyroidism

- Maintain seizure precautions.
- Keep tracheostomy tray and I.V. calcium gluconate available.

Cushing's syndrome defined

- Hyperactivity of the adrenal cortex that results in excessive secretion of glucocorticoids, particularly cortisol
- Causes a possible increase in mineralocorticoids and sex hormones

How Cushing's syndrome occurs

- Stimulation of the pituitary gland causes excessive corticotropin secretion
- Increased plasma cortisol occurs

- Adenoma or carcinoma of the pituitary gland
- Exogenous secretion of corticotropin by malignant neoplasms in the lungs or gallbladder
- Excessive or prolonged administration of glucocorticoids or corticotropin
- Adenoma or carcinoma of the adrenal cortex

Pathophysiology

- Hypothalamic stimulation of the pituitary gland causes excessive secretion of corticotropin
- Excessive secretion of corticotropin causes increased plasma cortisol
- Elevated blood cortisol levels don't diminish secretion of hypothalamic corticotropin-releasing hormone

Assessment findings

- Weight gain (see *Symptoms of cushingoid syndrome*)
- Hirsutism
- Amenorrhea
- Weakness and fatigue
- Pain in joints
- Ecchymosis
- Edema
- Hypertension
- Mood swings
- Fragile skin
- Purple striae on abdomen
- Poor wound healing
- Truncal obesity
- Buffalo hump
- Moon face
- Gynecomastia
- Enlarged clitoris
- Decreased libido
- Muscle wasting
- Recurrent infections
- Acne

Key test findings for Cushing's syndrome

- Dexamethasone suppression test: no decrease in 17-OHCS
- CT scan: pituitary or adrenal tumors
- Blood chemistry: increased cortisol, aldosterone, sodium, corticotropin, glucose; decreased potassium

Diagnostic test findings

- Dexamethasone suppression test: no decrease in 17-OHCS
- X-ray: pituitary or adrenal tumor; osteoporosis
- Angiography: pituitary or adrenal tumors
- CT scan: pituitary or adrenal tumors
- Urine chemistry: increased 17-OHCS and 17-KS; decreased specific gravity; glycosuria
- Blood chemistry: increased cortisol, aldosterone, sodium, corticotropin, glucose; decreased potassium
- Ultrasonography: pituitary or adrenal tumors
- Hematology: increased WBCs, RBCs; decreased eosinophils
- GTT: hyperglycemia

Symptoms of cushingoid syndrome

Long-term treatment with corticosteroids may produce an adverse effect called cushingoid syndrome – a condition marked by widespread systemic abnormalities and obvious fat deposits between the shoulders and around the waist.

In addition to the symptoms shown in the illustration, observe for signs of hypertension, renal disorders, hyperglycemia, tissue wasting, muscle weakness, and labile emotional state. The patient may also have amenorrhea and glycosuria.

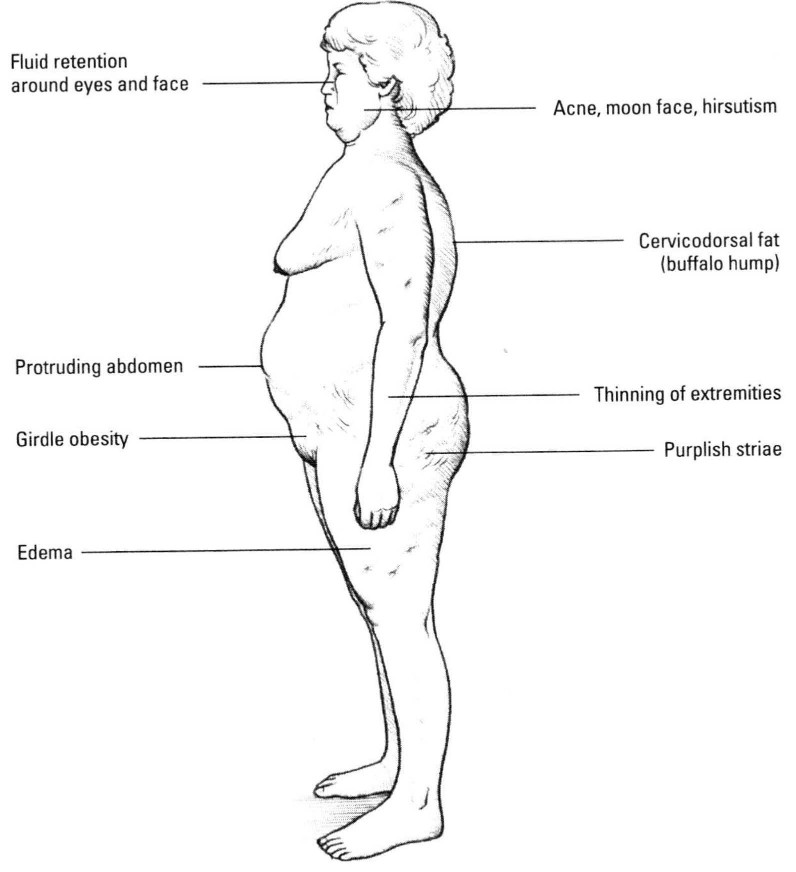

Key signs and symptoms of Cushing's syndrome

- Fluid retention around the eyes and face
- Protruding abdomen
- Girdle obesity
- Edema
- Acne
- Hirsutism
- Cervicodorsal fat
- Thinning of extremities
- Purplish striae

Medical management

- Diet: low-sodium, low-carbohydrate, low-calorie, high-potassium, and high-protein
- Activity: as tolerated
- Monitoring: vital signs, I/O, urine glucose and ketones, and specific gravity
- Laboratory studies: sodium, potassium, cortisol, BUN, glucose, WBCs, and RBCs
- Radiation therapy
- Diuretics: furosemide (Lasix), ethacrynic acid (Edecrin)

- Potassium supplements: potassium chloride (K-Lor), potassium gluconate (Kaon)
- Adrenal suppressants: metyrapone (Metopirone), aminoglutethimide (Cytadren)
- Hypoglycemics: rapid-acting (Lispro); short-acting (regular); intermediate-acting (NPH); long-acting (Lente, Lantus-insulin glargine); glyburide (DiaBeta, Micronase, Amaryl); glipizide (Glucotrol, Glucotrol XL)

Managing Cushing's syndrome with hypoglycemics

- Rapid-acting
- Short-acting
- Intermediate-acting
- Long-acting
- Glyburide
- Glipizide

Nursing interventions

- Maintain the patient's diet
- Assess fluid balance
- Monitor and record vital signs, I/O, specific gravity, blood glucose levels, urine glucose and ketones, and laboratory studies
- Assess edema
- Check for infections of skin, respiratory, and urinary tracts
- Protect the patient from falls and bruising
- Protect from infection
- Provide meticulous skin care
- Limit water intake
- Weigh the patient daily
- Administer medications, as prescribed
- Encourage the patient to express his feelings about changes in his body image and sexual function
- Provide rest periods
- Minimize environmental stress
- Provide postradiation nursing care
  - Provide prophylactic skin care
  - Monitor dietary intake
  - Provide rest periods
  - Assess for hypoglycemia
- Individualize home care instructions
  - Recognize the signs and symptoms of infection and fluid retention
  - Avoid exposure to people with infections
  - Monitor self for infection

Key nursing interventions for a patient with Cushing's syndrome

- Assess edema.
- Limit water intake.
- Weigh the patient daily.
- Protect from infection.
- Encourage the patient to express his feelings about changes in his body image and sexual function.

Home care instructions for a patient with Cushing's syndrome

- Recognize the signs and symptoms of infection and fluid retention.
- Avoid exposure to people with infections.
- Monitor for infection.

Complications

- Adrenal insufficiency
- Infection
- Peptic ulcers
- Hypertension
- Fractures
- Heart failure
- Psychosis
- Arrhythmias
- Diabetes mellitus
- Arteriosclerosis
- Nephrosclerosis

- **Surgical interventions**
  - Adrenalectomy
  - Hypophysectomy

ADDISON'S DISEASE

- **Definition**
  - Chronic hypoactivity of the adrenal cortex, resulting in insufficient secretion of glucocorticoids (cortisol) and mineralocorticoids (aldosterone)
- **Causes**
  - Idiopathic atrophy of adrenal glands
  - Surgical removal of adrenal glands
  - Autoimmune disease
  - Tuberculosis
  - Metastatic lesions from lung cancer
  - Pituitary hypofunction
  - Histoplasmosis
  - Trauma
- **Pathophysiology**
  - Autoimmune theory: body produces adrenocortical antibodies, resulting in adrenal hypofunction
  - Decreased aldosterone causes disturbances in sodium, water, and potassium metabolism
  - Decreased cortisol causes abnormal metabolism of fat, protein, and carbohydrate
- **Assessment findings**
  - Hypoglycemia
  - Weakness and lethargy
  - Bronzed skin pigmentation of nipples, scars, and buccal mucosa
  - Dehydration
  - Anorexia
  - Thirst
  - Decreased pubic and axillary hair
  - Orthostatic hypotension
  - Diarrhea
  - Nausea
  - Weight loss
  - Depression
- **Diagnostic test findings**
  - Blood chemistry: decreased HCT, Hb, cortisol, glucose, sodium, chloride, aldosterone; increased BUN, potassium
  - Urine chemistry: decreased 17-KS and 17-OHCS
  - Basal metabolic rate (BMR): decreased
  - Fasting serum glucose: hypoglycemia
  - ECG: prolonged PR and QT intervals

Addison's disease

- Chronic hypoactivity of the adrenal cortex
- Results in insufficient secretion of glucocorticoids and mineralocorticoids

Key causes of Addison's disease

- Idiopathic atrophy of adrenal glands
- Surgical removal of adrenal glands
- Autoimmune disease
- Tuberculosis

Key assessment findings in Addison's disease

- Hypoglycemia
- Weakness and lethargy
- Orthostatic hypotension
- Weight loss

Main medical treatment options for Addison's disease

- I.V. therapy
- Mineralocorticoids
- Glucocorticoids

Key home care instructions for a patient with Addison's disease

- Increase fluid intake in hot weather.
- Carry injectable dexamethasone.

Addisonian crisis characteristics

- Marked hypotension
- Cyanosis
- Abdominal cramps
- Diarrhea
- Costovertebral tenderness
- Fever
- Confusion
- Coma

Medical management

- Diet: high-carbohydrate, high-protein, high-sodium, low-potassium in small, frequent feedings before steroid therapy; high-potassium and low-sodium when on steroid therapy
- I.V. therapy: hydration, electrolyte replacement; saline lock
- Activity: bed rest
- Monitoring: vital signs, I/O, and specific gravity
- Laboratory studies: sodium, potassium, osmolality, cortisol, chloride, glucose, BUN, creatinine, Hb, and HCT
- I.V. saline
- Vasopressors: phenylephrine (Neo-Synephrine), norepinephrine (Levophed), dopamine (Intropin)
- Antacids: magnesium and aluminum hydroxide (Maalox), aluminum hydroxide gel (Gelusil)
- Mineralocorticoid (aldosterone): fludrocortisone (Florinef)
- Glucocorticoids: cortisone (Cortone), hydrocortisone (Solu-Cortef)

Nursing interventions

- Maintain the patient's diet
- Administer I.V. fluids
- Monitor and record vital signs, I/O, specific gravity, and laboratory studies
- Weigh the patient daily
- Administer medications, as prescribed
- Allay the patient's anxiety
- Protect the patient from falls
- Encourage fluid intake
- Assist with activities of daily living
- Maintain a quiet environment
- Individualize home care instructions
  - Avoid strenuous exercise, particularly in hot weather
  - Recognize the signs and symptoms of adrenal crisis
  - Increase fluid intake in hot weather
  - Carry injectable dexamethasone (Decadron)
  - Avoid using OTC drugs

Complications

- Addisonian crisis (adrenal crisis): marked hypotension, cyanosis, abdominal cramps, diarrhea, costovertebral tenderness, fever, confusion, coma
- Arrhythmias
- Hypovolemic shock
- Renal failure

Surgical interventions

- None

PHEOCHROMOCYTOMA

Definition
- Catecholamine-secreting neoplasm associated with hyperfunctioning adrenal medulla

Causes
- Genetics
- Pregnancy
- Trauma

Pathophysiology
- Tumor in the adrenal medulla secretes large amounts of catecholamines (epinephrine and norepinephrine)
- Increased catecholamines cause hypertension, increased BMR, and hyperglycemia

Assessment findings
- Labile malignant hypertension
- Throbbing headaches
- Diaphoresis
- Palpitations
- Tachycardia
- Excessive anxiety
- Hyperactivity
- Dilated pupils
- Cold extremities
- Weakness
- Weight loss
- Dyspnea
- Vertigo
- Angina
- Nausea
- Vomiting
- Anorexia
- Visual disturbances
- Polyuria
- Diarrhea
- Tinnitus
- Tremors

Diagnostic test findings
- CT scan: adrenal tumor
- Angiography: adrenal tumor
- Magnetic resonance imaging: adrenal tumor
- VMA: increased
- ECG: tachycardia
- Blood chemistries: increased BUN, creatinine, glucose, and catecholamines
- Urine chemistries: increased glucose and catecholamines

Pheochromocytoma defined

- Catecholamine-secreting neoplasm associated with hyperfunctioning adrenal medulla
- Increased catecholamines cause hypertension, increased BMR, and hyperglycemia

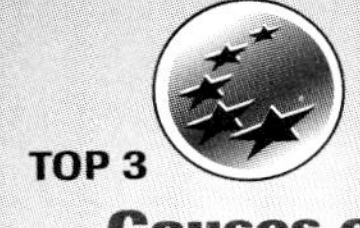

TOP 3

Causes of pheochromocytoma

1. Genetics
2. Pregnancy
3. Trauma

Key assessment findings in pheochromocytoma

- Labile malignant hypertension
- Throbbing headaches
- Diaphoresis
- Tachycardia

Main medication options for a patient with pheochromocytoma

- Alpha-adrenergic blockers
- Catecholamine inhibitor

Key interventions for a patient with pheochromocytoma

- Assess cardiovascular status.
- Monitor and record vital signs, I/O, orthostatic blood pressure, specific gravity, urine glucose and ketones, neurovital signs, and laboratory studies.
- Keep phentolamine (Regitine) available.

Surgical options for a patient with pheochromocytoma

- Adrenal medulla resection after administration of phentolamine
- Adrenalectomy

Medical management

- Diet: high-calorie, high-vitamin, and high-mineral with restricted use of stimulants such as caffeine beverages
- Activity: as tolerated
- Monitoring: vital signs, I/O, and urine glucose and ketones
- Position: semi-Fowler's
- Laboratory studies: BUN, creatinine, and glucose
- Sedative: lorazepam (Ativan)
- Alpha-adrenergic blockers: prazosin (Minipress), doxazosin (Cardura), terazosin (Hytrin)
- Beta-adrenergic blocker: propranolol (Inderal)
- Vasodilator: clonidine (Catapres), I.V. nitroglycerine
- Catecholamine inhibitor: metyrosine (Demser)

Nursing interventions

- Maintain the patient's diet
- Assess cardiovascular status
- Keep the patient in semi-Fowler's position
- Monitor and record vital signs, I/O, orthostatic blood pressure, specific gravity, urine glucose and ketones, neurovital signs, and laboratory studies
- Weigh the patient daily
- Administer medications, as prescribed
- Encourage the patient to express his feelings about fear of dying
- Protect the patient from falls
- Minimize environmental stress
- Provide rest periods
- Keep phentolamine (Regitine) available
- Provide postradiation nursing care
  - Provide skin and mouth care
  - Monitor dietary intake
  - Provide rest periods
- Individualize home care instructions
  - Stop smoking
  - Recognize the signs and symptoms of renal failure
  - Monitor blood pressure, urine glucose, and ketones daily

Complications

- Cardiac arrest
- Cerebral hemorrhage
- Blindness
- Renal failure
- MI
- Heart failure

Surgical interventions

- Adrenal medulla resection after administration of phentolamine (Regitine)
- Adrenalectomy

HYPERALDOSTERONISM (PRIMARY ALDOSTERONISM, CONN'S SYNDROME)

Definition
- Hypersecretion of aldosterone (mineralocorticoids) from adrenal cortex

Causes
- Adenoma of adrenal cortex
- Adrenal hyperplasia
- Adrenal carcinoma

Pathophysiology
- Aldosterone's primary effect on the renal tubules causes the kidneys to retain sodium and water and excrete potassium and hydrogen

Assessment findings
- Muscle weakness
- Polyuria
- Polydipsia
- Metabolic alkalosis
- Hypertension
- Postural hypotension
- Headache
- Paresthesia
- Pyelonephritis
- Nocturia
- Chvostek's sign: positive
- Trousseau's sign: positive

Diagnostic test findings
- Blood chemistry: decreased potassium; increased sodium, carbon dioxide
- Arterial blood gas (ABG) analysis: metabolic alkalosis
- Urine chemistry: increased aldosterone, protein, pH; decreased specific gravity

Medical management
- Diet: high-potassium, low-sodium
- Activity: as tolerated
- Monitoring: vital signs and I/O
- Laboratory studies: potassium, sodium, calcium, and ABG analysis
- Potassium salts: potassium chloride (KCl), potassium gluconate (Kaon)
- Diuretics: spironolactone (Aldactone), acetazolamide (Diamox)
- Calcium salts: calcium gluconate (Kalcinate), calcium carbonate (Os-Cal)

Nursing interventions
- Maintain the patient's diet, as tolerated
- Monitor and record vital signs, I/O, orthostatic blood pressure, specific gravity, and laboratory studies
- Monitor laboratory results: ABG analysis, sodium, potassium, and calcium
- Administer medications, as prescribed
- Allay the patient's anxiety

Hyperaldosteronism defined
- Hypersecretion of aldosterone from adrenal cortex

Key signs and symptoms of hyperaldosteronism
- Muscle weakness
- Headache
- Paresthesia
- Chvostek's sign: positive
- Trousseau's sign: positive

Key management options for hyperaldosteronism
- Potassium salts
- Diuretics

- Weigh the patient daily
- Provide a quiet environment
- Individualize home care instructions
  - Recognize the signs and symptoms of fluid overload and muscle irritability
  - Comply with medical follow-up

Key nursing interventions for a patient with hyperaldosteronism

- Assess fluid balance.
- Monitor laboratory results: ABG analysis, sodium, potassium, and calcium.
- Provide individualized home care instructions.

Complications

- Neuropathy
- Arrhythmias

Surgical intervention

- Adrenalectomy

DIABETES MELLITUS

Definition

- Chronic disorder of carbohydrate metabolism with subsequent alteration of protein and fat metabolism
- Results from a disturbance in the production, action, and rate of insulin use
- Five types of diabetes mellitus
  - Type 1 (insulin-dependent diabetes mellitus or ketosis-prone): usually develops in childhood
  - Type 2 (non-insulin-dependent diabetes mellitus or ketosis-resistant): usually develops after age 30
  - Gestational diabetes mellitus: occurs with pregnancy
  - Secondary diabetes: induced by trauma, surgery, pancreatic disease or medications; can be treated as type 1 or type 2
  - Maturity-onset diabetes: type 2 that develops in teens and young adults under age 30

Facts about diabetes mellitus

- Chronic disorder of carbohydrate metabolism with subsequent alteration of protein and fat metabolism
- Results from disturbance in insulin use
- Types include: type 1, type 2, gestational diabetes mellitus, secondary diabetes, and maturity-onset diabetes

Causes

- Failure of body to produce insulin
- Blockage of insulin supply
- Autoimmune disease
- Receptor defect in normally insulin-responsive cells
- Genetics
- Exposure to chemicals
- Hyperpituitarism
- Cushing's syndrome
- Hyperthyroidism
- Infection
- Surgery
- Stress
- Medications
- Pregnancy
- Trauma

Type 1 and type 2 diabetes mellitus defined

- Type 1: usually develops in childhood; insulin-dependent diabetes mellitus
- Type 2: usually develops after age 30; non-insulin-dependent diabetes mellitus

Pathophysiology

- Type 1 results from an inability to produce endogenous insulin by the beta cells in the islets of Langerhans in the pancreas
- Type 2 is a deficit in insulin release or an insulin-receptor defect in peripheral tissues
- Insulin deprivation of insulin-dependent cells leads to a marked decrease in the cellular rate of glucose uptake
- Glucogenesis increases because of decreased stimulation of glucose metabolism with resulting hyperglycemia and glycosuria
- Decreased insulin triggers release of free fatty acids that can't be metabolized and are released as ketone bodies in blood and urine
- Decreased insulin depresses protein synthesis, causing a release of amino acids that the liver converts into glucose and ketones
- The formation of urea results in overall nitrogen loss

Assessment findings

- Weight loss
- Anorexia
- Polyphagia
- Acetone breath
- Weakness
- Fatigue
- Dehydration
- Pain
- Paresthesia
- Polyuria
- Polydipsia
- Kussmaul's respirations
- Multiple infections and boils
- Flushed, warm, smooth, shiny skin
- Atrophic muscles
- Poor wound healing
- Mottled extremities
- Peripheral and visceral neuropathies
- Retinopathy
- Sexual dysfunction
- Blurred vision

Diagnostic test findings

- Blood chemistry: increased glucose, potassium, chloride, ketones, cholesterol, and triglycerides; decreased carbon dioxide; pH less than 7.4
- Urine chemistry: increased glucose, ketones
- Fasting serum glucose: increased
- GTT: hyperglycemia
- Postprandial blood glucose: hyperglycemia
- Glycosylated Hb assay: increased

Pathophysiology of diabetes mellitus

- Type 1: results from an inability of beta cells to produce endogenous insulin.
- Type 2: results from deficient insulin release or an insulin-receptor defect.
- Insulin deprivation leads to decrease in glucose uptake.
- Decreased insulin triggers release of free fatty acids that can't be metabolized and are released as ketone bodies in blood and urine.
- Decreased insulin depresses protein synthesis.
- Overall nitrogen loss occurs.

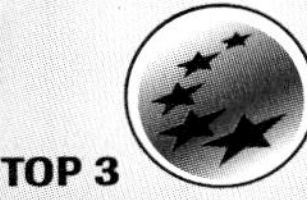

TOP 3

Assessment findings in diabetes mellitus

1. Polyphagia
2. Polyuria
3. Polydipsia

Key test findings in diabetes

- Fasting serum glucose: increased
- Postprandial blood glucose: hyperglycemia

Treating diabetes with diet and hypoglycemics

- Diet: individually prescribed diet based on ideal weight, metabolic activity, and personal activity levels
- Hypoglycemics: rapid-acting, short-acting, intermediate-acting, long-acting; glyburide; glipizide; metformin; pioglitazone; rosiglitazone; repaglinide

Key nursing interventions for a patient with diabetes mellitus

- Assess acid-base balance.
- Monitor and record vital signs, I/O, blood glucose levels, and laboratory studies.
- Provide meticulous skin and foot care.
- Monitor the patient for infection.
- Monitor wound healing.

Medical management

- Diet: individually prescribed diet based on ideal weight, metabolic activity, and personal activity levels
  - Use the American Diabetes Association's exchange list for meal planning to design a diet that will distribute an individual's caloric needs, carbohydrate, fat, and protein intake over 24 hours
  - Avoid refined and simple sugars and saturated fats
  - Limit cholesterol
  - Include high fiber and high complex carbohydrates
- Activity: as tolerated
- Monitoring: vital signs and I/O
- Laboratory studies: glucose, potassium, glycosylated Hb, and pH, and liver and renal function tests
- Hypoglycemics: rapid-acting (Lispro), short-acting (regular), intermediate-acting (NPH), long-acting (Ultralente, Lantus-insulin glargine); glyburide (DiaBeta, Micronase, Amaryl); glipizide (Glucotrol, Glucotrol XL); metformin (Glucophage); pioglitazone (Actos); rosiglitazone (Avandia); repaglinide (Prandin)
- Vitamin and mineral supplements

Nursing interventions

- Maintain the patient's diet
- Encourage fluids
- Assess acid-base balance
- Monitor and record vital signs, I/O, blood glucose levels, and laboratory studies
- Administer medications, as prescribed
- Encourage the patient to express his feelings about diet, medication regimen, and body image changes
- Encourage activity, as tolerated
- Weigh the patient weekly
- Provide meticulous skin and foot care
- Monitor the patient for infection
- Maintain a warm and quiet environment
- Monitor wound healing
- Observe for Somogyi phenomena and Sjögren's syndrome
- Provide information about the American Diabetes Association
- Foster independence
- Determine the patient's compliance to diet, exercise, and medication regimens
- Individualize home care instructions
  - Exercise regularly
  - Stop smoking
  - Recognize the signs and symptoms of hyperglycemia and hypoglycemia
  - Monitor self for infection, skin breakdown, changes in peripheral circulation, poor wound healing, and numbness in extremities

- Know and use proper dietary substitutions if unable to take prescribed diet because of illness
- Adjust diet and insulin for changes in work, exercise, trauma, infection, fever, and stress
- Demonstrate administration of hypoglycemics
- Demonstrate home blood glucose monitoring technique
- Complete daily skin and foot care
- Carry an emergency supply of glucose
- Seek counseling for sexual dysfunction and feelings about body image changes
- Avoid use of OTC medication
- Avoid alcohol
- Demonstrate use of the subcutaneous insulin infusion therapy (insulin pump)
- Adhere to the treatment regimen to prevent complications

Complications

- Ketoacidosis (diabetic coma): abdominal pain; acetone breath; altered consciousness; hot, flushed skin; Kussmaul's respirations; nausea; vomiting; hypotension; oliguria; tachycardia (see *Understanding DKA and HHNS,* page 296)
- Insulin reaction (hypoglycemia): hunger, weakness, hand tremors, pallor, tachycardia, diaphoresis, irritability, confusion, diplopia, slurred speech, headaches
- Infections
- Peripheral neuropathies
- Glaucoma
- Impotence
- CAD
- Gangrene
- Stroke
- Chronic renal failure
- Hyperosmolar hyperglycemic nonketotic syndrome: severe dehydration, severe hypotension, fever, stupor, and seizures
- Hypovolemia
- Diabetic retinopathy
- Peripheral vascular disease

Surgical interventions

- None

DIABETES INSIPIDUS

Definition

- Deficiency of ADH (vasopressin) that's secreted by the posterior lobe of the pituitary gland (neurohypophysis)

Causes

- Trauma to posterior lobe of pituitary gland

Home care instructions for a patient with diabetes mellitus

- Recognize the signs and symptoms of hyperglycemia and hypoglycemia.
- Monitor for infection, skin breakdown, changes in peripheral circulation, poor wound healing, and numbness in extremities.
- Adjust diet and insulin for changes in work, exercise, trauma, infection, fever, and stress.
- Demonstrate administration of hypoglycemics.
- Demonstrate home blood glucose monitoring technique.
- Carry an emergency supply of glucose.

Possible complications of diabetes mellitus

- Ketoacidosis
- Insulin reaction
- CAD
- Chronic renal failure

Diabetes insipidus defined

- Deficiency of ADH that's secreted by the posterior lobe of the pituitary gland
- Copious, dilute urine, and intense thirst result

Facts about DKA and HHNS

- Acute complications of hyperglycemic crisis
- DKA occurs most often in patients with type 1 diabetes
- HHNS occurs most often in patients with type 2 diabetes
- Insulin-deprived cells can't utilize glucose and the response is rapid metabolism of protein
- A loss of intracellular potassium and phosphorus occurs, along with excessive liberation of amino acids
- Amino acids are converted into urea and glucose by the liver
- Blood glucose levels become grossly elevated
- Increased serum osmotic diuresis occurs, creating a massive fluid loss and dehydration
- Dehydration is perpetuated, decreasing the glomerular filtration rate and reducing the amount of glucose excreted in urine
- Diminished glucose excretion raises blood glucose levels, producing hyperosmolarity and dehydration, which cause shock, coma, and death

Understanding DKA and HHNS

Diabetic ketoacidosis (DKA) and hyperosmolar hyperglycemic nonketotic syndrome (HHNS) are acute complications of hyperglycemic crisis that may occur with diabetes. If not treated properly, either may result in coma or death.

DKA occurs most often in patients with type 1 diabetes and may be the first evidence of the disease. HHNS occurs most often in patients with type 2 diabetes, but it also occurs in anyone whose insulin tolerance is stressed and in patients who have undergone certain therapeutic procedures, such as peritoneal dialysis, hemodialysis, tube feedings, or total parenteral nutrition.

Acute insulin deficiency (absolute in DKA; relative in HHNS) precipitates both conditions. Causes include illness, stress, infection and, in patients with DKA, failure to take insulin.

BUILDUP OF GLUCOSE

Inadequate insulin hinders glucose uptake by fat and muscle cells. Because the cells can't take in glucose to convert to energy, glucose accumulates in the blood. At the same time, the liver responds to the demands of the energy-starved cells by converting glycogen to glucose and releasing glucose into the blood, further increasing the blood glucose level. When this level exceeds the renal threshold, excess glucose is excreted in the urine.

Still, the insulin-deprived cells can't utilize glucose. Their response is rapid metabolism of protein, which results in loss of intracellular potassium and phosphorus and excessive liberation of amino acids. The liver converts these amino acids into urea and glucose.

As a result of these processes, blood glucose levels are grossly elevated. The aftermath is increased serum osmolarity and glycosuria (high amounts of glucose in the urine), leading to osmotic diuresis. Glucosuria is higher in HHNS than in DKA because blood glucose levels are higher in HHNS.

A DEADLY CYCLE

The massive fluid loss from osmotic diuresis causes fluid and electrolyte imbalances and dehydration. Water loss exceeds glucose and electrolyte loss, contributing to hyperosmolarity. This, in turn, perpetuates dehydration, decreasing the glomerular filtration rate and reducing the amount of glucose excreted in the urine. This leads to a deadly cycle: Diminished glucose excretion further raises blood glucose levels, producing hyperosmolarity and dehydration and finally causing shock, coma, and death.

DKA complication

All of these steps hold true for DKA and HHNS, but DKA involves an additional, simultaneous process that leads to metabolic acidosis. The absolute insulin deficiency causes cells to convert fats into glycerol and fatty acids for energy. The fatty acids can't be metabolized as quickly as they're released, so they accumulate in the liver, where they're converted into ketones (ketoacids). These ketones accumulate in the blood and urine and cause acidosis. Acidosis leads to more tissue breakdown, more ketosis, more acidosis, and eventually shock, coma, and death.

- Tumor of posterior lobe of pituitary gland
- Brain surgery
- Head injury

- Idiopathic
- Meningitis

Pathophysiology

- Decreased ADH reduces the ability of distal and collecting renal tubules to concentrate urine
- Copious, dilute urine, and intense thirst result

Assessment findings

- Polyuria (greater than 5 L/day)
- Polydipsia (4 to 40 L/day)
- Fatigue
- Dehydration
- Weight loss
- Muscle weakness and pain
- Headache
- Tachycardia

Diagnostic test findings

- Urine chemistry: specific gravity less than 1.004, osmolality 50 to 200 mOsm/kg
- Blood chemistry: decreased ADH by radioimmunoassay
- Water deprivation test: inability to concentrate urine

Medical management

- Diet: regular with restriction of foods that exert a diuretic effect
- I.V. therapy: hydration, electrolyte replacement; saline lock
- Activity: bed rest
- Monitoring: vital signs, CVP, and I/O
- Laboratory studies: potassium, sodium, BUN, creatinine, specific gravity, and osmolality
- Treatments: indwelling urinary catheter
- ADH stimulant: carbamazepine (Tegretol)
- ADH replacement: lypressin (Diapid nasal spray)

Nursing interventions

- Maintain the patient's diet
- Encourage fluids
- Administer I.V. fluids
- Maintain patency of indwelling urinary catheter
- Monitor and record vital signs, CVP, I/O, specific gravity, and laboratory studies
- Administer medications, as prescribed
- Allay the patient's anxiety
- Weigh the patient daily
- Individualize home care instructions
  - Recognize the signs and symptoms of dehydration
  - Increase fluid intake in hot weather
  - Carry medications on person at all times

Key assessment findings in diabetes insipidus

- Polyuria (greater than 5 L/day)
- Polydipsia (4 to 40 L/day)

Diagnostic urine chemistry findings in diabetes insipidus

- Specific gravity less than 1.004
- Osmolality 50 to 200 mOsm/kg

Key steps in managing diabetes insipidus

- I.V. therapy
- ADH replacements
- ADH stimulants

Facts about hyperpituitarism

- Hypersecretion of GH by the anterior pituitary gland
- GH-induced hypermetabolism causes hormone alterations

Key signs and symptoms of hyperpituitarism

- Coarse facial features
- Enlarged tongue
- Protruding jaw

Key test findings in hyperpituitarism

- X-rays: thickened long bones and skull
- Blood chemistry: increased phosphorus, prolactin, glucose, somatotropin; decreased FSH

Complications

- Dehydration
- Arrhythmias
- Hypovolemic shock

Surgical intervention

- Hypophysectomy, when etiology is tumor

HYPERPITUITARISM (ACROMEGALY)

Definition

- Hypersecretion of GH by the anterior pituitary gland (adenohypophysis)

Causes

- Prolactin-secreting benign adenomas
- GH-secreting tumors
- Cushing's syndrome caused by pituitary dysfunction
- LH-, FSH-, or TSH-secreting adenomas
- Adrenalectomy
- Pregnancy

Pathophysiology

- Excessive secretion of GH occurs after epiphyseal closing
- Excessive secretion of GH causes overdevelopment of cartilage, bone, soft tissue; thickens skin; and enlarges sweat glands, sebaceous glands, and gonads
- GH-induced hypermetabolism causes hormone alterations

Assessment findings

- Coarse facial features
- Enlarged tongue
- Protruding jaw
- Spiderlike fingers
- Wide hands and feet
- Weakness
- Impotence
- Infertility
- Thick skin and nails
- Diplopia
- Cranial nerve palsies
- Joint deformities
- Pain in joints
- Deepening of voice
- Diaphoresis
- Headache

Diagnostic test findings

- Insulin tolerance test: hyperglycemia
- CT scan: enlarged pituitary
- Visual fields: hemianopsia, diplopia

- X-rays: thickened long bones and skull
- Blood chemistry: increased phosphorus, prolactin, glucose, somatotropin; decreased FSH
- Urine chemistry: increased calcium, glucose

Medical management

- Activity: as tolerated
- Monitoring: vital signs and I/O
- Laboratory studies: glucose, potassium, and calcium
- Radiation therapy via transphenoidal implant
- Dopaminergics: levodopa (Larodopa), bromocriptine (Parlodel)
- Hormones: somatotropin (Humatrope), ethinyl estradiol (Estinyl), testosterone (Androgel), levothyroxine (Synthroid), liothyronine (Cytomel), diethylstilbestrol
- Glucocorticoids: cortisone (Cortone), hydrocortisone (Cortef), hydrocortisone sodium succinate (Solu-Cortef)
- Ergot alkaloid: methysergide (Sansert)
- Mineralocorticoid: fludrocortisone (Florinef)
- Cryosurgery
- Thermocoagulation
- Ultrasound therapy

Nursing interventions

- Monitor and record vital signs, I/O, urine glucose and ketones, blood glucose levels, and laboratory studies
- Administer medications, as prescribed
- Encourage the patient to express his feelings about changes in his body image and sexual dysfunction
- Maintain activity, as tolerated
- Provide skin care
- Position and support painful joints
- Protect the patient from falls
- Monitor for infection
- Provide postradiation nursing care
  - Provide prophylactic skin and mouth care
  - Monitor dietary intake
  - Provide rest periods
- Individualize home care instructions
  - Carry emergency adrenal hormone replacement drugs
  - Wear medical identification jewelry

Complications

- Blindness
- Vision disturbances
- Diabetes mellitus
- Cushing's syndrome
- Hyperthyroidism
- Hypertension
- Heart failure

Treating hyperpituitarism with medications

- Dopaminergics
- Hormones
- Glucocorticoids

Key nursing interventions for a patient with hyperpituitarism

- Monitor and record vital signs, I/O, urine glucose and ketones, blood glucose levels, and laboratory studies.
- Encourage the patient to express his feelings about changes in his body image and sexual dysfunction.
- Maintain activity, as tolerated.

Key home care instructions for a patient with hyperpituitarism

- Carry emergency adrenal hormone replacement drugs.
- Wear medical identification jewelry.

- Angina
- Cardiomyopathy
- Hyperparathyroidism
- Renal calculi
- Cardiac arrest

Surgical intervention

- Hypophysectomy

HYPOPITUITARISM (SIMMONDS' DISEASE)

Definition

- Hypofunction of anterior pituitary gland (adenohypophysis), resulting in insufficient or absent quantities of anterior pituitary gland hormones or target organ hormones

Causes

- Adenomas or carcinomas of pituitary gland
- Postpartum hemorrhage
- Head trauma
- Necrosis of pituitary gland (Sheehan's syndrome)
- Radiation of head
- Hypophysectomy
- Insufficient hypothalamic releasing factors

Pathophysiology

- Decreased pituitary function results in decreased amounts of GH, TSH, and corticotropin
- With progressive loss of pituitary function, levels of FSH and LH decrease

Assessment findings

- Lethargy
- Decreased strength
- Decreased tolerance for cold temperatures
- Hypothermia
- Hypotension
- Emaciation
- Decreased axillary and pubic hair
- Atrophy of gonads and thyroid
- Impotence
- Weight loss
- Pallor
- Decreased libido
- Amenorrhea
- Dry skin
- Decreased perspiration
- Recurrent infections
- Headaches

Characteristics of hypopituitarism

- Hypofunction of anterior pituitary gland
- Results in insufficient or absent quantities of anterior pituitary gland hormones or target organ hormones

Key signs and symptoms of hypopituitarism

- Lethargy
- Decreased tolerance for cold temperatures
- Hypotension
- Decreased axillary and pubic hair
- Atrophy of gonads and thyroid
- Impotence
- Weight loss
- Decreased libido

Diagnostic test findings

- Blood chemistry: decreased cortisol, growth hormone, corticotropin, TSH, LH, FSH, glucose, and gonadotropins
- RAIU: decreased
- Fasting serum glucose: decreased glucose
- GTT: decreased glucose
- Hematology: decreased Hb and HCT
- CT scan: adenohypophyseal tumor
- Visual fields: hemianopsia and loss of color vision
- Angiography: adenohypophyseal tumor
- Urine chemistry: decreased gonadotropins, 17-OHCS, and 17-KS
- Skull X-ray: adenohypophyseal tumor

Key test findings in hypopituitarism

- Blood chemistry: decreased cortisol, growth hormone, corticotropin, TSH, LH, FSH, glucose, and gonadotropins
- CT scan: adenohypophyseal tumor

Medical management

- Diet: high-protein
- Activity: as tolerated
- Monitoring: vital signs, I/O, and laboratory studies
- Radiation therapy
- Dopaminergics: levodopa (Larodopa), bromocriptine (Parlodel)
- Hormones: somatotropin (Humatrope), ethinyl estradiol (Estinyl), testosterone (Androgel), levothyroxine (Synthroid), liothyronine (Cytomel)
- Glucocorticoids: cortisone (Cortone), hydrocortisone (Cortef), hydrocortisone sodium succinate (Solu-Cortef)

Hormones used to manage hypopituitarism

- Somatotropin
- Ethinyl estradiol
- Testosterone
- Levothyroxine
- Liothyronine

Nursing interventions

- Maintain the patient's diet
- Monitor and record vital signs, I/O, urine glucose and ketones, and laboratory studies
- Administer medications, as prescribed
- Encourage the patient to express his feelings about changes in his body image and sexual dysfunction
- Maintain activity, as tolerated
- Prevent falls
- Monitor for infection
- Maintain a warm environment
- Provide skin care
- Allay the patient's anxiety
- Reinforce the need to eat
- Provide postradiation nursing care
  - Provide prophylactic skin care
  - Monitor dietary intake
  - Provide rest periods
- Individualize home care instructions
  - Recognize the signs and symptoms of dehydration
  - Avoid exposure to people with infections
  - Monitor self for infection

Key nursing interventions for a patient with hypopituitarism

- Encourage the patient to express his feelings about changes in his body image and sexual dysfunction.
- Monitor for infection.
- Maintain a warm environment.
- Reinforce the need to eat.

Home care instructions for a patient with hypopituitarism

- Recognize the signs and symptoms of dehydration.
- Avoid exposure to people with infections.
- Monitor for infection.

Complications

- Death

- Hypothyroidism
- Adrenal insufficiency

Surgical interventions
- Hypophysectomy
- Resection of pituitary gland

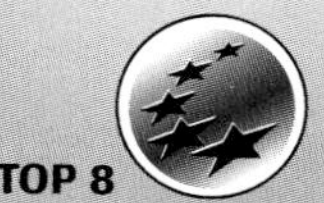

TOP 8

Items to study for your next test on the endocrine system

1. Functions of the thyroid gland and pancreas
2. Nursing interventions for a patient after thyroidectomy
3. Signs and symptoms of hyperthyroidism and hypothyroidism
4. Why thyrotoxic crisis occurs
5. Assessment findings in Cushing's syndrome
6. The difference between type 1 and type 2 diabetes mellitus
7. Signs and symptoms of hypoglycemia and hyperglycemia
8. Complications of diabetes mellitus, including DKA and HHNS

NCLEX CHECKS

It's never too soon to begin your NCLEX preparation. Now that you've reviewed this chapter, carefully read each of the following questions and choose the best answer. Then compare your responses to the correct answers.

1. A patient is diagnosed with hyperthyroidism. The nurse should expect to see which clinical signs and symptoms? (Select all that apply.)

- ☐ **A.** Anxiety
- ☐ **B.** Dry, flaky skin
- ☐ **C.** Hypothermia
- ☐ **D.** Increased blood pressure
- ☐ **E.** Tachycardia
- ☐ **F.** Weight gain

2. A patient with thyroid cancer undergoes a thyroidectomy. After surgery, the patient develops peripheral numbness, tingling, muscle twitching, and spasms. The nurse should administer:

- ☐ **A.** a thyroid supplement.
- ☐ **B.** an antispasmodic.
- ☐ **C.** a barbiturate.
- ☐ **D.** I.V. calcium gluconate.

3. A patient with intractable asthma develops Cushing's syndrome. This development is most likely attributed to long-term or excessive use of:

- ☐ **A.** prednisone.
- ☐ **B.** theophylline.
- ☐ **C.** metaproterenol (Alupent).
- ☐ **D.** cromolyn (Intal).

4. Which nursing diagnosis is most likely for a patient with an acute episode of diabetes insipidus?

- ☐ **A.** Imbalanced nutrition: More than body requirements
- ☐ **B.** Deficient fluid volume
- ☐ **C.** Impaired gas exchange
- ☐ **D.** Ineffective tissue perfusion: Cardiopulmonary

5. A patient with a parathyroid hormone (PTH) deficiency would most likely experience abnormal serum levels of:

- ☐ **A.** sodium and chloride.
- ☐ **B.** potassium and glucose.
- ☐ **C.** urea and uric acid.
- ☐ **D.** calcium and phosphorous.

6. A patient with newly diagnosed type 1 diabetes mellitus is learning about diabetic foot care. The nurse should instruct the patient to avoid:

- ☐ **A.** lotions.
- ☐ **B.** antiperspirants.
- ☐ **C.** foot soaks.
- ☐ **D.** nail files.

7. Following transsphenoidal hypophysectomy, the nurse notes clear drainage on the nasal dressing. Which of the following actions should the nurse take next?

- ☐ **A.** Have the patient blow his nose.
- ☐ **B.** Reinforce the nasal dressing.
- ☐ **C.** Test the drainage for glucose.
- ☐ **D.** Send a nasal culture to the laboratory.

8. Which statement by a patient following bilateral adrenalectomy indicates to the nurse that the patient understands discharge instructions?

- ☐ **A.** "I'll take steroids for two weeks."
- ☐ **B.** "I'll take steroids for life."
- ☐ **C.** "I'll take steroids until my symptoms subside."
- ☐ **D.** "I'll gradually taper the steroids."

9. Which of the following findings would the nurse expect in a patient with hypothyroidism?

- ☐ **A.** Exophthalmos
- ☐ **B.** Heat intolerance
- ☐ **C.** Weight loss
- ☐ **D.** Alopecia

10. A patient with diabetes mellitus exhibits tremors, tachycardia, and cold, clammy skin. The nurse should expect to treat the patient for which condition?

- ☐ **A.** Ketoacidosis
- ☐ **B.** Hyperosmolar hyperglycemic nonketotic syndrome (HHNS)
- ☐ **C.** Hypoglycemia
- ☐ **D.** Somogyi phenomenon

ANSWERS AND RATIONALES

1. CORRECT ANSWER: A, D, E

Hyperthyroidism is a hypermetabolic state with symptoms including anxiety, increased blood pressure, and tachycardia—all seen in sympathetic nervous system stimulation. Symptoms of dry, flaky skin, hypothermia, and weight gain are associated with a hypometabolic state of hypothyroidism.

2. CORRECT ANSWER: D

Removal of the thyroid gland can cause hyposecretion of parathyroid hormone, leading to calcium deficiency. Symptoms of calcium deficiency include muscle spasms, numbness, and tingling. Treatment includes immediate I.V. administration of calcium gluconate. Thyroid supplements are necessary following thyroidectomy but don't correct hypocalcemia. An antispasmodic doesn't treat the problem and a barbiturate isn't indicated.

3. CORRECT ANSWER: A
Cushing's syndrome results from long-term or excessive use of a glucocorticoid such as prednisone. Theophylline, metaproterenol, and cromolyn don't cause Cushing's syndrome.

4. CORRECT ANSWER: B
Diabetes insipidus causes a pronounced loss of intravascular volume; therefore, the most prominent risk to the patient is deficient fluid volume. The patient is at risk for imbalanced nutrition, impaired gas exchange, and ineffective tissue perfusion, but these risks stem from the deficient fluid volume.

5. CORRECT ANSWER: D
Because PTH regulates calcium and phosphorous metabolism, a PTH deficiency would affect calcium and phosphorous levels. PTH doesn't affect sodium, chloride, potassium, glucose, urea, and uric acid.

6. CORRECT ANSWER: C
Foot soaks macerate the skin and increase the risk for breaks in the skin. To moisturize the feet, use water-soluble lotions. Use nail files instead of nail clippers or scissors. When foot perspiration exists, use antiperspirants.

7. CORRECT ANSWER: C
The presence of glucose in the nasal drainage indicates leakage of cerebrospinal fluid. Following hypophysectomy, instruct the patient to avoid blowing his nose. You may reinforce the dressing, but not until you test the fluid for glucose. While infection can occur after surgery, clear drainage isn't indicative of infection.

8. CORRECT ANSWER: B
Following bilateral adrenalectomy, the patient requires lifelong glucocorticoid and mineralocorticoid replacement. The patient shouldn't stop taking steroids after two weeks or until his symptoms subside following removal of the adrenal glands. Because the patient requires steroids for life, they can't be tapered.

9. CORRECT ANSWER: D
The patient with hypothyroidism will have coarse hair and alopecia. Exophthalmos, heat intolerance, and weight loss are all associated with hyperthyroidism.

10. CORRECT ANSWER: C
Tremors, tachycardia, and cold, clammy skin are all signs of hypoglycemia. Ketoacidosis characteristics include abdominal pain, acetone breath, altered consciousness, Kussmaul's respirations, nausea, vomiting, oliguria, tachycardia, and hot, flushed skin. HHNS characteristics include severe dehydration, severe hypotension, fever, stupor, and seizures. Somogyi phenomena shows rebound hyperglycemia in which the person awakens with symptoms of hyperglycemia.

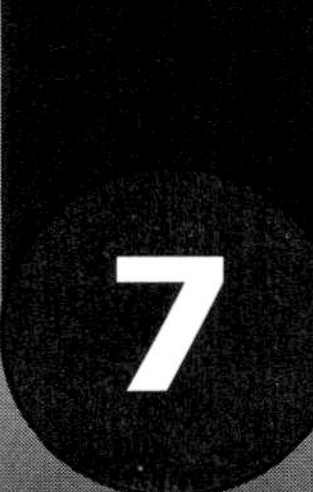

7 Renal and urologic system

LEARNING OBJECTIVES

After studying this chapter, you should be able to:

- Describe the psychosocial impact of renal and urologic disorders.
- Differentiate between modifiable and nonmodifiable risk factors in the development of a renal or urologic disorder.
- List three probable and three possible nursing diagnoses for any patient with a renal or urologic disorder.
- Identify nursing interventions for a patient with a renal or urologic disorder.
- Identify three teaching topics for a patient with a renal or urologic disorder.

CHAPTER OVERVIEW

Caring for the patient with a renal or urologic disorder requires a sound understanding of renal and urologic anatomy and physiology and fluid balance. A thorough assessment is essential to planning and implementing appropriate patient care. The assessment includes a complete history, a physical examination, diagnostic testing, identification of modifiable and nonmodifiable risk factors, and information related to the psychosocial impact of the disorder on the patient.

Nursing diagnoses focus primarily on altered urinary elimination and body image disturbance. Nursing interventions should include assessing patient hydration and urinary output, and helping the patient adjust to body image changes and possible sexual dysfunction. Patient teaching—a crucial nursing

Facts about the kidneys
- Two bean-shaped organs
- Four components:
  - Cortex: outer layer; contains glomeruli, proximal tubules, and distal tubules
  - Medulla: inner layer; contains loops of Henle and collecting tubules
  - Renal pelvis: collects urine
  - Nephron: functional unit; contains Bowman's capsule, glomerulus, and renal tubule

Ureter
- Extends from renal pelvis to bladder floor
- Transports urine from the kidney to the bladder

Facts about the bladder
- Muscular, distendible sac
- Stores urine

Urethra
- Extends from the bladder to the urinary meatus
- Transports urine

How urine is formed
- Blood from the renal artery is filtrated.
- Formed filtrate moves through the tubules of the nephron, which reabsorb and secrete electrolytes, water, glucose, amino acids, ammonia, and bicarbonate.
- Antidiuretic hormone and aldosterone control the reabsorption of water and electrolytes.

activity—involves providing information about medical follow-up, medication regimens, signs and symptoms of possible complications, and reduction of modifiable risk factors through adherence to dietary and fluid recommendations and restrictions.

ANATOMY AND PHYSIOLOGY

Kidneys (see *Structure of the kidneys*)
- Two bean-shaped organs
- Four components: cortex, medulla, renal pelvis, and nephron
  - Cortex
    - Makes up the outer layer of the kidney
    - Contains the glomeruli, proximal tubules of the nephron, and distal tubules of the nephron
  - Medulla
    - Makes up the inner layer of the kidney
    - Contains the loops of Henle and the collecting tubules
  - Renal pelvis
    - Collects urine from the calices
  - Nephron
    - Makes up the functional unit of the kidney
    - Contains the Bowman's capsule and the glomerulus
    - Contains the renal tubule, which consists of proximal convoluted tubule, loop of Henle, distal convoluted tubule, and collecting segments

Ureter
- This tubule extends from the renal pelvis to the bladder floor
- Transports urine from the kidney to the bladder
- Ureterovesical sphincter prevents reflux of urine from the bladder into the ureter

Bladder
- Muscular, distendible sac that stores urine
- Total capacity of approximately 1 L

Urethra
- This tubule extends from the bladder to the urinary meatus
- Urethra transports urine from the bladder to the urinary meatus

Urine formation
- Blood from the renal artery is filtrated across the glomerular capillary membrane in the Bowman's capsule
- Filtration requires adequate intravascular volume and adequate cardiac output
- Composition of formed filtrate is similar to blood plasma without proteins
- Formed filtrate moves through the tubules of the nephron, which reabsorb and secrete electrolytes, water, glucose, amino acids, ammonia, and bicarbonate

Structure of the kidneys

The illustration below shows the structures of the kidneys, along with the renal artery, adrenal gland, renal vein, and ureter.

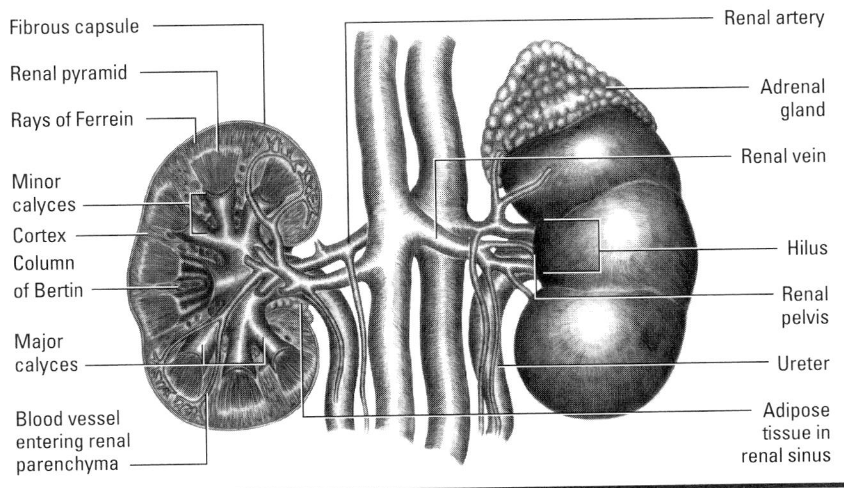

- Antidiuretic hormone and aldosterone control the reabsorption of water and electrolytes

- **Blood pressure control**
  - Blood pressure affects regulation of fluid volume by the kidney
  - Decreased blood pressure activates renin-angiotensin system
  - Renal disease can alter the renin-angiotensin system
- **Prostate gland**
  - This fibrous capsule is connected to and surrounds the male urethra
  - Prostate gland contains ducts that secrete the alkaline portion of seminal fluid and that open into the prostatic portion of the urethra

ASSESSMENT FINDINGS

- **History**
  - Changes in pattern of urination: frequency, nocturia, hesitancy, urgency, dribbling, incontinence, and retention
  - Changes in appearance of urine: dilute, concentrated, hematuria, and pyuria
  - Dysuria
  - Pain
  - Chills and fever
- **Physical examination**
  - Urine output changes: polyuria, oliguria, and anuria
  - Specific gravity abnormalities

Structures of the kidneys

- Fibrous capsule
- Renal pyramid
- Rays of Ferrein
- Minor calyces
- Cortex
- Column of Bertin
- Major calyces
- Blood vessel entering renal parenchyma
- Hilus
- Renal pelvis
- Adipose tissue in renal sinus

Blood pressure control

- Blood pressure affects regulation of the kidney's fluid volume
- Decreased blood pressure activates renin-angiotensin system

Prostate gland

- Fibrous capsule
- Connected to and surrounds the male urethra
- Contains ducts that secrete seminal fluid

Key assessment findings in a patient history

- Change in pattern of urination or appearance of urine
- Dysuria
- Pain
- Chills and fever

Key physical assessment findings
- Urine output changes
- Specific gravity abnormalities
- Hematuria
- Urine pH abnormalities

Urinalysis
- Laboratory test of urine
- Examines color, appearance, pH, specific gravity, protein, glucose, ketones, RBCs, WBCs, and casts
- Intervention: obtain first morning urine specimen

Urine culture and sensitivity
- Laboratory test of urine
- Detects bacteria
- Intervention: collect midstream sample in sterile container

24-hour urine collection
- Laboratory test of urine
- Samples collected over 24 hours to determine kidney function
- Intervention: instruct the patient to void and note time

Blood chemistry
- Laboratory test of blood sample
- Analysis for potassium, sodium, calcium, phosphorus, glucose, bicarbonate, BUN, creatinine, protein, albumin, and osmolality
- Intervention: check the site for bleeding after the procedure

- Hematuria
- Urine pH abnormalities
- Periorbital and peripheral edema
- Bladder distention
- Skin changes
- Intake and output (I/O) discrepancies
- Muscle tremors
- Pattern and character of respirations
- Enlargement of the prostate gland
- Temperature changes
- Weight changes
- Blood pressure changes

DIAGNOSTIC TESTS AND PROCEDURES

Urinalysis
- Definition and purpose
  - Laboratory test of urine
  - Microscopic examination for color, appearance, pH, specific gravity, protein, glucose, ketones, red blood cells (RBCs), white blood cells (WBCs), and casts
- Nursing interventions
  - Wash perineal area
  - Obtain first morning urine specimen

Urine culture and sensitivity
- Definition and purpose
  - Laboratory test of urine
  - Microscopic examination for bacteria
- Nursing interventions
  - Clean perineal area and urinary meatus with bacteriostatic solution
  - Collect midstream sample in sterile container

24-hour urine collection
- Definition and purpose
  - Laboratory test of urine
  - Quantitative analysis of samples collected over 24 hours to determine kidney function (see *Understanding the glomerular filtration rate*)
- Nursing interventions
  - Instruct the patient to void and note time (collection starts with the next voiding)
  - Place urine container on ice
  - Measure each voided urine
  - Instruct the patient to void at the end of the 24-hour period
  - Note medications that might alter tests results

Blood chemistry
- Definition and purpose

Understanding the glomerular filtration rate

The glomerular filtration rate (GFR) is the rate at which the glomeruli filter blood. The normal GFR is about 120 ml/minute. GFR depends on:
- permeability of capillary walls
- vascular pressure
- filtration pressure.

GFR AND CLEARANCE

Clearance is the complete removal of a substance from the blood. The most accurate measure of glomerular filtration is creatinine clearance. That's because creatinine is filtered by the glomeruli but not reabsorbed by the tubules.

EQUAL TO, GREATER THAN, OR LESS THAN

Here's more about how the GFR affects clearance measurements for a substance in the blood:
- If the tubules neither reabsorb nor secrete the substance – as happens with creatinine – clearance equals the GFR.
- If the tubules reabsorb the substance, clearance is less than the GFR.
- If the tubules secrete the substance, clearance exceeds the GFR.
- If the tubules reabsorb and secrete the substance, clearance may be less than, equal to, or greater than the GFR.

- – Laboratory test of blood sample
- – Analysis for potassium, sodium, calcium, phosphorus, glucose, bicarbonate, blood urea nitrogen (BUN), creatinine, protein, albumin, and osmolality
- Nursing interventions
  - – Withhold food and fluids before the procedure, as directed
  - – Check the site for bleeding after the procedure

Kidneys, ureters, bladder (KUB) X-ray

- Definition and purpose
  - – Noninvasive examination of the renal system
  - – Radiographic picture of the kidneys, ureters, and bladder
- Nursing interventions
  - – Schedule the X-ray before other examinations requiring contrast medium
  - – Ensure that the patient removes metallic belts

Excretory urography

- Definition and purpose
  - – Procedure using an injection of a radiopaque dye
  - – Fluoroscopic examination of kidneys, ureters, and bladder
- Nursing interventions before the procedure
  - – Note the patient's allergies to iodine, seafood, and radiopaque dyes
  - – Withhold food and fluids after midnight
  - – Administer laxatives, as prescribed

Characteristics of the GFR

- The rate at which glomeruli filter blood
- Normal GFR is 120 ml/minute
- Depends on permeability of capillary walls, vascular pressure, and filtration pressure

How GFR affects clearance of substances in the blood

- If tubules neither reabsorb or secrete the substance, clearance equals the GFR.
- If tubules reabsorb the substance, clearance is less than the GFR.
- If tubules secrete the substance, clearance exceeds GFR.
- If tubules reabsorb and secrete the substance, clearance may be less than, equal to, or greater than GFR.

KUB X-ray

- Noninvasive examination of the renal system
- Radiographic picture of the kidneys, ureters, and bladder
- Intervention: schedule the X-ray before other examinations that require contrast medium

Excretory urography

- Injection of radiopaque dye
- Fluoroscopic examination of the kidneys, ureters, and bladder
- Intervention: note the patient's allergies before the procedure

- Inform the patient about possible throat irritation, flushing of the face, and feelings of warmth
- Nursing interventions after the procedure
  - Instruct the patient to drink at least 1 qt (1 L) of fluids
  - Check the venipuncture site for bleeding

Cystoscopy

- Procedure using cystoscope
- Provides visualization of the bladder
- Intervention: check the patient's urine for blood clots after the procedure

Cystoscopy

- Definition and purpose
  - Procedure using a cystoscope
  - Direct visualization of the bladder
- Nursing interventions before the procedure
  - Withhold food and fluids
  - Allay the patient's anxiety
  - Place obtained written informed consent in the patient's chart
  - Administer enemas and medications, as prescribed
- Nursing interventions after the procedure
  - Administer analgesics and sitz baths, as prescribed
  - Monitor I/O and vital signs
  - **Check the patient's urine for blood clots**
  - Encourage fluids

Renal angiography

- Procedure using injection of radiopaque dye through a catheter
- Radiographic examination of the renal arterial supply
- Intervention: note the patient's allergies before the procedure

Renal angiography

- Definition and purpose
  - Procedure using an injection of a radiopaque dye through a catheter
  - Radiographic examination of the renal arterial supply
- Nursing interventions before the procedure
  - Allay the patient's anxiety
  - Inform the patient about a possible warm feeling after dye is injected
  - Place obtained written informed consent in the patient's chart
  - Withhold food and fluids after midnight
  - Instruct the patient to void immediately before the procedure
  - Administer enemas, as prescribed
  - **Note the patient's allergies to iodine, seafood, and radiopaque dyes**
- Nursing interventions after the procedure
  - Assess vital signs and peripheral pulses
  - Inspect the catheter insertion site for bleeding
  - Encourage fluids

Renal scan

- Procedure using an I.V. injection of a radioisotope
- Visual imaging of blood flow distribution
- Intervention: assess the patient for signs of delayed allergic reaction

Renal scan

- Definition and purpose
  - Procedure using an I.V. injection of a radioisotope
  - Visual imaging of blood flow distribution to the kidneys
- Nursing interventions before the procedure
  - Assist with administering radioisotope as necessary
  - Check the patient's history for allergies
- Nursing interventions after the procedure
  - **Assess the patient for signs of delayed allergic reaction, such as itching and hives**

- Wear gloves when caring for incontinent patients, and double-bag linens

Renal biopsy

- Definition and purpose
  - Percutaneous procedure to remove a small amount of renal tissue
  - Histologic evaluation
- Nursing interventions before the procedure
  - Assess baseline clotting studies and vital signs
  - Withhold food and fluids after midnight
  - Place obtained written informed consent in the patient's chart
- Nursing interventions after the procedure
  - Monitor and record vital signs, hemoglobin (Hb) and hematocrit (HCT)
  - Check biopsy site for bleeding

Cystourethrogram

- Definition and purpose
  - Procedure calling for the insertion of a catheter and the introduction of radiopaque dye
  - Visualization of the bladder and ureters
- Nursing interventions before the procedure
  - Allay the patient's anxiety
  - **Note the patient's allergies to iodine, seafood, and radiopaque dyes before the procedure**
  - Advise the patient about voiding requirements during the procedure
- Nursing interventions after the procedure
  - Monitor voiding
  - Monitor for urinary tract infection (UTI)

Cystometrogram (CMG)

- Definition and purpose
  - Procedure to test the urinary bladder using a catheter
  - Graphic recording of the pressures exerted at varying phases of filling of the bladder
- Nursing interventions before the procedure
  - Allay the patient's anxiety
  - Advise the patient about voiding requirements during the procedure
- Nursing interventions after the procedure
  - Monitor voiding
  - Observe for persistent hematuria
  - Monitor for UTI

Hematologic studies

- Definition and purpose
  - Laboratory test of blood sample
  - Analysis of blood sample for WBCs, RBCs, erythrocyte sedimentation rate, platelets, prothrombin time (PT), partial thromboplastin time (PTT), Hb, and HCT
- Nursing interventions

Renal biopsy

- Percutaneous procedure to remove renal tissue
- Histologic evaluation
- Intervention: check biopsy site for bleeding after the procedure

Cystourethrogram

- Procedure in which a catheter and radiopaque dye is inserted
- Visualizes the bladder and ureters
- Intervention: note the patient's allergies before the procedure

Cystometrogram

- Procedure to test urinary bladder
- Records pressures exerted at phases of bladder filling
- Intervention: advise the patient about voiding requirements during the procedure

Hematologic studies

- Laboratory tests of blood samples
- Analyzes for WBCs, RBCs, erythrocyte sedimentation rate, platelets, PT, PTT, Hb, and HCT
- Intervention: check the venipuncture site for bleeding after the procedure

– Explain the purpose of the procedure
– Check the venipuncture site for bleeding

PSYCHOSOCIAL IMPACT OF RENAL AND UROLOGIC DISORDERS

- **Developmental impact**
  - Body image changes
  - Feeling of lack of control over body functions
  - Fear of rejection
  - Embarrassment from changes in body function and structure
  - Decreased self-esteem
- **Economic impact**
  - Cost of renal dialysis and organ transplant
  - Cost of hospitalizations and follow-up care
  - Cost of medications
  - Cost of special diet
  - Disruption of employment
- **Occupational and recreational impact**
  - Restrictions in physical activity
  - Changes in leisure activity
- **Social impact**
  - Changes in eating patterns
  - Social isolation
  - Changes in elimination patterns and modes
  - Changes in sexual function

Key psychosocial impacts of renal and urologic disorders

- Costs associated with hospitalizations, medications, and special diet
- Disruption of employment
- Restrictions in physical activity
- Social isolation
- Changes in activities, eating patterns, elimination patterns, and sexual function

RISK FACTORS

- **Modifiable risk factors**
  - Diet: high-sodium, high-calcium
  - Exposure to chemical and environmental pollutants
  - Smoking
  - Contact sports
  - Culturally based reluctance to discuss hygiene and health habits
- **Nonmodifiable risk factors**
  - History of renal dysfunction
  - History of hypertension
  - Aging
  - Family history of renal disease

Key risk factors for renal and urologic disorders

- High-sodium, high-calcium diet
- Exposure to pollutants
- Smoking
- History of renal dysfunction
- History of hypertension

Key modifiable risk factors

- Diet
- Smoking
- Exposure to pollutants

NURSING DIAGNOSES

- **Probable nursing diagnoses**
  - Risk for deficient fluid volume
  - Excess fluid volume

- Impaired urinary elimination
- Acute pain
- Ineffective sexuality patterns
- Disturbed body image
- Situational low self-esteem

Possible nursing diagnoses
- Risk for impaired skin integrity
- Noncompliance
- Risk for activity intolerance
- Anticipatory grieving
- Impaired gas exchange

KIDNEY TRANSPLANTATION

Description
- Implantation of a donated kidney in a person who requires dialysis during the last stage of renal disease

Preoperative nursing interventions
- Complete patient and family preoperative teaching
  - Determine the patient's understanding of the procedure
  - Describe the operating room, postanesthesia care unit (PACU), and preoperative and postoperative routines
  - Demonstrate postoperative turning, coughing, deep breathing, splinting, and range-of-motion (ROM) exercises
  - Explain the postoperative need for drainage tubes, surgical dressings, oxygen therapy, I.V. therapy, and pain control
- Complete a preoperative checklist
- Administer preoperative medications, as prescribed
- Allay the patient's and his family's anxiety about surgery
- Document the patient's history and physical assessment data
- Verify histocompatibility tests
- Administer immunosuppressive drugs, as prescribed, for 2 days before the transplantation
- Maintain protective isolation
- Administer transfusion therapy, as prescribed
- Administer I.V. therapy, as prescribed
- Monitor urinary output
- Verify that hemodialysis was completed 24 hours before transplant

Postoperative nursing interventions
- Assess cardiac and respiratory status and fluid balance
- Assess pain and administer postoperative analgesics, as prescribed
- Assess for return of peristalsis; give solid foods and liquids, as tolerated
- Administer I.V. fluids and transfusion therapy, as prescribed
- Allay the patient's anxiety
- Inspect the surgical dressing and change, as directed
- Reinforce turning, coughing, and deep breathing, and splinting of incision

Key probable nursing diagnoses
- Risk for deficient fluid volume
- Excess fluid volume
- Impaired urinary elimination
- Acute pain

Kidney transplantation defined
- Implantation of a donated kidney in a person who requires dialysis during the last stage of renal disease

Key nursing interventions before kidney transplantation
- Verify histocompatibility tests.
- Administer immunosuppressive drugs for 2 days before the transplantation.
- Maintain protective isolation.
- Verify that hemodialysis was completed 24 hours before the transplantation.

Key interventions after kidney transplantation

- Assess cardiac and respiratory status and fluid balance.
- Monitor and record vital signs, I/O, CVP, laboratory studies, urine for blood, ECG, specific gravity, daily weight, pulse oximetry, and creatinine levels.
- Monitor and maintain position and patency of drainage tubes.
- Administer immunosuppressive agents with synthetic prostaglandins.
- Administer corticosteroids, as prescribed.
- Monitor for infection.
- Administer ALG and ATG, as prescribed.
- Prepare for hemodialysis.

Key home care instructions for a patient with a kidney transplant

- Recognize the signs and symptoms of rejection.
- Avoid contact sports.
- Complete incision care daily.

Key surgical complications of a kidney transplantation

- Renal graft rejection
- GI hemorrhage
- Acute renal failure

- Keep the patient in semi-Fowler's position
- Provide incentive spirometry, intermittent positive pressure breathing
- Maintain activity: as tolerated; increase walking
- Monitor and record vital signs, I/O, central venous pressure (CVP), laboratory studies, urine for blood, electrocardiogram (ECG), specific gravity, daily weight, pulse oximetry, and serum creatinine levels
- Monitor and maintain position and patency of drainage tubes: indwelling urinary catheter, nasogastric (NG), wound drainage
- Isolation precautions: protective
- Encourage the patient to express his feelings about chronicity of illness, fear of dying, guilt
- Administer antifungals, as prescribed
- Administer immunosuppressive agents with synthetic prostaglandins, as prescribed
- Administer corticosteroids, as prescribed
- **Assess for organ rejection**
- Monitor for infection
- Provide mouth and skin care
- Administer antibiotics, as prescribed
- Administer antilymphocytic globulin (ALG) and antithymocyte globulin (ATG), as prescribed
- Prepare for hemodialysis
- Avoid prolonged periods of sitting
- Promote live donor and recipient relationship
- Monitor for depression
- Monitor for edema of the scrotum, labia, or thigh ipsilateral to the graft
- Assess the allograft site for pain and edema
- Individualize home care instructions
  - Recognize the signs and symptoms of rejection
  - Avoid contact sports
  - Complete incision care daily
  - Adhere to a low-sodium and low-protein diet
  - Monitor stool for occult blood

Surgical complications

- Renal graft rejection
- GI hemorrhage
- Acute renal failure
- Bladder and ureter fistulas
- Candidiasis of mouth
- Hypertension
- Stroke
- Gastric ulcer
- Liver failure
- Depression
- Psychosis
- Heart failure
- Hypovolemia

KIDNEY SURGERY

Description
- Nephrectomy: surgical removal of the entire kidney
- Lithotomy: surgical removal of renal calculi

Preoperative nursing interventions
- Complete patient and family preoperative teaching
  - Determine the patient's understanding of the procedure
  - Describe the operating room, PACU, and preoperative and postoperative routines
  - Demonstrate postoperative turning, coughing, deep breathing, splinting, and leg and ROM exercises
  - Explain the postoperative need for drainage tubes, surgical dressings, oxygen therapy, I.V. therapy, and pain control
- Complete a preoperative checklist
- Administer preoperative medications, as prescribed
- Allay the patient's and his family's anxiety about surgery
- Document the patient's history and physical assessment data
- Administer antibiotics, as prescribed

Postoperative nursing interventions
- Assess cardiac, respiratory, and neurologic status and fluid balance
- Assess pain and administer analgesics, as prescribed
- Assess for return of peristalsis; give solid foods, as tolerated, with increased fluids
- Administer I.V. fluids and transfusion therapy, as prescribed
- Allay the patient's anxiety
- Inspect the surgical dressing and change it, as directed
- Reinforce turning, coughing, and deep breathing, and splinting of incision
- Keep the patient in semi-Fowler's position
- Provide incentive spirometry
- Maintain activity: as tolerated; active and passive ROM exercises; increase walking
- Monitor and record vital signs, I/O, CVP, laboratory studies, urine for blood, daily weight, specific gravity, and pulse oximetry
- Monitor and maintain position and patency of drainage tubes: NG, indwelling urinary catheter, wound drainage, nephrostomy, suprapubic, ureteral
- Encourage the patient to express his feelings about changes in his body image and a fear of dying
- Administer antibiotics, as prescribed
- Administer stool softeners, as prescribed
- **Don't irrigate or manipulate the nephrostomy tube**
- Apply antiembolism stockings
- Individualize home care instructions
  - Recognize the signs and symptoms of renal failure
  - Complete incision care daily

2 types of kidney surgery
- Nephrectomy: surgical removal of the entire kidney
- Lithotomy: surgical removal of renal calculi

Key nursing interventions before kidney surgery
- Complete patient and family preoperative teaching.
- Administer preoperative medications and antibiotics, as prescribed.

Key nursing interventions after kidney surgery
- Assess cardiac, respiratory, and neurologic status and fluid balance.
- Administer I.V. fluids and transfusion therapy, as prescribed.
- Monitor and record vital signs, I/O, CVP, laboratory studies, urine for blood, daily weight, specific gravity, and pulse oximetry.
- Monitor and maintain position and patency of drainage tubes: NG, indwelling urinary catheter, wound drainage, nephrostomy, suprapubic, ureteral.
- Administer antibiotics, as prescribed.
- Individualize home care instructions.

- Avoid using over-the-counter (OTC) medications
- Increase fluid intake, especially cranberry juice
- Avoid lifting, straining, horseback riding, and contact sports
- Void frequently

TURP

- Insertion of a resectoscope into the urethra to excise prostatic tissue

Suprapubic prostatectomy

- Low abdominal incision into the bladder to the anterior aspect of the prostate to remove large tumors of the prostate

Retropubic prostatectomy

- Low midline incision below the bladder into prostatic capsule to remove a mass in the pelvic area

Perineal prostatectomy

- Incision through the perineum to remove the prostate and surrounding tissue

Key nursing steps before prostate surgery

- Complete patient and family preoperative teaching.
- Administer preoperative medications and antibiotics, as prescribed.

Surgical complications

- Hemorrhage
- Atelectasis
- Pneumothorax
- Pneumonia
- Paralytic ileus

PROSTATE SURGERY

Description

- Transurethral resection of prostate (TURP): insertion of a resectoscope into the urethra to excise prostatic tissue
- Suprapubic prostatectomy: low abdominal incision into the bladder to the anterior aspect of the prostate to remove large tumors of the prostate
- Retropubic prostatectomy: low midline incision below the bladder into prostatic capsule to remove a mass in the pelvic area
- Perineal prostatectomy: incision through the perineum to remove the prostate and surrounding tissue

Preoperative nursing interventions

- Complete patient and family preoperative teaching
  - Determine the patient's understanding of the procedure
  - Describe the operating room, PACU, and preoperative and postoperative routines
  - Demonstrate postoperative turning, coughing, deep breathing, splinting, and leg and ROM exercises
  - Explain the postoperative need for drainage tubes, surgical dressings, oxygen therapy, I.V. therapy, and pain control
- Complete a preoperative checklist
- Administer preoperative medications, as prescribed
- Allay the patient's and his family's anxiety about surgery
- Document the patient's history and physical assessment data
- Administer antibiotics, as prescribed

Postoperative nursing interventions

- Assess cardiac and respiratory status and fluid balance
- Assess pain and administer postoperative analgesics, as prescribed
- Assess for return of peristalsis; provide a high-protein, high-fiber, acid-ash diet, as tolerated, with increased fluids
- Administer I.V. fluids
- Allay the patient's anxiety
- Inspect the surgical dressing and change it, as directed
- Reinforce turning, coughing, and deep breathing, and splinting of incision
- Keep the patient in semi-Fowler's position

- Provide incentive spirometry
- Maintain activity: as tolerated, progressive ambulation
- Monitor and record vital signs, I/O, laboratory studies, urine for blood, stool counts, and pulse oximetry
- Monitor and maintain position and patency of drainage tubes: NG, indwelling urinary catheter, wound drainage, suprapubic
- Encourage the patient to express his feelings about changes in his body image and fear of sexual dysfunction
- Administer stool softeners, as prescribed
- Maintain closed continuous bladder irrigation
- Administer antibiotics, as prescribed
- Provide treatment: sitz baths
- Administer anticholinergics, as prescribed
- Administer antispasmodics, as prescribed
- Avoid giving enemas and taking temperature rectally
- Administer urinary antiseptics, as prescribed
- Monitor urinary patterns after removal of catheters
- Individualize home care instructions
  - Recognize the signs and symptoms of bleeding and urinary tract obstruction
  - Complete incision care daily
  - Avoid using OTC medications
  - Avoid Valsalva's maneuver, lifting, exercising vigorously, or prolonged sitting in the car
  - Increase fluid intake
  - Complete perineal strengthening exercises daily
  - Avoid alcohol and caffeine
- Avoid Valsalva's maneuver, lifting, exercising vigorously, or prolonged sitting in the car
- Increase fluid intake

Surgical complications

- Hemorrhage
- Shock
- Infection
- Epididymitis
- Impotence

URINARY DIVERSION

Description

- Ureterosigmoidostomy: ureters are excised from the bladder and implanted into the sigmoid colon; urine flows through the colon and is excreted through the rectum
- Nephrostomy: percutaneous insertion of catheter into kidney
- Ileal conduit: ureters are implanted into a segment of the ileum that has been resected from the intestinal tract with the formation of an abdominal stoma

Key nursing steps after prostate surgery

- Assess cardiac and respiratory status and fluid balance.
- Monitor and record vital signs, I/O, laboratory studies, urine for blood, stool counts, and pulse oximetry.
- Monitor and maintain position and patency of drainage tubes: NG, indwelling urinary catheter, wound drainage, suprapubic.
- Maintain closed continuous bladder irrigation.
- Administer antibiotics, as prescribed.
- Provide sitz baths.
- Monitor urinary patterns after removal of catheters.

Ureterosigmoidostomy defined

- Ureters are excised from the bladder and implanted into the sigmoid colon.
- Urine flows through the colon and is excreted through the rectum.

Nephrostomy defined

- Percutaneous insertion of a catheter into kidney

Ileal conduit defined

- Ureters are implanted into a segment of the ileum that has been resected from the intestinal tract with the formation of an abdominal stoma.

- Cutaneous ureterostomy: ureters are excised from the bladder and brought through the abdominal wall to create a stoma

Preoperative nursing interventions

- Complete patient and family preoperative teaching
  - Determine the patient's understanding of the procedure
  - Describe the operating room, PACU, and preoperative and postoperative routines
  - Demonstrate postoperative turning, coughing, deep breathing, splinting, and ROM exercises
  - Explain the postoperative need for drainage tubes, surgical dressings, oxygen therapy, I.V. therapy, and pain control
- Complete a preoperative checklist
- Administer preoperative medications, as prescribed
- Allay the patient's and his family's anxiety about surgery
- Document the patient's history and physical assessment data
- Administer bowel preparation, as prescribed

Postoperative nursing interventions

- Assess renal status and fluid balance
- Assess pain and administer postoperative analgesics, as prescribed
- Assess for return of peristalsis; provide acid-ash diet, as tolerated, with increased fluids; avoid giving milk and dairy products
- Administer I.V. fluids
- Allay the patient's anxiety
- Inspect the surgical dressing and change it, as directed
- Reinforce turning, coughing, deep breathing, and splinting of incision
- Keep the patient in semi-Fowler's position
- Provide incentive spirometry
- Maintain activity: as tolerated, increased walking
- Monitor and record vital signs, I/O, laboratory studies, daily weight, specific gravity, and pulse oximetry
- Monitor and maintain position and patency of drainage tubes: NG, indwelling urinary catheter, wound drainage
- Encourage the patient to express his feelings about changes in his body image, embarrassment, and sexual dysfunction
- Administer antibiotics, as prescribed
- Administer antispasmodics, as prescribed
- Apply and change ostomy bags
- Provide skin care, particularly around the stoma
- Apply antiembolism stockings
- Individualize home care instructions
  - Recognize the signs and symptoms of stomal stenosis
  - Complete stoma and skin care daily
  - Use ostomy bags and leg bags
  - Increase fluid intake
  - Avoid enemas and laxatives
  - Empty urinary diversion appliances frequently

Cutaneous ureterostomy defined

- Ureters are excised from the bladder and brought through the abdominal wall to create a stoma.

Key nursing interventions before urinary diversion

- Complete patient and family preoperative teaching.
- Administer preoperative medications and bowel preparation, as prescribed.
- Document the patient's history and physical assessment data.

Key nursing interventions after urinary diversion

- Assess renal status and fluid balance.
- Encourage the patient to express his feelings about changes in his body image, embarrassment, and sexual dysfunction.
- Administer antibiotics, as prescribed.
- Apply and change ostomy bags.
- Provide skin care, particularly around the stoma.

Surgical complications

- Chronic renal failure
- Infection
- Urinary and rectal fistulas
- Hemorrhage
- Peritonitis
- Ureteral obstruction
- Stomal stenosis
- Bowel obstruction
- Renal calculi

Key surgical complications of urinary diversion

- Chronic renal failure
- Infection
- Urinary and rectal fistulas
- Hemorrhage

CYSTITIS

Definition

- Inflammation of the urinary bladder related to a superficial infection that doesn't extend to the bladder mucosa

Cystitis defined

- Inflammation of the urinary bladder related to a superficial infection that doesn't extend to the bladder mucosa

Causes

- Stagnation of urine in the bladder
- Obstruction of the urethra
- Sexual intercourse
- Incorrect aseptic technique during catheterization
- Incorrect perineal care
- Kidney infection
- Radiation
- Diabetes mellitus
- Pregnancy

Pathophysiology

- Bacterial infection from a secondary source spreads to the bladder, causing an inflammatory response
- Cell destruction from trauma to the bladder wall, particularly the trigone area, initiates an acute inflammatory reaction

Assessment findings

- Frequency of urination
- Urgency of urination
- Burning or pain on urination
- Lower abdominal discomfort
- Dark, odoriferous urine
- Flank tenderness or suprapubic pain
- Nocturia
- Low-grade fever
- Urge to bear down on urination
- Dysuria
- Dribbling

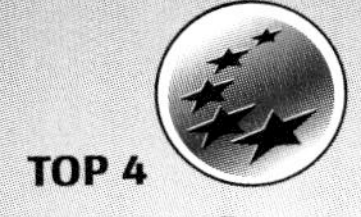

TOP 4

Signs and symptoms of cystitis

1. Frequency of urination
2. Urgency of urination
3. Burning or pain on urination
4. Low-grade fever

Diagnostic test findings

- Urine culture and sensitivity: positive identification of organisms (*Escherichia coli, Proteus vulgaris, Streptococcus faecalis*)

Key teaching topics for a patient with a renal or urologic disorder

- Keeping follow-up appointments
- Smoking cessation
- Medication therapy
- Infection control measures
- Dietary restrictions
- Fluid intake recommendations and restrictions

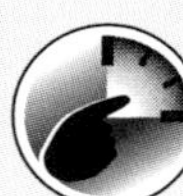

TIME-OUT FOR TEACHING

Patients with renal or urologic disorders

Be sure to include the following topics in your teaching plan for patients with renal or urologic disorders.

- Follow-up appointments
- Smoking cessation
- Optimal body weight maintenance
- Medication therapy, including the action, adverse effects, and scheduling of medications
- Infection control measures, including avoiding exposure to people with infections and monitoring self for infection
- Dietary recommendations and restrictions
- Fluid intake recommendations and restrictions
- Signs and symptoms of renal failure
- Rest and activity patterns, including limitations or restrictions
- Signs and symptoms of urinary tract infection
- Community agencies and resources for supportive services

Key diagnostic test findings in cystitis

- Urine culture and sensitivity: positive identification of organisms
- Urine chemistry: hematuria, pyuria, increased protein, leukocytes, specific gravity

- Urine chemistry: hematuria, pyuria; increased protein, leukocytes, specific gravity
- Cystoscopy: obstruction or deformity

Medical management

- Diet: acid-ash diet with increased intake of fluids and vitamin C
- Activity: as tolerated
- Monitoring: vital signs and I/O
- Laboratory studies: specific gravity, urine culture and sensitivity
- Treatment: sitz baths
- Antibiotics: co-trimoxazole (Bactrim), cephalexin (Keflex)
- Analgesic: oxycodone (Tylox)
- Urinary antiseptic: phenazopyridine (Pyridium)
- Antipyretic: acetaminophen (Tylenol)

Key steps in the medical management of cystitis

- Acid-ash diet with increased intake of fluids and vitamin C
- Antibiotics, such as co-trimoxazole and cephalexin

Nursing interventions

- Maintain the patient's diet
- Encourage fluids (cranberry or orange juice) to 3 qt (3 L)/day
- Assess renal status
- Monitor and record vital signs, I/O, and laboratory studies
- Administer medications, as prescribed
- Allay the patient's anxiety
- Maintain treatments: sitz baths, perineal care
- Encourage voiding every 2 to 3 hours
- Individualize home care instructions (for teaching tips, see *Patients with renal or urologic disorders*)
  - Avoid coffee, tea, alcohol, and cola
  - Increase fluid intake to 3 qt (3 L)/day using orange juice and cranberry juice

  - Void every 2 to 3 hours and after intercourse
  - Perform perineal care correctly
  - Avoid bubble baths, vaginal deodorants, and tub baths

Complications
- Chronic cystitis
- Urethritis
- Pyelonephritis

Surgical interventions
- None

GLOMERULONEPHRITIS

Definition
- Inflammation of the capillary loops in the glomeruli of the kidney

Causes
- Injected serum proteins
- Systemic lupus erythematosus (SLE)
- Group A beta-hemolytic streptococcal infection

Pathophysiology
- Antigen-antibody complexes are filtered and trapped within the glomeruli, causing inflammation
- Inflammation occludes the glomeruli, causing decreased glomerular filtration and retention of protein wastes and electrolytes

Assessment findings
- Bradycardia
- Pharyngitis and tonsillitis
- Peripheral and periorbital edema
- Lethargy and malaise
- Anorexia
- Elevated temperature
- Hypertension
- Tea-colored urine
- Flank pain
- Dyspnea
- Vision disturbances
- Dizziness
- Oliguria
- Seizures
- Weight loss
- Dehydration

Diagnostic test findings
- Urine chemistry: increased RBCs, WBCs, protein, casts, specific gravity
- Blood chemistry: increased BUN, creatinine; decreased protein, creatinine clearance, C-reactive protein, albumin

Key nursing interventions for the patient with cystitis
- Maintain the patient's diet.
- Encourage fluids to 3 qt/day.
- Encourage voiding every 2 to 3 hours.

Facts about glomerulonephritis
- Inflammation of the capillary loops in the glomeruli of the kidney
- Inflammation causes decreased glomerular filtration and retention of protein wastes and electrolytes

Key assessment findings in glomerulonephritis
- Pharyngitis and tonsillitis
- Peripheral and periorbital edema
- Lethargy and malaise
- Oliguria

Key test findings in glomerulonephritis
- Urine chemistry: increased RBCs, WBCs, protein, casts, specific gravity
- Blood chemistry: increased BUN, creatinine; decreased protein, creatinine clearance, C-reactive protein, albumin

- Hematology: decreased Hb, HCT; increased erythrocyte sedimentation rate
- Renal biopsy: inflammation of the glomerular capillaries

Medical management

- Diet: high-carbohydrate, high-vitamin, with restricted intake of sodium, protein, potassium, and fluids
- I.V. therapy: saline lock
- Activity: bed rest
- Monitoring: vital signs, I/O, and ECG
- Laboratory studies: BUN, creatinine, specific gravity, sodium, potassium, glucose, Hb, and HCT
- Antibiotics: penicillin V potassium (Pen-Vee K), ampicillin (Omnipen)
- Antihypertensives: diazoxide (Hyperstat), hydralazine (Apresoline)
- Cardiac glycoside: digoxin (Lanoxin)
- Immunosuppressants: cyclophosphamide (Cytoxan), azathioprine (Imuran)
- Antacids: magnesium and aluminum hydroxide (Maalox), aluminum hydroxide gel (AlternaGEL)
- Corticosteroid: prednisone (Deltasone)
- Diuretics: chlorthalidone (Hygroton), furosemide (Lasix)
- Peritoneal dialysis and hemodialysis (see *Types of dialysis*)
- Anticoagulants: warfarin (Coumadin), heparin (Lipo-Hepin)
- Precaution: seizure
- Plasmapheresis

Nursing interventions

- Maintain the patient's diet
- Restrict fluids
- Reinforce turning, coughing, and deep breathing
- Assess renal, respiratory, cardiovascular, and neurologic status as well as fluid balance
- Monitor and record vital signs, I/O, ECG, laboratory studies, urine glucose and ketones, hematuria, weight, and specific gravity
- Administer medications, as prescribed
- Encourage the patient to express his feelings about changes in his body image
- Maintain seizure precautions
- Protect the patient from falls
- Monitor for bleeding and infection
- Provide skin and mouth care
- Individualize home care instructions
  - Limit physical activity
  - Restrict protein and sodium intake
  - **Monitor blood pressure and urine protein**

Complications

- Metabolic acidosis
- Chronic renal failure
- Hypertensive encephalopathy
- Heart failure

Main treatment options for glomerulonephritis

- High-carbohydrate, high-vitamin diet, with restricted intake of sodium, protein, potassium, and fluids
- Bed rest
- Antihypertensives
- Diuretics

Key nursing interventions for a patient with glomerulonephritis

- Assess renal, respiratory, cardiovascular, and neurologic status as well as fluid balance.
- Monitor and record vital signs, I/O, ECG, laboratory studies, urine glucose and ketones, hematuria, weight, and specific gravity.
- Monitor for bleeding and infection.

Common complications of glomerulonephritis

- Metabolic acidosis
- Chronic renal failure
- Hypertensive encephalopathy

Types of dialysis

The two types of dialysis used to treat chronic renal failure and other conditions are hemodialysis and peritoneal dialysis.

REMOVING WASTE

Hemodialysis removes toxic wastes and other impurities from the blood. Blood is removed from the body through a surgically created access site, pumped through a filtration unit to remove toxins, and then returned to the body. The extracorporeal dialyzer works through osmosis, diffusion, and filtration. Specially trained nurses perform hemodialysis.

Nursing actions

- Monitor the venous access site for bleeding. If bleeding is excessive, maintain pressure on the site.
- Don't use the arm for blood pressure monitoring, I.V. catheter insertion, or venipuncture.
- At least four times daily, auscultate the access site for bruits and palpate for thrills.

USING THE BODY

Peritoneal dialysis removes toxins from the blood, but unlike hemodialysis, it uses the patient's peritoneal membrane as a semipermeable dialyzing membrane. Hypertonic dialyzing solution is instilled through a catheter inserted into the peritoneal cavity. By diffusion, excessive concentrations of electrolytes and uremic toxins in the blood move across the peritoneal membrane and into the dialysis solution. Next, by osmosis, excessive water in the blood does the same.

After appropriate dwelling time, the dialysis solution is drained, taking toxins and wastes with it. The patient is trained to perform this procedure.

Nursing actions

- Check the patient's weight, and report a gain.
- Using aseptic technique, change the catheter dressing every 24 hours and whenever it becomes wet or soiled.
- Calculate the patient's fluid balance at the end of each dialysis session or after 8 hours in a longer session. Include oral and I.V. fluid intake as well as urine output and wound drainage. Record and report any significant imbalance, either positive or negative.

- Nephrotic syndrome
- Pulmonary edema

Surgical interventions

- None

PYELONEPHRITIS

Definition

- Inflammation of renal pelvis

Causes

- Enteric bacteria
- Ureterovesical reflux
- Urinary tract obstruction

How hemodialysis works

- Blood is removed from the body through a surgically created access site, pumped through a filtration unit to remove toxins, and then returned to the body.
- Extracorporeal dialyzer works through osmosis, diffusion, and filtration.
- It should be performed by specially-trained nurses.

How peritoneal dialysis works

- Hypertonic dialyzing solution is instilled through a catheter inserted into the peritoneal cavity.
- By diffusion, excessive concentrations of electrolytes and uremic toxins in the blood move across the peritoneal membrane and into the dialysis solution.
- By osmosis, excessive water in the blood does the same.
- Dialysis solution is drained, taking toxins and waste with it.
- It should be performed by the patient.

Pyelonephritis highlights

- Inflammation of renal pelvis
- Occurs when a bacterial infection spreads causing cell destruction from trauma

- Pregnancy
- Trauma
- UTI
- Incorrect aseptic technique
- Diabetes mellitus
- Staphylococcal or streptococcal infections

Pathophysiology
- Bacterial infection from a secondary source spreads to the renal pelvis, causing an inflammatory response
- Cell destruction from trauma to the renal pelvis initiates an inflammatory reaction

Assessment findings
- Elevated temperature
- Chills
- Nausea and vomiting
- Flank pain
- Chronic fatigue
- Bladder irritability
- Hypertension
- Dysuria
- Burning on urination
- Frequency of urination
- Urgency of urination
- Headache
- Anorexia
- Weight loss
- Odoriferous, concentrated urine

Diagnostic test findings
- Excretory urography: atrophy, blockage, or deformity of kidney
- Urine culture and sensitivity: bacteria
- Urine chemistry: pyuria, hematuria; leukocytes, WBCs, and casts; specific gravity greater than 1.025; albuminuria
- Hematology: increased WBCs
- 24-hour urine collection: decreased creatinine clearance

Medical management
- Diet: soft, high-calorie, low-protein
- I.V. therapy: saline lock, electrolyte and fluid replacement
- Activity: as tolerated
- Monitoring: vital signs, I/O, urine pH, and specific gravity
- Laboratory studies: WBCs, urine protein, and urine culture and sensitivity
- Treatments: warm, moist compresses to flank
- Fluid intake: 3 qt (3 L)/day
- Analgesic: meperidine (Demerol)
- Antibiotics: cefazolin (Ancef), cefoxitin (Mefoxin), co-trimoxazole (Bactrim)
- Urinary antiseptic: phenazopyridine (Pyridium)

Key signs and symptoms of pyelonephritis
- Elevated temperature
- Chills
- Nausea and vomiting
- Flank pain

Key urine test findings
- Culture and sensitivity: bacteria
- Chemistry: pyuria, hematuria; leukocytes, WBCs, and casts; specific gravity greater than 1.025; albuminuria

Key steps in managing pyelonephritis
- 3 qt fluid/day
- Antibiotics

- Antiemetic: prochlorperazine (Compazine)
- Alkalinizers: potassium acetate, sodium bicarbonate
- Sedative: oxazepam (Serax)
- Peritoneal dialysis and hemodialysis

Nursing interventions
- Maintain the patient's diet
- Encourage fluids to 3 qt (3 L)/day
- Assess renal status and fluid balance
- Monitor and record vital signs, I/O, laboratory studies, daily weight, specific gravity, and urine for blood, protein, and pH
- Administer medications, as prescribed
- Allay the patient's anxiety
- Provide hot, moist compresses and warm baths
- Prevent chilling
- Provide rest periods
- Provide skin, mouth, and perineal care
- Encourage frequent voiding
- Individualize home care instructions
  - Void frequently
  - Return to the physician immediately if symptoms reoccur
  - Take prescribed medications for entire duration of prescription

Complications
- Chronic renal failure
- Hypertension
- Septicemia

Surgical interventions
- None

Key nursing steps in pyelonephritis
- Encourage fluids to 3 qt/day.
- Assess renal status and fluid balance.
- Monitor and record vital signs, I/O, laboratory studies, daily weight, specific gravity, and urine for blood, protein, and pH.
- Encourage frequent voiding.
- Provide individualized home care instructions.

RENAL CALCULI

Definition
- Stones in kidneys, ureters, or bladder

Causes
- Diet high in calcium, vitamin D, milk, protein, oxalate, alkali
- Gout
- Hyperparathyroidism
- UTI
- Urinary stasis
- Dehydration
- Idiopathic
- Immobility
- Genetics
- Hypercalcemia
- Urinary tract obstruction
- Leukemia
- Polycythemia vera

Renal calculi defined
- Stones in kidneys, ureters, or bladder

Key causes of renal calculi
- Diet high in calcium, vitamin D, protein, oxalate, alkali
- Gout
- Hyperparathyroidism
- UTI

Facts about renal calculi

- Crystalline substances that are normally dissolved and excreted in the urine form precipitates
- The stones are composed of calcium phosphate, oxalate, or uric acid

A close look at renal calculi

Renal calculi vary in size and type. Small calculi may remain in the renal pelvis or pass down the ureter as shown below. A staghorn calculus, shown in the second illustration, is a cast of the innermost part of the kidney – the calyx and renal pelvis. A staghorn calculus may develop from a calculus that stays in the kidney.

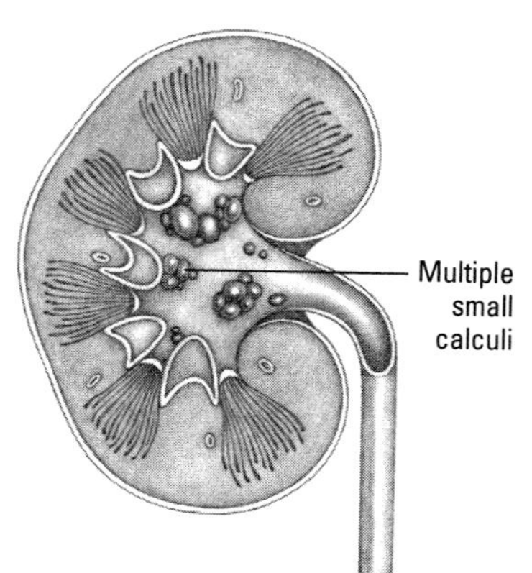

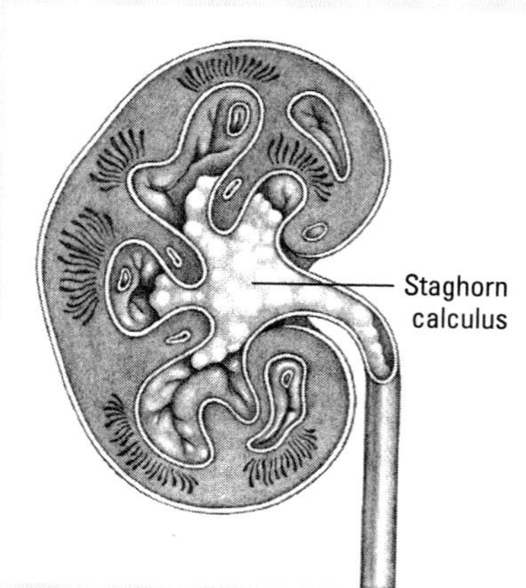

TOP 3

Assessment findings in renal calculi

1. Flank pain
2. Costovertebral tenderness
3. Cool, moist skin

Diagnostic test findings for renal calculi

- KUB: stones
- Excretory urography: stones

- Chemotherapy

Pathophysiology

- Crystalline substances that normally are dissolved and excreted in the urine form precipitates (see *A close look at renal calculi*)
- Stones are composed of calcium phosphate, oxalate, or uric acid

Assessment findings

- Flank pain
- Costovertebral tenderness
- Cool, moist skin
- Renal colic
- Frequency of urination
- Urgency of urination
- Diaphoresis
- Chills and fever
- Pallor
- Nausea and vomiting
- Syncope
- Dysuria

Diagnostic test findings

- KUB: stones
- Excretory urography: stones
- Urine chemistry: acidic or alkaline urine, pyuria, proteinuria, hematuria, presence of WBCs, increased specific gravity

- Cystoscopy: visualization of stones
- 24-hour urine collection: increased uric acid, oxalate, calcium, phosphorus, creatinine
- Blood chemistry: increased calcium, phosphorus, creatinine, BUN, uric acid, protein, alkaline phosphatase

Medical management

- Diet
  - For calcium stones — acid-ash with limited intake of calcium and milk products
  - For oxalate stones — alkaline-ash with limited intake of foods high in oxalate (cola, tea)
  - For uric acid stones — alkaline-ash with limited intake of foods high in purine
- I.V. therapy: saline lock, fluid replacement
- Activity: as tolerated
- Monitoring: vital signs, I/O, and urine pH vital signs
- Laboratory studies: creatinine, BUN, phosphorus, calcium, and protein
- Treatments: strain urine, moist heat to flank, hot baths
- Encourage fluids to 3 qt (3 L)/day
- Antigout agent: sulfinpyrazone (Anturane)
- Analgesic: meperidine (Demerol)
- Antibiotics: cefazolin (Ancef), cefoxitin (Mefoxin)
- Antiemetic: prochlorperazine (Compazine)
- Acidifiers: ammonium chloride, methenamine (Mandelamine)
- Alkalinizers: potassium acetate, sodium bicarbonate
- Chemolysis
- Electrohydraulic lithotripsy
- Ultrasonic lithotripsy
- Laser impulse
- Extracorporeal shock wave lithotripsy (ESWL)
- Percutaneous nephrostolithotomy
- Prevention of cystinuria: tiopronin (Thiola)

Nursing interventions

- Maintain the patient's diet
- Encourage fluids to 3 qt (3 L)/day
- Assess renal status
- Monitor and record vital signs, I/O, daily weight, specific gravity, laboratory studies, and urine pH
- Administer medications, as prescribed
- Allay the patient's anxiety
- Continue straining urine and giving warm baths and warm soaks to flank
- Assess pain
- Individualize home care instructions
  - **Increase fluid intake, especially during hot weather, illness, and exercise**
  - Void when urge is felt

Managing renal calculi with special diets

- Calcium stones – acid-ash with limited intake of calcium and milk products
- Oxalate stones – alkaline-ash with limited intake of foods high in oxalate (cola, tea)
- Uric acid stones – alkaline-ash with limited intake of foods high in purine

Key ways to manage renal calculi

- Diet
- Strain urine, moist heat to flank, hot baths
- ESWL

Key nursing interventions for a patient with renal calculi

- Encourage fluids to 3 qt/day.
- Assess renal status.
- Continue straining urine.

– Test urine pH
– Increase fluids at night and void frequently

Complications
- Chronic UTI
- Renal obstruction
- Ureterovesical reflux
- Hydronephrosis
- Pyelonephritis

Surgical intervention
- Lithotomy

Acute renal failure defined
- Sudden inability of the kidneys to regulate fluid and electrolyte balance and remove toxic products from the body

Key causes of acute renal failure
- Heart failure
- Cardiogenic shock
- Hemorrhage
- Burns
- Septicemia

Pathophysiology of acute renal failure
- Decreased perfusion of the kidney causes decreased blood flow and glomerular filtrate, ischemia, and oliguria
- Damaged nephrons can't absorb or secrete water, electrolytes, glucose, amino acids, ammonia, and bicarbonate
- May develop into chronic renal failure

ACUTE RENAL FAILURE

Definition
- Sudden inability of the kidneys to regulate fluid and electrolyte balance and remove toxic products from the body

Causes
- Heart failure
- Cardiogenic shock
- Hemorrhage
- Burns
- Septicemia
- Hypotension
- Acute tubular necrosis
- Acute vasoconstriction
- Endocarditis
- Malignant hypertension
- Diabetes mellitus
- Dehydration
- Tumor
- Blood transfusion reaction
- Cardiopulmonary bypass
- Nephrotoxins: antibiotics, X-ray dyes, pesticides, anesthetics
- Renal calculi
- Benign prostatic hyperplasia (BPH)
- Acute glomerulonephritis
- Trauma
- Congenital deformity
- Anaphylaxis
- Collagen diseases
- Aortic aneurysm repair

Pathophysiology
- Decreased perfusion of the kidney results in decreased blood flow and glomerular filtrate, ischemia, and oliguria
- Damaged nephrons are unable to absorb and secrete water, electrolytes, glucose, amino acids, ammonia, and bicarbonate

- Disorder may progress from anuric or oliguric phase through diuretic phase to convalescence phase to recovery of function
- Disorder may develop into chronic renal failure

Assessment findings

- Urine output less than 400 ml/day for 1 to 2 weeks followed by diuresis (3 to 5 L/day) for 2 to 3 weeks
- Lethargy
- Drowsiness
- Stupor
- Coma
- Irritability
- Headache
- Costovertebral pain
- Circumoral numbness
- Tingling extremities
- Anorexia
- Restlessness
- Weight gain
- Nausea and vomiting
- Pallor
- Epistaxis
- Ecchymosis
- Diarrhea or constipation
- Stomatitis
- Thick, tenacious sputum

Diagnostic test findings

- Blood chemistry: increased potassium, phosphorus, magnesium, BUN, creatinine, and uric acid; decreased calcium, carbon dioxide, and sodium
- Hematology: decreased Hb, HCT, erythrocytes; increased PT and PTT
- Urine chemistry: albuminuria, proteinuria, increased sodium; casts, RBCs, and WBCs; specific gravity greater than 1.025, then fixed at less than 1.010
- Excretory urography: decreased renal perfusion and function
- Phenolsulfonphthalein (PSP): decreased
- Arterial blood gas (ABG) analysis: metabolic acidosis

Medical management

- Diet: low-protein, increased-carbohydrate, moderate-fat, and moderate-calorie, with potassium, sodium, and phosphorus intake regulated according to serum levels
- I.V. therapy: electrolyte replacement, hypertonic glucose and insulin to treat hyperkalemia, saline lock
- Position: semi-Fowler's
- Activity: bed rest, active and passive ROM and isometric exercises
- Monitoring: vital signs, I/O, ECG, and CVP
- Laboratory studies: BUN, creatinine, phosphorus, calcium, potassium, sodium, Hb, HCT, and specific gravity
- Nutritional support: total parental nutrition (TPN)

Key assessment findings in acute renal failure

- Urine output less than 400 ml/day for 1 to 2 weeks followed by diuresis (3 to 5 L/day) for 2 to 3 weeks
- Weight gain

Blood chemistry findings in acute renal failure

- Increased potassium, phosphorus, magnesium, BUN, creatinine, and uric acid
- Decreased calcium, carbon dioxide, and sodium

Urine chemistry findings in acute renal failure

- Albuminuria, proteinuria, increased sodium
- Casts, RBCs, and WBCs
- Specific gravity greater than 1.025, then fixed at less than 1.010

Key treatment options for acute renal failure

- Continuous arteriovenous hemofiltration
- Fluids: restrict intake to amount needed to replace fluid loss
- Antibiotics

Key nursing interventions for a patient with acute renal failure

- Maintain the patient's diet.
- Restrict fluids.
- Monitor and record vital signs, I/O, CVP, daily weight, specific gravity, laboratory studies, stool for occult blood, and urine glucose and ketones.
- Monitor for arrhythmias.
- Maintain seizure precautions.
- Observe for uremic frost.

- Treatments: indwelling urinary catheter, incentive spirometry, cooling blanket
- **Fluids: restrict intake to amount needed to replace fluid loss**
- Transfusion therapy: packed RBCs
- Antibiotics: cefazolin (Ancef), cefoxitin (Mefoxin)
- Analgesic: oxycodone (Tylox)
- Diuretics: furosemide (Lasix), mannitol (Osmitrol)
- Antacid: aluminum hydroxide gel (AlternaGEL)
- Antiemetic: prochlorperazine (Compazine)
- Cation exchange resins: sodium polystyrene sulfonate (Kayexalate)
- Chelating agent: dimercaprol (BAL in Oil)
- Beta-adrenergic: dopamine (Intropin)
- Anticonvulsant: phenytoin (Dilantin)
- Peritoneal dialysis and hemodialysis
- Antipyretic: acetaminophen (Tylenol)
- Precaution: seizure
- Alkalinizing agent: sodium bicarbonate
- Continuous arteriovenous hemofiltration

Nursing interventions

- Maintain the patient's diet
- Restrict fluids
- Administer I.V. fluids
- Assess fluid balance, respiratory, cardiovascular, and neurologic status
- Keep the patient in semi-Fowler's position
- Monitor and record vital signs, I/O, CVP, daily weight, specific gravity, laboratory studies, stool for occult blood, and urine glucose and ketones
- Administer TPN
- Administer medications, as prescribed
- Encourage the patient to express his feelings about changes in his body image
- Monitor for arrhythmias
- Provide cooling blanket
- Monitor the patient for infection
- Maintain a quiet environment
- **Maintain seizure precautions**
- Monitor the patient for bleeding
- Protect the patient from falls
- Encourage turning, coughing, and deep breathing
- Allay the patient's anxiety
- **Observe for uremic frost**
- Provide skin and mouth care using plain water
- Monitor neurovital signs
- Individualize home care instructions
  - Avoid using OTC medications
  - Maintain a quiet environment

Complications

- Chronic renal failure
- Pressure ulcers
- Contractures
- Atelectasis
- GI hemorrhage
- Convulsions
- Arrhythmias
- Cardiac arrest
- Pericarditis
- Potassium intoxication
- Pulmonary edema
- Pulmonary infection
- Heart failure
- Hypertension
- Anemia
- Metabolic acidosis
- Peripheral neuropathy
- Hypocalcemia

Surgical interventions

- None

CHRONIC RENAL FAILURE

Definition

- Progressive, irreversible destruction of kidneys, resulting in loss of renal function

Causes

- Recurrent UTI
- Exacerbations of nephritis
- Urinary tract obstructions
- Diabetes mellitus
- Hypertension
- Congenital abnormalities
- SLE
- Nephrotoxins
- Dehydration

Pathophysiology

- Scarred nephrons are unable to absorb and secrete water, glucose, amino acids, ammonia, bicarbonate, and electrolytes
- First stage: renal reserve is diminished, but metabolic wastes don't accumulate although renal damage exists
- Second stage: renal insufficiency occurs and metabolic wastes begin to accumulate; kidneys are less able to correct metabolic imbalances

Key complications of acute renal failure

- Chronic renal failure
- Pressure ulcers
- Contractures
- Atelectasis
- GI hemorrhage

Chronic renal failure highlights

- Progressive, irreversible destruction of kidneys
- Results in loss of renal function

3 stages of chronic renal failure

- First stage: renal reserve is diminished but metabolic wastes don't accumulate
- Second stage: renal insufficiency occurs and metabolic wastes begin to accumulate
- Third stage: uremia occurs with decreased urine output and metabolic waste accumulation increases

- Third stage: uremia occurs with decreased urine output; increased accumulation of metabolic wastes; and disturbed fluid, electrolyte, and acid-base balances

Key signs of chronic renal failure

- Pruritus
- Decreased urine output
- Lethargy
- Weight gain

Assessment findings

- Muscle twitching
- Paresthesia
- Bone pain
- Pruritus
- Decreased urine output
- Stomatitis
- Lethargy
- Seizures
- Brittle nails and hair
- Kussmaul's respirations
- Uremic frost
- Ecchymosis
- Weight gain

Blood chemistry findings in chronic renal failure

- Increased BUN, creatinine, phosphorus, lipids
- Decreased calcium, carbon dioxide, albumin

Diagnostic test findings

- Urine chemistry: proteinuria; increased WBCs, sodium; decreased and fixed specific gravity
- Blood chemistry: increased BUN, creatinine, phosphorus, lipids; decreased calcium, carbon dioxide, albumin
- ABG analysis: metabolic acidosis
- Hematology: decreased Hb, HCT, platelets
- Glucose tolerance test: decreased

Key treatment options for a patient with chronic renal failure

- Low-protein, low-sodium, low-potassium, low-phosphorus, high-carbohydrate, and high-calorie diet
- Fluid limitations
- Diuretics
- Antacids
- Antiemetics
- Cation exchange resins
- Peritoneal dialysis and hemodialysis
- Calcium supplements

Medical management

- Diet: low-protein, low-sodium, low-potassium, low-phosphorus, with high-calorie and high-carbohydrate
- Dietary restrictions: limit fluids
- I.V. therapy: saline lock
- Activity: as tolerated
- Monitoring: vital signs and I/O
- Laboratory studies: BUN, creatinine, potassium, sodium, Hb, HCT, glucose, albumin, and platelets
- Treatment: tepid baths
- Transfusion therapy: platelets
- Antibiotics: cefazolin (Ancef), cefoxitin (Mefoxin)
- Analgesic: oxycodone (Tylox)
- Diuretic: furosemide (Lasix)
- Antacids: aluminum hydroxide gel (AlternaGEL), magnesium and aluminum hydroxide (Maalox)
- Antiemetic: prochlorperazine (Compazine)
- Cation exchange resin: sodium polystyrene sulfonate (Kayexalate)
- Chelating agent: dimercaprol (BAL)
- Beta-adrenergic: dopamine (Intropin)
- Anticonvulsant: phenytoin (Dilantin)

- Peritoneal dialysis and hemodialysis
- Antipyretic: acetaminophen (Tylenol)
- Precautions: seizure
- Alkalinizing agent: sodium bicarbonate
- Cardiac glycoside: digoxin (Lanoxin)
- Stool softener: docusate (Colace)
- Antiarrhythmic: procainamide (Pronestyl)
- Antianemics: ferrous sulfate (Feosol), iron dextran (Imferon), epoetin alfa (recombinant human erythropoietin, Epogen)
- Vitamins: pyridoxine (vitamin B_6), ascorbic acid (vitamin C)
- Calcium supplement: calcium carbonate (Os-Cal)

Nursing interventions

- Maintain the patient's diet
- Restrict fluids
- Assess renal, respiratory, and cardiovascular status and fluid balance
- Monitor and record vital signs, I/O, ECG, specific gravity, daily weight, laboratory studies, neurovital signs, neurovascular checks, urine for glucose and ketones, and urine, stool, and emesis for occult blood
- Administer medications, as prescribed
- Encourage the patient to express his feelings about chronicity of illness
- Provide treatment: tepid baths
- Maintain a cool and quiet environment
- Provide skin and mouth care using plain water
- Maintain seizure precautions
- Monitor for ecchymosis
- Monitor for infection
- Avoid giving the patient I.M. injections
- Protect the patient from falls
- Individualize home care instructions
  - Maintain a quiet environment
  - Complete skin and mouth care daily

Complications

- Arrhythmias
- GI bleeding
- Heart failure
- Pericardial effusion
- Hyperphosphatemia
- Pleural effusion
- Dehydration
- Hyperparathyroidism
- Renal osteodystrophy
- Uremia
- Hypocalcemia

Surgical intervention

- Kidney transplantation

Key nursing interventions for a patient with chronic renal failure

- Restrict fluids.
- Assess renal, respiratory, and cardiovascular status and fluid balance.
- Monitor and record vital signs, I/O, ECG, specific gravity, daily weight, laboratory studies, neurovital signs, neurovascular checks, urine for glucose and ketones, and urine, stool, and emesis for occult blood.
- Avoid giving the patient I.M. injections.
- Protect the patient from falls.

TOP 5

Complications of chronic renal failure

1. Arrhythmias
2. GI bleedling
3. Heart failure
4. Pericardial effusion
5. Hyperphosphatemia

BLADDER CANCER

Definition
- Malignant tumor that ulcerates mucosal lining of the bladder

Causes
- Exposure to industrial chemicals
- Cigarette smoking
- Chronic bladder irritation
- Radiation
- Excessive intake of coffee, phenacetin, sodium, saccharin, sodium cyclamate
- Drug induced: cyclophosphamide (Cytoxan)

Pathophysiology
- Unregulated cell growth and uncontrolled cell division in bladder's transitional epithelium around trigone result in the development of a neoplasm
- Tumor metastasizes to ureters, prostate gland, vagina, rectum, and periaortic lymph nodes

Assessment findings
- Painless hematuria
- Dysuria
- Frequency of urination
- Anuria
- Urgency of urination
- Chills
- Flank or pelvic pain
- Elevated temperature
- Peripheral edema

Diagnostic test findings
- Cystoscopy: mass
- Excretory urography: mass or obstruction
- KUB: mass or obstruction
- Cytologic exam: cytology positive for malignant cells
- Urine chemistry: hematuria
- Hematology: decreased RBCs, Hb, HCT

Medical management
- I.V. therapy: saline lock
- Activity: as tolerated
- Monitoring: vital signs and I/O
- Laboratory studies: Hb and HCT
- Radiation therapy
- Chemotherapy
- Treatment: indwelling urinary catheter
- Transfusion therapy: packed RBCs
- Sedative: oxazepam (Serax)
- Antispasmodic: phenazopyridine (Pyridium)

Key facts about bladder cancer
- Tumor that ulcerates mucosal lining of the bladder
- Tumor metastasizes to ureters, prostate gland, vagina, rectum, and periaortic lymph nodes

Key signs of bladder cancer
- Painless hematuria
- Frequency of urination

Key treatment options for bladder cancer
- Radiation therapy
- Chemotherapy

- Antineoplastics: 5-fluorouracil (Adrucil), methotrexate (Rheumatrex), bleomycin (Blenoxane), thiotepa (Thioplex), doxorubicin (Adriamycin)
- Antiemetics: prochlorperazine (Compazine), ondansetron (Zofran)

Nursing interventions
- Maintain the patient's diet
- Encourage fluids
- Administer I.V. fluids
- Assess renal status
- Monitor and record vital signs, I/O, and laboratory studies
- Administer medications, as prescribed
- Encourage the patient to express his feelings about a fear of dying
- Provide postchemotherapeutic and postradiation nursing care
  - Provide prophylactic skin, mouth, and perineal care
  - Monitor dietary intake
  - Administer antiemetics and antidiarrheals, as prescribed
  - Monitor the patient for bleeding, infection, and electrolyte imbalance
  - Provide rest periods
- Individualize home care instructions
  - Provide information about the American Cancer Society
  - Seek help from community agencies and resources for supportive services

Complications
- Ureteral obstruction
- Vesicorectal and vesicovaginal fistulas

Surgical interventions
- Depends on location and progress of tumor
- Ureterosigmoidostomy
- Ileal conduit
- Cutaneous ureterostomy
- Cystectomy
- Transurethral resection of bladder tumor

BENIGN PROSTATIC HYPERPLASIA

Definition
- Hyperplasia of the lateral and subcervical lobes of the prostate gland that results in enlargement of the structure

Causes
- Unknown
- Hormonal

Pathophysiology
- Enlarged prostate gland compresses urethra, resulting in urinary obstruction and retention
- Obstruction causes hydroureter and hydronephrosis

Nursing interventions after chemotherapy and radiation

- Provide prophylactic skin, mouth, and perineal care.
- Monitor dietary intake.
- Administer antiemetics and antidiarrheals, as prescribed.
- Monitor the patient for bleeding, infection, and electrolyte imbalance.
- Provide rest periods.

Key surgical options for a patient with bladder cancer

- Depends on location and progress of tumor
- Ureterosigmoidostomy
- Ileal conduit

Benign prostatic hyperplasia defined

- Hyperplasia of the lateral and subcervical lobes of the prostate gland
- Results in enlargement of the structure

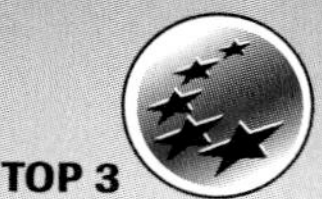

TOP 3

Assessment findings in benign prostatic hyperplasia

1. Urgency, frequency, and burning on urination
2. Decreased force and amount of stream
3. Hesitancy

Key test findings in benign prostatic hyperplasia

- Digital rectal examination: enlarged prostate gland by palpation
- Cystoscopy: enlarged prostate gland, obstructed urine flow, and urinary stasis

Key steps in managing benign prostatic hyperplasia

- Fluids
- Indwelling urinary catheter
- Antibiotics

Key nursing interventions for benign prostatic hyperplasia

- Encourage fluids.
- Maintain position and patency of indwelling urinary catheter.
- Provide hot baths.

Assessment findings

- Nocturia
- Urgency, frequency, and burning on urination
- Decreased force and amount of stream
- Hesitancy
- Dysuria
- Urine retention
- UTI
- Dribbling

Diagnostic test findings

- Digital rectal examination: enlarged prostate gland by palpation
- Urine chemistry: bacteria, hematuria, alkaline pH, increased specific gravity
- Blood chemistry: increased BUN, creatinine
- PSP: decreased
- Excretory urography: urethral obstruction, hydronephrosis
- Cystoscopy: enlarged prostate gland, obstructed urine flow, urinary stasis
- CMG: abnormal pressure recordings
- Urinary flow rate determination: volume small, flow pattern prolonged, peak flow low

Medical management

- Diet: encourage fluids
- Position: semi-Fowler's
- Activity: as tolerated
- Monitoring: vital signs and I/O
- Laboratory studies: BUN and creatinine
- Treatments: indwelling urinary catheter, hot baths, intermittent self-catheterization
- Antibiotics: co-trimoxazole (Bactrim), cephalexin (Keflex)
- Analgesic: oxycodone (Tylox)
- Urinary antiseptic: phenazopyridine (Pyridium)
- Antianxiety: oxazepam (Serax)
- Alpha-blocker: phenoxybenzamine (Dibenzyline)
- Alpha-adrenergic antagonists: prazosin (Minipress), terazosin (Hytrin)

Nursing interventions

- Encourage fluids
- Assess fluid balance
- Keep the patient in semi-Fowler's position
- Monitor and record: vital signs, I/O, and laboratory studies
- Administer medications, as prescribed
- Encourage the patient to express his feelings about changes in his body image and fear of sexual dysfunction
- Maintain position and patency of indwelling urinary catheter to straight drainage
- Maintain activity, as tolerated
- Provide hot baths
- Provide privacy while urinating

- Monitor for UTI
- Individualize home care instructions
  - Recognize the signs and symptoms of urine retention
  - Adhere to medical follow-up
  - Perform intermittent self-catheterization and document time and amount of flow sheet

Complications
- Chronic renal failure
- Hydronephrosis
- Hydroureter
- Renal calculi
- Cystitis

Surgical interventions
- Suprapubic cystotomy with insertion of suprapubic catheter
- TURP
- Prostatectomy
- Transurethral dilation of prostate gland

Key complications of benign prostatic hyperplasia

- Chronic renal failure
- Hydronephrosis
- Hydroureter

PROSTATIC CANCER

Definition
- Malignant tumor of the prostate gland

Causes
- No known etiology
- Associated risk factors: family history, age, black race, vasectomy, increased dietary fat

Pathophysiology
- Unregulated cell growth and uncontrolled cell division result in the development of a neoplasm
- Obstruction of urine flow occurs when the tumor encroaches on the bladder neck
- Metastasis commonly occurs to bone, lymph nodes, brain, and lungs

Prostatic cancer highlights

- Malignant tumor of the prostate gland
- No known etiology
- Metastasis commonly occurs to bone, lymph nodes, brain, and lungs

Assessment findings
- Difficulty and frequency of urination
- Urine retention
- Decreased size and force of urinary stream
- Hematuria

Assessment findings in prostatic cancer

- Difficulty and frequency of urination
- Urine retention
- Decreased size and force of urinary stream
- Hematuria

Diagnostic test findings
- Digital rectal examination: palpable firm nodule in gland or diffuse induration in posterior lobe
- Serum acid phosphatase level: increased
- Radioimmunoassay for acid phosphatase: increased
- Prostate-specific antigen (PSA): increased
- Transurethral ultrasound studies: mass or obstruction
- Prostate biopsy: cytology positive for cancer cells

Key treatment options for prostatic cancer

- Radiation therapy; radiation implant
- Chemotherapy
- NSAIDs
- Estrogen therapy

Key nursing interventions for prostatic cancer

- Assess renal and fluid status.
- Maintain patency of the urinary catheter.
- Encourage the patient to express his feelings about the changes in his body image and fear of sexual dysfunction.
- Assess pain.
- Provide postchemotherapeutic and postradiation nursing care.

Key nursing interventions after chemotherapy and radiation

- Provide prophylactic skin, mouth, and perineal care.
- Monitor dietary intake.
- Administer antiemetics and antidiarrheals, as prescribed.
- Provide rest periods.

- Excretory urograms: mass or obstruction

Medical management

- Diet: high-protein
- Dietary restrictions: caffeine, spicy foods
- Activity: as tolerated
- Monitoring: vital signs and I/O
- Laboratory studies: BUN, creatinine, PSA
- I.V. therapy: saline lock
- Analgesics: oxycodone (Tylox), meperidine (Demerol)
- Corticosteroid: prednisone (Deltasone)
- Nonsteroidal anti-inflammatory drugs (NSAIDs): indomethacin (Indocin), ibuprofen (Motrin), sulindac (Clinoril)
- Stool softener: docusate (Colace)
- Radiation therapy
- Chemotherapy
- Estrogen therapy: diethylstilbestrol (Stilphostrol)
- Radiation implant
- Antineoplastics: doxorubicin (Adriamycin), cisplatin (Platinol)
- Immunosuppressant: cyclophosphamide (Cytoxan)
- Nitrogen mustard: estramustine (Emcyt)
- Treatment: suprapubic or transurethral catheter
- Antiemetics: prochlorperazine (Compazine), ondansetron (Zofran)

Nursing interventions

- Maintain the patient's diet
- Monitor fluid intake
- Assess renal and fluid status
- Monitor and record vital signs, I/O, and laboratory studies
- Administer medications, as prescribed
- Allay the patient's anxiety
- Maintain patency of the urinary catheter
- Encourage the patient to express his feelings about the changes in his body image and fear of sexual dysfunction
- Encourage ambulation
- Assess pain
- Provide postchemotherapeutic and postradiation nursing care
  - Provide prophylactic skin, mouth, and perineal care
  - Monitor dietary intake
  - Administer antiemetics and antidiarrheals, as prescribed
  - Provide rest periods
- Individualize home care instructions
  - Provide information about the American Cancer Society
  - Seek help from community agencies and resources for supportive services
  - Monitor effect of impotency on sexual activities
  - Avoid prolonged sitting, standing, and walking
  - Avoid straining during exercise and lifting

- Urinate frequently
- Avoid coffee and cola beverages
- Decrease fluid intake during evening hours
- Perform perineal exercises
- Complete catheter care, as directed
- Monitor self for bloody urine, pain, burning, frequency, decreased urine output, and loss of bladder control
- Use walker or cane, if needed

Complications

Metastatic cancer (bone, lymph nodes, brain, and lung)

Surgical interventions

- Radical prostatectomy
- Bilateral orchiectomy
- Cryosurgery
- Transurethral resection

NEUROGENIC BLADDER DYSFUNCTION

Definition

- An interruption of normal bladder innervation
- Three types of neurogenic bladder may occur: spastic, flaccid, and mixed

Causes

- Acute infectious diseases such as transverse myelitis
- Cerebral disorders (stroke, brain tumor, Parkinson's disease, multiple sclerosis, dementia)
- Chronic alcoholism
- Collagen diseases such as SLE
- Disorders of peripheral innervation
- Distant effects of cancer such as primary oat cell carcinoma of the lung
- Heavy metal toxicity
- Herpes zoster
- Metabolic disturbances (hypothyroidism, porphyria, or uremia)
- Sacral agenesis
- Spinal cord disease or trauma
- Vascular diseases such as atherosclerosis

Pathophysiology

- Spastic neurogenic bladder: caused by an upper motor neuron (above S2 to S4), with spontaneous contractions of detrusor muscles, elevated intravesical voiding pressure, bladder wall hypertrophy with trabeculation, and urinary sphincter spasms
- Flaccid neurogenic bladder: caused by a lower motor neuron lesion (below S2 to S4), with decreased intravesical pressure, increased bladder capacity and large residual urine retention, and poor detrusor contraction
- Mixed neurogenic bladder: the result of cortical damage from some disorder or trauma

Neurogenic bladder dysfunction

- An interruption of normal bladder innervation
- Three types: spastic, flaccid, and mixed

Facts about flaccid neurogenic bladder

- Caused by lower motor neuron lesion
- Greatly distended bladder with an accompanying feeling of bladder fullness

Facts about spastic neurogenic bladder

- Caused by upper motor neuron lesion
- Involuntary or frequent scanty urination without a feeling of bladder fullness

Facts about mixed neurogenic bladder

- Results from cortical damage from some disorder or trauma
- Dulled perception of bladder fullness

Using urodynamic studies for neurogenic bladder dysfunction

- Consists of cystometry, uroflometry, urethral pressure profiles, and sphincter electromyelography
- Evaluates how well the bladder stores urine, bladder emptying, and the rate of urine movement out of the bladder during voiding

Main medical options for neurogenic bladder dysfunction

- Treatments: Valsalva's maneuver, indwelling urinary catheter, intermittent self-catheterization, Credé's maneuver
- Antispasmodics
- Alpha-adrenergic blockers

Key nursing interventions for a patient with neurogenic bladder dysfunction

- Use strict aseptic technique for inserting and maintaining indwelling urinary catheter.
- Assess for signs and symptoms of infection.
- Arrange for consult with enterostomal therapist, if urinary diversion is performed.

Assessment findings

- Flaccid neurogenic bladder
  - Overflow incontinence
  - Diminished anal sphincter tone
  - Greatly distended bladder with an accompanying feeling of bladder fullness
- Spastic neurogenic bladder
  - Involuntary or frequent scanty urination without a feeling of bladder fullness
  - Possible spontaneous spasms of the arms and legs
  - Increased anal sphincter tone
- Mixed neurogenic bladder
  - Dulled perception of bladder fullness
  - Diminished ability to empty the bladder
  - Urgency that can't be controlled

Diagnostic test findings

- Voiding cystourethrography: evaluates bladder neck function, vesicoureteral reflux, and continence
- Urodynamic studies: consist of cystometry, uroflometry, urethral pressure profiles, and sphincter electromyelography; evaluates how well the bladder stores urine, bladder emptying, and the rate of urine movement out of the bladder during voiding
- Retrograde urethrography: reveals presence of strictures and diverticula

Medical management

- Diet: regular diet, encourage fluids
- Activity: as tolerated
- Monitoring: vital signs and I/O
- Treatments: Valsalva's maneuver, indwelling urinary catheter, intermittent self-catheterization, Credé's maneuver
- Antispasmodics: propantheline (Pro-Banthine), flavoxate (Urispas), dicyclomine
- Alpha-adrenergic blockers: terazosin (Hytrin), doxazosin (Cardura)

Nursing interventions

- Maintain the patient's diet
- Monitor fluid intake
- Assess renal status
- Monitor and record vital signs, I/O, and laboratory studies
- Administer medications, as prescribed
- Allay the patient's anxiety
- Use strict aseptic technique for inserting and maintaining indwelling urinary catheter
- Assess for signs and symptoms of infection
- Arrange for consult with enterostomal therapist, if urinary diversion is performed
- Provide individualized home care instructions
  - Recognize and report signs and symptoms of infection

  - Take measures to prevent UTI
  - Increase fluid intake
  - Perform Credé's maneuver and intermittent self-catheterization
  - Follow dietary measures to prevent renal calculi

- **Complications**
  - UTI
  - Urolithiasis
  - Renal failure
- **Surgical interventions**
  - Transurethral resection of the bladder neck, urethral dilation, or external sphincterotomy
  - Urinary diversion

NCLEX CHECKS

It's never too soon to begin your NCLEX preparation. Now that you've reviewed this chapter, carefully read each of the following questions and choose the best answer. Then compare your responses to the correct answers.

1. The nurse is caring for a patient with acute renal failure. The nurse should expect hypertonic glucose and insulin infusions to be used to treat:

☐ **A.** hypernatremia.
☐ **B.** hypokalemia.
☐ **C.** hyperkalemia.
☐ **D.** hypercalcemia.

2. A patient with fever and urinary urgency is asked to provide a urine specimen for culture and sensitivity. The nurse should instruct the patient to collect the specimen from the:

☐ **A.** first stream of urine from the bladder.
☐ **B.** middle stream of urine from the bladder.
☐ **C.** final stream of urine from the bladder.
☐ **D.** full volume of urine from the bladder.

3. The nurse is teaching a patient with chronic renal failure about foods to avoid. It would be accurate for her to teach the patient to avoid foods high in:

☐ **A.** monosaccharides.
☐ **B.** disaccharides.
☐ **C.** iron.
☐ **D.** protein.

4. The nurse is developing a care plan for a 36-year-old male patient hospitalized with renal calculi. Which intervention should you include in his plan?

☐ **A.** Maintain bed rest.
☐ **B.** Increase dietary purines.
☐ **C.** Restrict fluids.
☐ **D.** Strain all urine.

5. A patient's diagnostic test results show an increased prostate-specific antigen (PSA). This test is used to screen for which disorder?________________

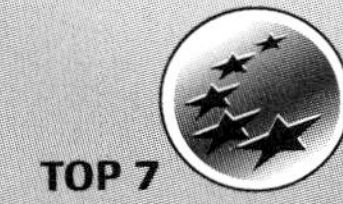

TOP 7

Items to study for your next test on the renal and urologic system

1. Structures of the kidneys and their functions
2. Glomerular filtration rate
3. Nursing interventions for the patient undergoing kidney transplantation
4. Types of urinary diversion surgeries
5. Differences between hemodialysis and peritoneal dialysis
6. Signs and symptoms of renal calculi
7. How acute renal failure and chronic renal failure happen

6. Which of the following factors can contribute renal calculi formation?

- ☐ **A.** Hypocalcemia
- ☐ **B.** Changes in urine pH
- ☐ **C.** Hypothyroidism
- ☐ **D.** Hypertension

7. For a patient with renal calcium stones, the nurse should provide instruction on which of the following diets?

- ☐ **A.** Acid-ash with limited intake of calcium and milk products
- ☐ **B.** Alkaline-ash with limited intake of foods high in oxalate
- ☐ **C.** Alkaline-ash with limited intake of foods high in purine
- ☐ **D.** Low cholesterol diet with limited intake of saturated fats

8. Which of the following assessment findings would the nurse expect in a patient with flaccid neurogenic bladder?

- ☐ **A.** Greatly distended bladder with a feeling of bladder fullness
- ☐ **B.** Involuntary or frequent scanty urination without a feeling of bladder fullness
- ☐ **C.** Dulled perception of bladder fullness
- ☐ **D.** Spontaneous spasms of the arms and legs

9. A patient is scheduled to perform a 24-hour urine test beginning at 8 a.m. on the first day and ending at 8 a.m. on the second day. The nurse should instruct the patient to:

- ☐ **A.** discard the second-day 8 a.m. sample.
- ☐ **B.** discard the first and last samples.
- ☐ **C.** discard the first-day 8 a.m. sample.
- ☐ **D.** retain the first-day 8 a.m. sample.

10. A patient is scheduled for an ileal conduit. The nurse knows the patient understands the procedure when he states:

- ☐ **A.** "I'll pass urine from my rectum."
- ☐ **B.** "Urine will flow out a catheter."
- ☐ **C.** "Urine will come out an abdominal stoma."
- ☐ **D.** "Urine will flow from my urethra."

ANSWERS AND RATIONALES

1. CORRECT ANSWER: C

Hyperkalemia is a common complication of acute renal failure. The administration of glucose and regular insulin infusions can temporarily prevent cardiac arrest by moving potassium into the cells and reducing serum potassium levels. Hypernatremia, hypokalemia, and hypercalcemia don't usually occur with acute renal failure and aren't treated with glucose and insulin infusions.

2. CORRECT ANSWER: B

The midstream specimen is recommended because it is less likely to be contaminated with microorganisms from the external genitalia than other specimens. It isn't necessary to collect a full volume of urine for a urine culture and sensitivity.

3. CORRECT ANSWER: D
Proteins are typically restricted in patients with chronic renal failure because of their metabolites. Iron and carbohydrates aren't restricted.

4. CORRECT ANSWER: D
All urine should be strained through gauze or a urine strainer to catch any stones passed. The stone's composition can then be analyzed. Ambulation may aid the movement of the stone down the urinary tract. A patient at risk for uric acid stones should follow a low-purine diet to reduce uric acid levels. Encourage fluid intake to help flush the stones out of the urinary tract.

5. CORRECT ANSWER: PROSTATE CANCER
PSA measurement is widely used as a screening test for prostatic cancer.

6. CORRECT ANSWER: B
Urine that's consistently acidic or alkaline provides a favorable medium for stone formation.

7. CORRECT ANSWER: A
A patient with calcium stones should follow an acid-ash diet with limited intake of calcium and milk products. An alkaline-ash diet with limited intake of foods high in oxalate is appropriate for a patient with oxalate stones. A patient with uric acid stones should follow an alkaline-ash diet with limited intake of foods high in purine. A patient with coronary artery disease should follow a low cholesterol diet with limited intake of saturated fats.

8. CORRECT ANSWER: A
A patient with flaccid neurogenic bladder will have a greatly distended bladder with an accompanying feeling of bladder fullness, overflow incontinence, and diminished anal sphincter tone. With spastic neurogenic bladder, the patient will experience involuntary or frequent scanty urination without a feeling of bladder fullness, possible spontaneous spasms of the arms and legs, and increased anal sphincter tone. In mixed neurogenic bladder, the patient has a dulled perception of bladder fullness, a diminished ability to empty the bladder, and urgency that can't be controlled.

9. CORRECT ANSWER: C
In a 24-hour urine test, discard the first sample and retain the last sample. Therefore, the nurse should instruct the patient to discard the first-day 8 a.m. urine sample and retain the second-day 8 a.m. sample.

10. CORRECT ANSWER: C
In an ileal conduit, the ureters are implanted into a segment of the ileum that has been resected from the intestinal tract with the formation of an abdominal stoma. In an ureterosigmoidostomy the ureters are excised from the bladder and implanted into the sigmoid colon. Urine then flows through the colon and is excreted through the rectum. With a nephrostomy, a catheter is inserted percutaneously into the kidney. Normal urine flow occurs through the urethra.

8

Musculoskeletal system

LEARNING OBJECTIVES

After studying this chapter, you should be able to:

- Describe the psychosocial impact of musculoskeletal disorders.
- Differentiate between modifiable and nonmodifiable risk factors in the development of a musculoskeletal disorder.
- List three probable and three possible nursing diagnoses for a patient with a musculoskeletal disorder.
- Identify nursing interventions for a patient with a musculoskeletal disorder.
- Identify three teaching topics for a patient with a musculoskeletal disorder.

CHAPTER OVERVIEW

Caring for the patient with a musculoskeletal disorder requires a sound understanding of musculoskeletal anatomy and physiology as well as body mechanics. A thorough assessment is essential to planning and implementing appropriate patient care. The assessment includes a complete history, physical examination, diagnostic testing, identification of modifiable and nonmodifiable risk factors, and information related to the psychosocial impact of the disorder on the patient.

Nursing diagnoses focus primarily on impaired physical mobility and altered peripheral tissue perfusion. Nursing interventions are designed to maintain the patient's ability to carry out the activities of daily living (ADLs) and prevent further injury. Patient teaching — a crucial nursing activity — involves providing information about medical follow-up, medication regimens, signs and symptoms of possible complications, and reduction of modifiable risk factors, such as using proper body mechanics, preventing falls, and participating in body flexibility and strength regimens.

ANATOMY AND PHYSIOLOGY REVIEW

- **Skeleton**
  - Consists of 206 bones (long, short, flat, or irregular)
  - Stores calcium, magnesium, and phosphorus; marrow produces red blood cells (RBCs)
  - Works with muscles to provide support, locomotion, and protection of internal organs
- **Skeletal muscles**
  - Provide body movement and posture by tightening and shortening
  - Attach to bones by tendons
  - Begin contracting with the stimulus of a muscle fiber by a motor neuron
  - Derive energy for muscle contraction from hydrolysis of adenosine triphosphate to adenosine diphosphate and phosphate
  - Retain some contraction to maintain muscle tone
  - Relax with the breakdown of acetylcholine by cholinesterase
- **Ligaments**
  - Tough bands of collagen fibers that connect bones
  - Encircle a joint to add strength and stability
- **Tendons**
  - Nonelastic collagen cords
  - Connect muscles to bones
- **Joints**
  - Articulation of two bone surfaces
  - Provide stabilization and permit locomotion; degree of joint movement is called *range of motion* (ROM)
- **Synovium**
  - Membrane that lines a joint's inner surfaces
  - Secretes synovial fluid and antibodies
  - Reduces friction in joints (in conjunction with cartilage)
- **Cartilage**
  - Serves as a smooth surface for articulating bones
  - Absorbs shock to joints
  - Atrophies with limited ROM or in the absence of weight bearing
- **Bursa**
  - Fluid-filled sac
  - Serves as padding to reduce friction
  - Facilitates the motion of body structures that rub against each other

Key facts about the skeleton

- 206 bones
- Stores calcium, magnesium, and phosphorus
- Marrow produces RBCs
- Functions include support, locomotion, and protection of internal organs

Key facts about skeletal muscles

- Provide body movement and posture
- Attach to bones by tendons
- Retain some contraction for muscle tone

Key facts about joints

- Articulation of two bone surfaces
- Provide stabilization
- Permit locomotion
- ROM is degree of joint movement

Key facts about bursa

- Fluid-filled sac
- Serves as padding
- Facilitates motion of body structures

Key physical findings in disorders of the musculoskeletal system
- Skeletal deformity
- Limited ROM
- Inflammation
- Edema

Electromyography
- Test of muscle activity
- Graphical recording of the muscle
- Intervention: explain to the patient that it's a nonpainful procedure

Arthroscopy
- Visualization of a joint after local anesthesia injection
- Intervention: apply a pressure dressing to the injection site after the procedure

ASSESSMENT FINDINGS

History
- Pain
- Numbness
- Joint stiffness
- Swelling
- Fatigue
- Fever
- Difficulty with movement

Physical examination
- Abnormal vital signs
- Inflammation
- Edema
- Skin breakdown
- Skeletal deformity
- Limited ROM
- Poor posture
- Muscle weakness and rigidity
- Abnormal skin color and temperature
- Paresthesia
- Nodules
- Erythema
- Tophi
- Abnormal peripheral pulses
- Muscle spasms

DIAGNOSTIC TESTS AND PROCEDURES

Electromyography (EMG)
- Definition and purpose
  - Test of muscle activity
  - Graphical recording of the muscle at rest and during contraction
- Nursing interventions
  - Explain that the patient will be asked to flex and relax muscles during the procedure
  - Explain that the procedure may cause some minor discomfort but isn't painful
  - Administer analgesics as prescribed, after the procedure

Arthroscopy
- Definition and purpose
  - Direct visualization of a joint after injection of local anesthesia
- Nursing interventions before the procedure
  - Administer prophylactic antibiotics as prescribed
  - Explain the procedure, skin preparation, and use of local anesthetics
- Nursing interventions after the procedure

Neurovascular checks

Fractures may cause nerve or arterial damage, producing any or all of the five Ps: pain, pallor, paralysis, paresthesia, and pulselessness. When performing a neurovascular check, compare findings bilaterally and above and below the fracture.

PAIN
Ask the patient if he's having pain. Assess the location, severity, and quality of the pain as well as anything that seems to relieve or worsen it. Pain that's unrelieved by a narcotic or that worsens when the limb is elevated (elevation reduces circulation and worsens ischemia) may indicate compartment syndrome.

PALLOR
Paleness, discoloration, and coolness of the injured site may indicate neurovascular compromise from decreased blood supply to the area. Check capillary refill time. Tissues should return to normal color within 3 seconds. Palpate skin temperature with the back of your hand.

PARALYSIS
Note deficits in movement or strength. If the patient can't move the affected area or if movement causes severe pain and muscle spasms, he might have nerve or tendon damage. For a femoral fracture, assess peroneal nerve injury by checking for sensation over the top of the foot between the first and second toes.

PARESTHESIA
Ask the patient about changes in sensation, such as numbness or tingling. Check for loss of sensation by touching the injured area with the tip of an open safety pin or the point of a paper clip. Abnormal sensation or loss of sensation indicates neurovascular involvement.

PULSELESSNESS
Palpate peripheral pulses distal to the injury, noting rate and quality. If a pulse is decreased or absent, blood supply to the area is reduced.

5 P's of fractures in a neurovascular check

- Pain
- Pallor
- Paralysis
- Paresthesia
- Pulselessness

- **Apply a pressure dressing to the injection site**
- Monitor neurovascular status (see *Neurovascular checks*)
- Apply ice to the affected joint
- Limit weight bearing or joint use until allowed by the physician
- Administer analgesics as prescribed

Arthrocentesis

- Definition and purpose
  - Needle aspiration of synovial fluid from a joint under local anesthesia to examine a specimen or remove the fluid
- Nursing interventions before the procedure
  - Administer prophylactic antibiotics as prescribed
  - Explain the procedure to the patient
- Nursing interventions after the procedure
  - **Maintain a pressure dressing on the aspiration site**
  - Monitor neurovascular status
  - Apply ice to the affected area
  - Limit weight bearing or joint use until allowed by the physician
  - Administer analgesics as prescribed

Arthrocentesis

- Needle aspiration of synovial fluid from a joint
- Used to examine a specimen or remove fluid
- Intervention: maintain a pressure dressing on the aspiration site after the procedure

Bone scan

- Procedure using an I.V. injection of an isotope
- Provides visual imaging of bone metabolism
- Intervention: explain that the patient will be required to drink several glasses of fluid to enhance excretion of isotope not absorbed by bone tissue

Myelogram

- Fluoroscopic procedure using an injection of radiopaque dye
- Allows visualization of the subarachnoid space, spinal cord, and vertebral bodies
- Intervention: before the procedure, note the patient's allergies

X-ray examination

- Noninvasive examination of bones and joints
- Intervention: before the procedure, make sure the patient isn't pregnant to prevent possible fetal damage from radiation exposure

Blood chemistry

- Blood test
- Analyzes levels of potassium, calcium, BUN, protein, LE, anti-DNA, and other factors
- Intervention: monitor the venipuncture site for bleeding after the procedure

Bone scan

- Definition and purpose
  - Procedure using I.V. injection of a radioisotope
  - Visual imaging of bone metabolism
- Nursing interventions before the procedure
  - Determine the patient's ability to lie still during the scan
  - Advise the patient that radioisotope will be injected intravenously
  - Explain that the patient will be required to drink several glasses of fluid during the waiting period to enhance excretion of isotope not absorbed by bone tissue

Myelogram

- Definition and purpose
  - Procedure using an injection of radiopaque dye by lumbar puncture
  - Fluoroscopic visualization of the subarachnoid space, spinal cord, and vertebral bodies
- Nursing interventions before the procedure
  - **Note the patient's allergies to iodine, seafood, and radiopaque dyes**
  - Inform the patient about possible throat irritation and flushing of the face from the injection
- Nursing interventions after the procedure
  - Maintain bed rest, with the head of the bed between 15 to 30 degrees
  - Inspect the insertion site for bleeding
  - Monitor neurovital signs
  - Encourage fluids

X-ray examination

- Definition and purpose
  - Noninvasive radiographic examination of bones and joints
- Nursing interventions
  - Use caution when moving a patient with a suspected fracture
  - Explain the procedure to the patient
  - **Make sure the patient isn't pregnant to prevent possible fetal damage from radiation exposure**

Blood chemistry

- Definition and purpose
  - Laboratory test of a blood sample
  - Analysis for potassium, sodium, calcium, phosphorus, glucose, bicarbonate, blood urea nitrogen (BUN), creatinine, protein, albumin, osmolality, creatine kinase, serum aspartate aminotransferase, aldolase, rheumatoid factor, complement fixation, lupus erythematosus (LE) cell preparation test, antinuclear antibody (ANA), anti-DNA, and C-reactive protein
- Nursing interventions
  - Withhold food and fluid before the procedure
  - Monitor the venipuncture site for bleeding after the procedure

- **Hematologic studies**
  - Definition and purpose
    - Laboratory test of a blood sample
    - Analysis for white blood cells (WBCs), RBCs, platelets, prothrombin time, partial thromboplastin time, erythrocyte sedimentation rate (ESR), hemoglobin (Hb), and hematocrit (HCT)
  - Nursing interventions
    - Note current drug therapy to anticipate possible interference with test results
    - Assess the venipuncture site for bleeding after the procedure

Hematologic studies

- Blood test
- Analyzes for substances, such as WBCs, RBCs, Hb, and HCT
- Intervention: note current drug therapy to anticipate possible interference with test results

PSYCHOSOCIAL IMPACT OF MUSCULOSKELETAL DISORDERS

- **Developmental impact**
  - Decreased self-esteem
  - Fear of rejection
  - Changes in body image
  - Embarrassment from changes in body structure and function
  - Dependence
- **Economic impact**
  - Disruption or loss of employment
  - Cost of vocational retraining
  - Cost of hospitalizations
  - Cost of home health care
  - Cost of special equipment
- **Occupational and recreational impact**
  - Restrictions in work activity
  - Changes in leisure activity
  - Restrictions in physical activity
- **Social impact**
  - Social isolation
  - Changes in role performance

Key impacts of musculoskeletal disorders

- Decreased self-esteem
- Dependence
- Disruption or loss of employment
- Economic impact: cost of hospitalizations, home health care, cost of special equipment

RISK FACTORS

- **Modifiable risk factors**
  - Occupations that require heavy lifting or use of machinery
  - Occupational or recreational activities that include repetitive motion of joints
  - Vegetarian diets
  - Medication history
  - Stress
  - Contact sports
  - Obesity

Key modifiable risk factors in musculoskeletal disorders

- Occupations that require heavy lifting, use of machinery, or repetitive motion
- Vegetarian diets
- Contact sports
- Obesity

Key nonmodifiable risk factors in musculoskeletal disorders

- Aging
- Menopause
- Family history

Key probable nursing diagnoses

- Impaired physical mobility
- Ineffective tissue perfusion
- Impaired skin integrity

3 types of joint surgery

- Arthrodesis – surgical removal of cartilage from joint surfaces to fuse a joint into a functional position
- Synovectomy – removal of the synovial membrane from a joint, using an arthroscope, to reduce pain
- Arthroplasty (total joint replacement) – surgical replacement of a joint with a metal, plastic, or porous prosthesis

Nonmodifiable risk factors

- Aging
- Menopause
- Family history of musculoskeletal illness
- History of musculoskeletal injury
- History of immune disorders

NURSING DIAGNOSES

Probable nursing diagnoses

- Impaired physical mobility
- Ineffective tissue perfusion: peripheral
- Impaired skin integrity
- Acute pain
- Toileting self-care deficit
- Feeding self-care deficit
- Bathing or hygiene self-care deficit

Possible nursing diagnoses

- Sexual dysfunction
- Powerlessness
- Constipation
- Disturbed body image
- Social isolation
- Risk for disuse syndrome
- Chronic pain

JOINT SURGERY

Description

- Arthrodesis — surgical removal of cartilage from joint surfaces to fuse a joint into a functional position
- Synovectomy — removal of the synovial membrane from a joint, using an arthroscope, to reduce pain
- Arthroplasty (total joint replacement) — surgical replacement of a joint with a metal, plastic, or porous prosthesis

Preoperative nursing interventions

- Complete patient and family preoperative teaching
  - Determine the patient's understanding of the procedure
  - Describe the operating room, postanesthesia care unit (PACU), and preoperative and postoperative routines
  - Demonstrate postoperative turning, coughing, deep breathing, splinting, and ROM exercises
  - Explain the postoperative need for drainage tubes, surgical dressings, oxygen therapy, I.V. therapy, and pain control
- Complete a preoperative checklist
- Administer preoperative medications as prescribed

Adduction versus abduction

Here's an easy way to keep adduction and abduction straight:

Adduction is moving a limb toward the body's midline; think of it as adding two things together.

Abduction is moving a limb away from the body's midline; think of it as taking something away, like abducting, or kidnapping.

- Allay the patient's and family's anxiety about surgery
- Document the patient's history and physical assessment data
- Administer antibiotics as prescribed

Postoperative nursing interventions

- Assess cardiac and respiratory status
- Assess pain and administer postoperative analgesic as prescribed
- Administer I.V. fluids and transfusion therapy as prescribed
- Allay the patient's anxiety
- Inspect the surgical dressing and change as directed
- Reinforce turning, coughing, and deep breathing
- Keep the patient in semi-Fowler's position
- Provide incentive spirometry
- Maintain activity: active and passive ROM for unaffected limbs and isometric exercises as tolerated
- Monitor vital signs, intake and output (I/O), laboratory studies, neurovascular checks, and pulse oximetry
- Monitor and maintain the position and patency of wound drainage tubes
- Encourage the patient to express his feelings about limited mobility
- Assess movement limitations
- Elevate the affected extremity
- Administer antibiotics as prescribed
- Assess for return of peristalsis
- Give solid foods and liquids as tolerated
- Administer stool softeners as prescribed
- Provide routine cast care (arthrodesis)
- Provide specific care for total knee replacement
  - Maintain continuous passive motion
  - Apply a knee immobilizer before getting the patient out of bed
  - Administer anticoagulants as prescribed
- Provide specific care for total hip replacement
  - Maintain hips in abduction (see *Adduction versus abduction*)
  - **Limit hip flexion to 90 degrees when sitting**
  - Turn to the affected or unaffected side as ordered
  - Avoid sitting in low or soft chairs
  - **Don't allow the patient to cross his legs; possible dislodgment of the prosthesis or dislocation may occur**
  - Have patient use an elevated toilet seat
  - Administer anticoagulants as prescribed

Adduction vs. abduction

- Adduction: moving a limb toward the body's midline
- Abduction: moving a limb away from the body's midline

Key nursing interventions for a patient before joint surgery

- Assess cardiac and respiratory status.
- Inspect the surgical dressing and change as directed.
- Maintain activity.
- Monitor vital signs, I/O, laboratory studies, neurovascular checks, and pulse oximetry.
- Maintain activity.
- Elevate the affected extremity.

Key nursing interventions after total hip replacement

- Maintain hips in abduction.
- Limit hip flexion to 90 degrees when sitting.
- Don't allow the patient to cross his legs; possible dislodgment of the prosthesis or dislocation may occur.
- Administer anticoagulants as prescribed.

External fixation defined

- Fracture immobilization in which transfixing pins are inserted through the bone above and below the fracture
- It's then attached to a rigid external metal frame

Key nursing steps before external fixation

- Monitor for fracture complications.
- Maintain the position of the affected extremity with sandbags and pillows.
- Maintain traction or splint.

Key nursing steps after external fixation

- Assess pain and administer postoperative analgesics as prescribed.
- Check wound and pin sites for infection.
- Provide pin care.
- Maintain balanced suspension traction.
- Don't readjust traction clamps.

- Individualize home care instructions
  - Avoid jogging, jumping, and lifting as prescribed
  - Complete incision care daily as prescribed
  - Continue cast care as directed

Surgical complications

- Infection
- Hemorrhage

EXTERNAL FIXATION

Description

- Fracture immobilization in which transfixing pins are inserted through the bone above and below the fracture and then attached to a rigid external metal frame

Preoperative nursing interventions

- Complete patient and family preoperative teaching
  - Determine the patient's understanding of the procedure
  - Describe the operating room, PACU, and preoperative and postoperative routines
  - Demonstrate postoperative turning, coughing, deep breathing, splinting, and ROM exercises
  - Explain the postoperative need for drainage tubes, surgical dressings, oxygen therapy, I.V. therapy, and pain control
- Complete a preoperative checklist
- Administer preoperative medications as prescribed
- Allay the patient's and family's anxiety about surgery
- Document the patient's history and physical assessment data
- Monitor for fracture complications
- Maintain the position of the affected extremity with sandbags and pillows
- Maintain traction or splint

Postoperative nursing interventions

- Assess pain and administer postoperative analgesics as prescribed
- Assess for return of peristalsis; give solid foods and liquids as tolerated
- Administer I.V. fluids
- Allay the patient's anxiety
- Reinforce turning, coughing, and deep breathing
- Keep the patient in semi-Fowler's position
- Provide incentive spirometry
- Maintain activity: active and passive ROM for unaffected limbs, isometric exercises (strengthening and increasing muscle tone by contracting muscles against resistance either from other muscles or a stationary object), and quadriceps setting as tolerated
- Monitor vital signs, I/O, laboratory studies, and neurovascular checks
- Encourage the patient to express his feelings about changes in his body image
- Check wound and pin sites for infection

- Provide pin care
- Maintain balanced suspension traction
- Don't readjust traction clamps
- Individualize home care instructions
  - Attend physical therapy sessions
  - Maintain fixator as set
  - Complete pin care daily as directed

Surgical complications

- Infection of wound and pin sites
- Osteomyelitis
- Hemorrhage
- Chronic pain

AMPUTATION

Description

- Surgical removal of all or part of a limb
- Two types of amputation
  - Closed (flap)
  - Open (guillotine)

Preoperative nursing interventions

- Complete patient and family preoperative teaching
  - Determine the patient's understanding of the procedure
  - Describe the operating room, PACU, and preoperative and postoperative routines
  - Demonstrate postoperative turning, coughing, deep breathing, splinting, and ROM exercises
  - Explain the postoperative need for drainage tubes, surgical dressings, oxygen therapy, I.V. therapy, and pain control
- Complete a preoperative checklist
- Administer preoperative medications as prescribed
- Allay the patient's and family's anxiety about surgery
- Document the patient's history and physical assessment data
- Administer antibiotics as prescribed
- Prepare the patient for the possibility of phantom limb sensation or phantom pain

Postoperative nursing interventions

- Assess cardiac and respiratory status
- Assess pain and administer postoperative analgesics as prescribed
- Administer I.V. fluids and transfusion therapy as prescribed
- Allay the patient's anxiety
- Inspect the ace wrap surgical dressing and change as directed
- Reinforce turning, coughing, and deep breathing
- Keep the patient in semi-Fowler's position
- Assess for return of peristalsis; give solid foods and liquids as tolerated
- Provide incentive spirometry

Key facts about amputation

- Surgical removal of all or part of a limb
- Two types: closed and open

Key nursing steps before amputation

- Complete patient and family preoperative teaching.
- Prepare the patient for the possibility of phantom limb sensation or phantom pain.
- Allay the patient's and family's anxiety about surgery.

- Maintain activity: active and passive ROM for unaffected limbs and isometric exercises as tolerated
- Monitor vital signs, I/O, laboratory studies, neurovascular checks, and pulse oximetry
- Monitor and maintain the position and patency of wound drainage tubes
- **Encourage the patient to express his feelings about changes in his body image and phantom limb sensation and pain**
- Administer antibiotics as prescribed
- Elevate the affected extremity for 24 hours only
- Rewrap the stump before getting the patient out of bed
- Prevent hip flexion
- Inspect the stump for bleeding, infection, and edema
- Maintain a rigid dressing for the stump prosthesis
- Irrigate the wound and change the ace wrap stump dressing as directed
- Reinforce physical therapy attendance
- Provide trapeze
- Individualize home care instructions
  - Recognize the signs and symptoms of skin breakdown
  - Complete stump care daily
  - Use of a prosthesis
  - Maintain a stump-conditioning program
  - Avoid using powder or lotion on the stump
  - Demonstrate proper wrapping of the stump
  - Protect the stump from injury

Surgical complications

- Hemorrhage
- Infection
- Contractures
- Skin breakdown

Key nursing steps after amputation

- Assess cardiac and respiratory status.
- Assess pain and administer postoperative analgesics as prescribed.
- Inspect the ace wrap surgical dressing and change as directed.
- Monitor vital signs, I/O, laboratory studies, neurovascular checks, and pulse oximetry.
- Elevate the affected extremity for 24 hours only.
- Rewrap the stump before getting the patient out of bed.
- Prevent hip flexion.
- Inspect the stump for bleeding, infection, and edema.
- Maintain a rigid dressing for the stump prosthesis.
- Provide trapeze.
- Encourage the patient to express his feelings about changes in his body image and phantom limb sensation and pain.

RELEASE OF TRANSVERSE CARPAL LIGAMENT

Description

- Surgical ligation of the transverse carpal ligament to relieve compression of the median nerve in the carpal canal of the wrist

Preoperative nursing interventions

- Complete patient and family preoperative teaching
  - Determine the patient's understanding of the procedure
  - Describe the operating room, PACU, and preoperative and postoperative routines
  - Demonstrate postoperative turning, coughing, deep breathing, splinting, and ROM exercises
  - Explain the postoperative need for drainage tubes, surgical dressings, oxygen therapy, I.V. therapy, and pain control
- Complete a preoperative checklist
- Administer preoperative medications as prescribed

Release of transverse carpal ligament defined

- Surgical ligation of the transverse carpal ligament
- Performed to relieve compression of the median nerve in the carpal canal of the wrist

- Allay the patient's and family's anxiety about surgery
- Document the patient's history and physical assessment data
- Use a splint to increase the patient's comfort

Postoperative nursing interventions

- Assess pain and administer postoperative analgesics as prescribed
- Assess for return of peristalsis; give solid foods and liquids as tolerated
- Administer I.V. fluids
- Allay the patient's anxiety
- Inspect the surgical dressing and change as directed
- Reinforce turning, coughing, and deep breathing
- Keep the patient in semi-Fowler's position
- Provide incentive spirometry
- Maintain activity: active and passive ROM and isometric exercises to affected and unaffected extremities as tolerated
- Monitor vital signs, I/O, laboratory studies, and neurovascular checks
- Elevate the hand and apply ice
- Administer steroids as prescribed
- Administer antibiotics as prescribed
- Assist with activities of daily living (ADLs)
- Prevent injury to the affected hand
- Apply splint
- Reinforce immobilization of the affected hand
- Individualize home care instructions
  - Continue active ROM exercises of the affected hand
  - Avoid heavy lifting
  - Use a splint
  - Monitor the affected hand for return of sensation and motor function
  - Complete incision care daily as directed

Surgical complications

- Infection
- Paralysis

OPEN REDUCTION INTERNAL FIXATION (ORIF) OF THE HIP

Description

- Surgical reduction and stabilization of a fracture, using orthopedic devices or hardware, such as Austin Moore prosthesis, Smith-Petersen nail, Jewett nail, intramedullary nails, and compression screws

Preoperative nursing interventions

- Complete patient and family preoperative teaching
  - Determine the patient's understanding of the procedure
  - Describe the operating room, PACU, and preoperative and postoperative routines
  - Demonstrate postoperative turning, coughing, deep breathing, splinting, and ROM exercises

Key nursing steps before release of transverse carpal ligament

- Demonstrate postoperative turning, coughing, deep breathing, splinting, and ROM exercises.
- Administer preoperative medications as prescribed.
- Use a splint to increase the patient's comfort.

Key nursing steps after release of transverse carpal ligament

- Assess pain and administer postoperative analgesics as prescribed.
- Inspect the surgical dressing and change as directed.
- Elevate the hand and apply ice.
- Reinforce immobilization of the affected hand.

ORIF of the hip defined

- Surgical reduction and stabilization of a fracture using orthopedic devices or hardware
- Types of orthopedic devices and hardware include Austin Moore prosthesis, Smith-Petersen nail, Jewett nail, intramedullary nails, and compression screws

- Explain the postoperative need for drainage tubes, surgical dressings, oxygen therapy, I.V. therapy, and pain control
- Complete a preoperative checklist
- Administer preoperative medications as prescribed
- Allay the patient's and family's anxiety about surgery
- Document the patient's history and physical assessment data
- Monitor the patient for fracture complications
- Keep the affected extremity in position with sandbags and pillows
- Maintain traction or splint

Postoperative nursing interventions

- Assess cardiac and respiratory status
- Assess pain and administer postoperative analgesics as prescribed
- Assess for return of peristalsis; give solid foods and liquids as tolerated
- Administer I.V. fluids and transfusion therapy as prescribed
- Allay the patient's anxiety
- Inspect the surgical dressing and change as directed
- Reinforce turning, coughing, and deep breathing
- Keep the patient in semi-Fowler's position: no higher than 30 degrees
- Provide incentive spirometry
- Maintain activity: bed rest, active and passive ROM for unaffected limbs, isometric exercises, and progressive ambulation
- Monitor vital signs, I/O, laboratory studies, neurovascular checks, and pulse oximetry
- Monitor and maintain the position and patency of drainage tubes
- Use abductor pillow and trochanter rolls
- Turn the patient to the affected or unaffected side as ordered
- Maintain a high-fiber, low-calcium diet with increased fluid intake
- Apply antiembolism or pneumatic stockings
- Administer anticoagulants as prescribed
- Administer antibiotics as prescribed
- Administer stool softeners as prescribed
- Use a fracture bedpan
- Provide heel and elbow protectors
- Individualize home care instructions
  - Avoid jogging, jumping, lifting, crossing the legs, and sitting in soft or low chairs
  - Complete incision care daily as directed
  - Apply antiembolism stockings
  - Use an elevated toilet seat

Surgical complications

- Osteomyelitis
- Hemorrhage
- Thrombophlebitis
- Pneumonia
- Avascular necrosis
- Pulmonary embolism

Key nursing interventions before ORIF

- Monitor the patient for fracture complications.
- Keep the affected extremity in position with sandbags and pillows.
- Maintain traction or splint.

Key nursing interventions after ORIF

- Assess cardiac and respiratory status.
- Assess pain and administer postoperative analgesics as prescribed.
- Inspect the surgical dressing and change as directed.
- Keep the patient in semi-Fowler's position: no higher than 30 degrees.
- Provide incentive spirometry.
- Monitor vital signs, I/O, laboratory studies, neurovascular checks, and pulse oximetry.
- Use abductor pillow and trochanter rolls.
- Apply antiembolism or pneumatic stockings.
- Administer anticoagulants as prescribed.
- Administer stool softeners as prescribed.

LAMINECTOMY

Description

- Surgical excision of vertebral posterior arch

Preoperative nursing interventions

- Complete patient and family preoperative teaching
  - Determine the patient's understanding of the procedure
  - Describe the operating room, PACU, and preoperative and postoperative routines
  - Demonstrate postoperative turning, coughing, deep breathing, splinting, and ROM exercises
  - Explain the postoperative need for drainage tubes, surgical dressings, oxygen therapy, I.V. therapy, and pain control
- Complete a preoperative checklist
- Administer preoperative medications as prescribed
- Allay the patient's and family's anxiety about surgery
- Document the patient's history and physical assessment data
- Teach the patient the logrolling technique
- Administer antibiotics as prescribed

Postoperative nursing interventions

- Assess neurologic and neurovascular status
- Assess pain and administer postoperative analgesics as prescribed
- Assess for return of peristalsis; give solid foods and liquids as tolerated
- Administer I.V. fluids
- Allay the patient's anxiety
- Inspect surgical dressings for drainage of cerebrospinal fluid (CSF) and blood
- Reinforce turning, coughing, and deep breathing
- Keep the patient in a flat position
- Provide incentive spirometry
- Maintain activity: active and passive ROM and isometric exercises
- Monitor vital signs, I/O, laboratory studies, and neurovascular checks
- Turn the patient by logrolling
- Prevent flexion of the neck after cervical laminectomy
- Administer muscle relaxants as prescribed
- Administer corticosteroids as prescribed
- Administer stool softeners as prescribed
- Individualize home care instructions
  - Avoid lifting, driving, stooping, tub bathing, and repetitive bending as prescribed
  - Wear a supportive brace
  - Complete exercises for the lower back daily
  - Sleep on the side, with hips and knees flexed
  - Sleep on a firm mattress
  - Monitor lower extremities for numbness and decreased circulation
  - Monitor ability to void

Laminectomy defined

- Surgical excision of vertebral posterior arch

Key nursing steps before laminectomy

- Complete patient and family preoperative teaching.
- Teach the patient the logrolling technique.
- Administer antibiotics as prescribed.

Key nursing steps after laminectomy

- Assess neurologic and neurovascular status.
- Inspect surgical dressings for drainage of CSF and blood.
- Keep the patient in a flat position.
- Turn the patient by logrolling.
- Prevent flexion of the neck after cervical laminectomy.
- Administer muscle relaxants, corticosteroids, and stool softeners, as prescribed.

– Complete incision care daily as directed

Surgical complications

- Urine retention
- Motor and sensory deficits
- Infection
- Muscle spasm
- Paralytic ileus

Spinal fusion highlights

- Stabilization of spinous processes
- Uses bone chips from iliac crest or Harrington rod metallic implant

SPINAL FUSION

Description

- Stabilization of spinous processes with bone chips from iliac crest or Harrington rod metallic implant

Preoperative nursing interventions

- Complete patient and family preoperative teaching
  - Determine the patient's understanding of the procedure
  - Describe the operating room, PACU, and preoperative and postoperative routines
  - Demonstrate postoperative turning, coughing, deep breathing, splinting, and ROM exercises
  - Explain the postoperative need for drainage tubes, surgical dressings, oxygen therapy, I.V. therapy, and pain control
- Complete a preoperative checklist
- Administer preoperative medications as prescribed
- Allay the patient's and family's anxiety about surgery
- Document the patient's history and physical assessment data
- Administer antibiotics as prescribed
- Teach the patient the logrolling technique

Key nursing interventions before spinal fusion

- Demonstrate postoperative turning, coughing, deep breathing, and ROM exercises
- Explain the postoperative need for drainage tubes, surgical dressings, oxygen therapy, I.V. therapy, and pain control.
- Teach the patient the logrolling technique.

Postoperative nursing interventions

- Assess cardiac, respiratory, and neurologic status
- Assess pain and administer postoperative analgesics as prescribed
- Assess for return of peristalsis; give solid foods and liquids as tolerated
- Administer I.V. fluids
- Allay the patient's anxiety
- Inspect the surgical dressing and change as directed
- Reinforce turning, coughing, and deep breathing
- Maintain the patient in the supine position
- Provide incentive spirometry
- Maintain activity: active and passive ROM and isometric exercises
- Monitor vital signs, I/O, and laboratory studies
- Check neurovascular status: color, temperature, pulses, movement, and sensation in extremities
- Administer antipyretics as prescribed
- Administer antibiotics as prescribed
- Administer corticosteroids as prescribed
- Turn the patient every 2 hours using the logrolling technique

Key nursing interventions after spinal fusion

- Assess cardiac, respiratory, and neurologic status.
- Inspect the surgical dressing and change as directed.
- Check neurovascular status: color, temperature, pulses, movement, and sensation in extremities.
- Administer antibiotics, corticosteroids, and stool softeners, as prescribed.
- Turn the patient every 2 hours using the logrolling technique.

- Administer muscle relaxants as prescribed
- Administer stool softeners as prescribed
- Individualize home care instructions
  - Avoid lifting, driving, stooping, tub bathing, repetitive bending, and prolonged sitting as prescribed
  - Walk regularly
  - Note spinal flexion limitations
  - Complete exercises for the lower back daily
  - Sleep on the side with hips and knees flexed
  - Sleep on a firm mattress
  - Monitor lower extremities for numbness and decreased circulation
  - Monitor ability to void
  - Complete incision care daily as directed

Surgical complications

- Urine retention
- Infection
- Muscle spasm
- Motor and sensory deficits
- Paralytic ileus

Key home care instructions for patients after spinal fusion

- Avoid lifting, driving, stooping, tub bathing, repetitive bending, and prolonged sitting as prescribed.
- Sleep on the side with hips and knees flexed.
- Sleep on a firm mattress.
- Monitor lower extremities for numbness and decreased circulation.

RHEUMATOID ARTHRITIS

Definition

- Systemic inflammatory disease that affects the synovial lining of the joints

Causes

- Unknown
- Autoimmune disease
- Genetic transmission (increases susceptibility to the disease)

Pathophysiology

- Inflammation of the synovial membranes is followed by formation of pannus, an inflammatory exudate, and destruction of cartilage, bone, and ligaments
- Pannus is replaced by fibrotic tissue and calcification, which causes subluxation of the joint

Assessment findings

- Fatigue
- Anorexia
- Malaise
- Elevated body temperature
- Painful, swollen joints
- Limited ROM
- Subcutaneous nodules
- Symmetrical joint swelling (mirror image of affected joints)
- Morning stiffness
- Paresthesia of the hands and the feet
- Crepitus

Key facts about rheumatoid arthritis

- Systemic inflammatory disease that affects the synovial lining of the joints
- Inflammation is followed by formation of pannus and destruction of cartilage, bone, and ligaments
- Pannus is replaced by fibrotic tissue and calcification

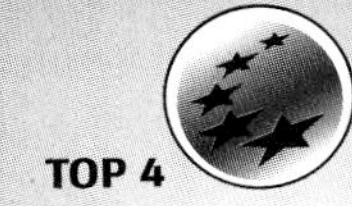

TOP 4

Assessment findings in rheumatoid arthritis

1. Painful, swollen joints
2. Symmetrical joint swelling
3. Morning stiffness
4. Crepitus

- Pericarditis
- Splenomegaly
- Leukopenia
- Enlarged lymph nodes

Diagnostic test findings

- X-rays: joint space narrowing, bone erosions
- Hematology: increased ESR, WBCs, platelets
- Gamma globulin: increased immunoglobulin (Ig) M, IgG
- Synovial fluid analysis: increased WBCs, decreased viscosity, opaque
- Latex fixation test: positive rheumatoid factor
- Tumor necrosis factor: elevated
- ANA test: positive

Key test findings in rheumatoid arthritis

- Latex fixation test: positive rheumatoid factor
- ANA test: positive

Medical management

- Activity: as tolerated
- Monitoring: vital signs and I/O
- Analgesic: aspirin
- Nonsteroidal anti-inflammatory drugs (NSAIDs): indomethacin (Indocin), ibuprofen (Motrin), sulindac (Clinoril), piroxicam (Feldene), flurbiprofen (Ansaid), diclofenac (Voltaren), naproxen (Naprosyn), diflunisal (Dolobid), celecoxib (Celebrex)
- Biologic response modifiers: infliximab (Remicade), etanercept (Enbrel)
- Glucocorticoids: prednisone (Deltasone), hydrocortisone (Cortef)
- Antacids: magnesium and aluminum hydroxide (Maalox), aluminum hydroxide gel (Gelusil)
- Gold therapy: gold sodium thiomalate (Aurolate)
- Physical therapy
- Heat therapy
- Cold therapy
- Plasmapheresis
- Laboratory studies: ESR, WBCs
- Antirheumatic: hydroxychloroquine (Plaquenil)
- Antimetabolite: methotrexate (Rheumatrex)

Medications to help manage rheumatoid arthritis

- NSAIDs
- Biologic response modifiers
- Glucocorticoids
- Heat therapy
- Cold therapy
- Antirheumatics

Nursing interventions

- Assess neuromuscular status
- Keep joints extended
- Monitor and record vital signs, I/O, and laboratory studies
- Administer medications as prescribed
- Encourage the patient to express his feelings about changes in his body image and self-esteem
- Provide skin care
- Minimize environmental stress
- Check joints for swelling, pain, and redness
- Provide passive ROM exercises
- Provide warm compresses and paraffin dips (heat therapy) as prescribed
- Individualize home care instructions (for teaching tips, see *Patients with musculoskeletal disorders*)

Key nursing interventions for a patient with rheumatoid arthritis

- Administer medications as prescribed.
- Encourage the patient to express his feelings about changes in his body image and self-esteem.
- Check joints for swelling, pain, and redness.

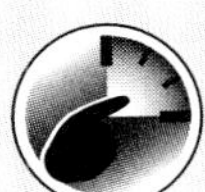

TIME-OUT FOR TEACHING

Patients with musculoskeletal disorders

Be sure to include the following topics in your teaching plan when caring for patients with musculoskeletal disorders.

- Follow-up appointments
- Optimal body weight maintenance
- Medication therapy, including the action, adverse effects, and scheduling
- Use of assistive and adaptive devices, such as crutches, a walker, or a cane
- Signs and symptoms of soft tissue and bone infection
- Rest and activity patterns, including activity limitations or restrictions
- Signs and symptoms of motor, sensory, and circulatory deficits
- Safe environment
- Change in activities of daily living to compensate for limited range-of-motion
- Proper body mechanics and correct posture
- Dietary recommendations and restrictions
- Community agencies and resources for supportive services
- Exercises for extremities
- Signs and symptoms of skin breakdown and contractures

– Provide information about the Arthritis Foundation
– Identify ways to reduce stress
– Avoid cold, stress, and infection
– Avoid unproven remedies
– Promote a quiet environment
– Complete skin and foot care daily

Medical complication

- Carpal tunnel syndrome

Surgical interventions

- Joint replacement
- Synovectomy

OSTEOARTHRITIS (DEGENERATIVE JOINT DISEASE)

Definition

- Degeneration of articular cartilage, usually affecting the weight-bearing joints (spine, knees, hips)

Causes

- Aging
- Obesity
- Joint trauma
- Congenital abnormalities

Pathophysiology

- Cartilage softens with age, narrowing the joint space
- Normal use thins and erodes cartilage

Key teaching topics for a patient with a musculoskeletal disorder

- Medication therapy
- Use of an assistive or adaptive device
- Signs and symptoms of motor, sensory, and circulatory deficits

Osteoarthritis defined

- Degeneration of articular cartilage
- Cartilage flakes enter the synovial lining, which fibroses and limits joint movement
- Usually affects the weight-bearing joints (spine, knees, hips)

Causes of osteoarthritis

- Aging
- Obesity
- Joint trauma
- Congenital abnormalities

What happens to nodes in osteoarthritis

- Initially painless
- Redness
- Swelling
- Tenderness
- Impaired sensation
- Impaired dexterity

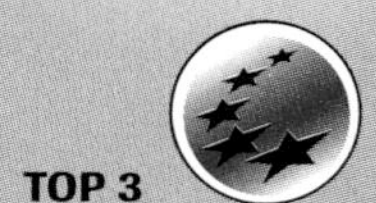

Signs and symptoms of osteoarthritis

1. Enlarged, edematous joints
2. Joint stiffness
3. Heberden's nodes and Bouchard's nodes

Key diagnostic test findings in osteoarthritis

- X-rays: joint deformities or bone spurs
- Hematology: increased ESR

Key ways to manage osteoarthritis

- Heat therapy
- Cold therapy
- Canes, walkers
- NSAIDs

Digital joint deformities

Osteoarthritis of the interphalangeal joints produces irreversible changes in the distal joints (Heberden's nodes, left) and proximal joints (Bouchard's nodes, right). Initially painless, these nodes gradually progress to or suddenly flare up as redness, swelling, tenderness, and impaired sensation and dexterity.

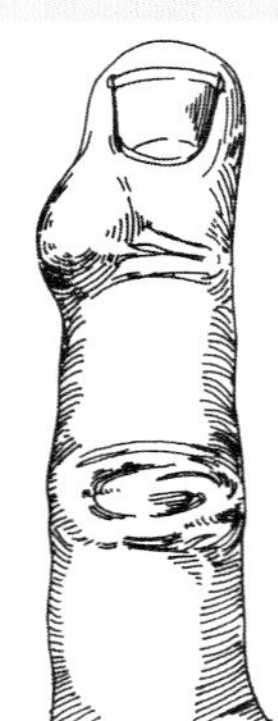

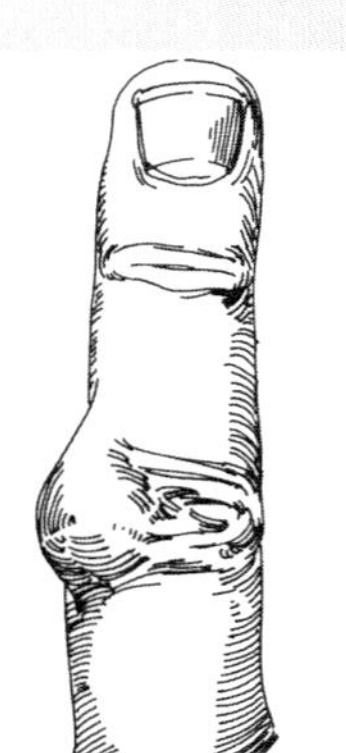

- Cartilage flakes enter the synovial lining, which fibroses, thus limiting joint movement

Assessment findings

- Pain relieved by resting joints
- Joint stiffness
- Heberden's nodes and Bouchard's nodes (see *Digital joint deformities*)
- Limited ROM
- Crepitation (a grating sensation associated with degenerative joint disease that can be heard or felt; it's best detected by palpation of the affected joint)
- Increased pain in damp, cold weather
- Enlarged, edematous joints
- Smooth, taut, shiny skin

Diagnostic test findings

- X-rays: joint deformity, narrowing of joint space, bone spurs
- Arthroscopy: bone spurs, narrowing of joint space
- Hematology: increased ESR

Medical management

- Diet: low-calorie if not at optimal weight
- Activity: as tolerated
- Monitoring: vital signs and I/O
- Heat therapy
- Cold therapy
- Isometric exercises, strengthening exercises, aerobic exercises
- Weight reduction
- Canes, walkers
- Analgesic: aspirin
- NSAIDs: indomethacin (Indocin), ibuprofen (Motrin), sulindac (Clinoril), piroxicam (Feldene), flurbiprofen (Ansaid), diclofenac (Voltaren), naproxen (Naprosyn), diflunisal (Dolobid), rofecoxib (Vioxx)

Nursing interventions

- Maintain the patient's diet
- Assess musculoskeletal status
- Keep joints extended
- Monitor and record vital signs and I/O
- Administer medications as prescribed
- Assess for increased bleeding or bruising
- Urge the patient to express his feelings about changes in his body image
- Provide skin care
- Provide rest periods
- Determine degree of joint mobility
- Maintain calorie count
- Assess pain and provide analgesics, as indicated
- Provide moist compresses and paraffin baths (heat therapy) as prescribed
- Teach proper body mechanics
- Provide passive ROM exercises
- Individualize home care instructions
  - Provide information about the Arthritis Foundation
  - Avoid jogging, jumping, and lifting
  - Identify ways to reduce stress
  - Complete skin and foot care daily

Medical complications

- Contractures

Surgical interventions

- Synovectomy
- Arthrodesis
- Joint replacement

GOUTY ARTHRITIS

Definition

- Inflammatory joint disease caused by the deposit of uric acid crystals

Causes

- Genetics
- Decreased uric acid excretion
- Chronic renal failure
- Myxedema
- Polycythemia vera
- Hyperparathyroidism

Pathophysiology

- End product of purine metabolism is uric acid
- Abnormal purine metabolism results in decreased secretion of urates and increased blood levels of uric acid
- Uric acid forms a precipitate in areas where blood flow is slowest
- Genetic defect in purine metabolism can cause overproduction of uric acid

Key nursing interventions in osteoarthritis

- Assess musculoskeletal status.
- Assess for increased bleeding or bruising.
- Assess pain and provide analgesics, as indicated.

Gouty arthritis defined

- Inflammatory joint disease
- Caused by the deposit of uric acid crystals

Common causes of gouty arthritis

- Genetics
- Decreased uric acid excretion
- Chronic renal failure

Signs of the final stages of gout

- Painful polyarthritis
- Large, subcutaneous, tophaceous deposits in cartilage, synovial membranes, tendons, and soft tissue
- Shiny, thin, and taut skin over the tophus

Key assessment findings in gouty arthritis

- Joint pain
- Redness and swelling in joints
- Tophi in great toe, ankle, and outer ear

Diagnostic test findings in gouty arthritis

- Hematology: increased ESR
- Blood chemistry: increased uric acid
- Synovial fluid analysis: sodium urate crystals

Key steps in the medical management of gouty arthritis

- Low-purine, alkaline-ash diet
- Uricosuric agents
- Antigout agents

Gouty deposits

The final stage of gout is marked by painful polyarthritis, with large, subcutaneous, tophaceous deposits in cartilage, synovial membranes, tendons, and soft tissue. The skin over the tophus is shiny, thin, and taut.

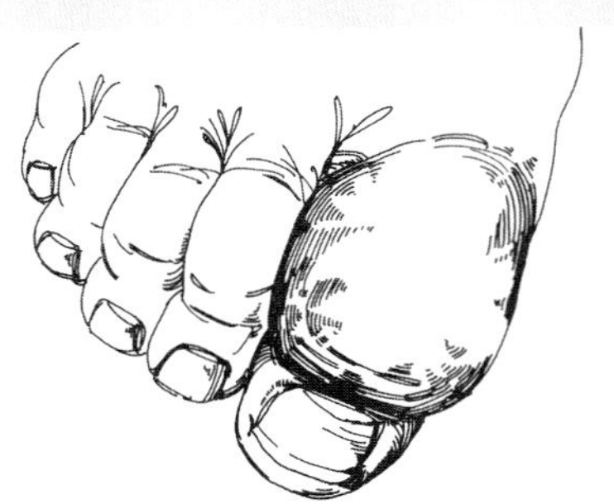

Assessment findings

- Joint pain
- Redness and swelling in joints
- Tophi in great toe, ankle, and outer ear (see *Gouty deposits*)
- Malaise
- Tachycardia
- Elevated skin temperature

Diagnostic test findings

- Hematology: increased ESR
- Blood chemistry: increased uric acid
- Synovial fluid analysis: sodium urate crystals

Medical management

- Diet: low-purine, alkaline-ash
- Dietary recommendations: increase fluid intake to 3 qt (3 L)/day
- Dietary restrictions: no shellfish, liver, sardines, anchovies, and kidneys; limited alcohol
- Activity: as tolerated
- Monitoring: vital signs and I/O
- Laboratory studies: uric acid, ESR
- Exercise program, including passive and active ROM exercises and ambulation as tolerated
- Uricosuric agents: probenecid (Probalan), sulfinpyrazone (Anturane)
- Xanthine-oxidase inhibitor: allopurinol (Zyloprim)
- Antigout: colchicine
- Analgesic: aspirin
- NSAIDs: indomethacin (Indocin), ibuprofen (Motrin), sulindac (Clinoril), piroxicam (Feldene), flurbiprofen (Ansaid), diclofenac (Voltaren), naproxen (Naprosyn), diflunisal (Dolobid)

Nursing interventions

- Maintain the patient's diet
- Encourage fluids to 3 qt (3 L)/day

- Assess integumentary status
- Monitor and record vital signs, I/O, and laboratory studies
- Administer medications as prescribed
- Allay the patient's anxiety
- Provide skin care
- Check joints for pain, edema, and ROM
- Provide a bed cradle
- Reinforce exercise of joints; show the patient how to perform the exercises
- Individualize home care instructions
  - Provide information about the Arthritis Foundation
  - Recognize signs and symptoms of gout
  - Limit alcohol intake
  - Avoid fasting
  - Identify ways to reduce stress
  - Complete skin and foot care daily

Medical complications
- Renal calculi
- Cartilage damage

Surgical interventions
- None

OSTEOMYELITIS

Definition
- Bacterial infection of bone and soft tissue

Causes
- *Staphylococcus aureus*
- Hemolytic streptococcus
- Open trauma
- Infection

Pathophysiology
- Organism reaches bone through an open wound or via the bloodstream
- Infection causes bone destruction
- Bone fragments necrose (sequestra)
- New bone cells form over the sequestrum during healing, resulting in nonunion

Assessment findings
- Malaise
- Elevated body temperature
- Bone pain
- Tachycardia
- Localized edema and redness
- Muscle spasms
- Increased pain with movement

Key nursing interventions in gouty arthritis

- Encourage fluids to 3 qt (3 L)/day.
- Monitor and record vital signs, I/O, and laboratory studies.
- Administer medications as prescribed.
- Provide a bed cradle.

Characteristics of osteomyelitis

- Bacterial infection of bone and soft tissue
- Infection causes bone destruction
- Bone fragments necrose
- New bone cells form, causing nonunion

Key symptoms of osteomyelitis

- Bone pain
- Localized edema and redness

Common test findings for osteomyelitis

- Blood cultures: positive identification of organism
- Hematology: increased WBCs, ESR
- Wound culture: positive identification of organism

Common ways to manage osteomyelitis

- Antibiotics
- Cast or splint for the affected body part

Key nursing interventions for a patient with osteomyelitis

- Maintain the patency of wound irrigation.
- Change dressings and irrigate wound using strict sterile aseptic technique.
- Monitor and record vital signs, I/O, and laboratory studies.
- Provide cast and splint care.

Diagnostic test findings

- Blood cultures: positive identification of organism
- Hematology: increased WBCs, ESR
- Wound culture: positive identification of organism
- Bone biopsy: positive
- Bone scan: positive

Medical management

- Diet: high-calorie, high-vitamin C and D, high-protein, and high-calcium
- I.V. therapy: saline lock
- Activity: bed rest
- Monitoring: vital signs, I/O, and neurovascular checks
- Laboratory studies: WBCs, ESR
- Nutritional support: total parenteral nutrition (TPN)
- Special care: wound and skin
- Antibiotic: ciprofloxacin (Cipro)
- Analgesic: oxycodone (Tylox)
- Continuous wound irrigation
- Heat therapy
- Cast or splint for the affected body part
- Antipyretic: aspirin

Nursing interventions

- Maintain the patient's diet
- Encourage fluids to 3 qt (3 L)/day
- Administer I.V. fluids
- Assess integumentary status
- Maintain the patency of wound irrigation
- Change dressings and irrigate wound using strict sterile technique
- Monitor and record vital signs, I/O, and laboratory studies
- Administer TPN
- Administer medications as prescribed
- Encourage the patient to express his feelings about changes in his body image
- Provide skin care
- Turn the patient every 2 hours
- Immobilize the affected body part
- Maintain proper body alignment
- Maintain bed rest
- Provide cast and splint care
- Assess pain
- Individualize home care instructions
  - Recognize the signs and symptoms of fractures
  - Avoid exposure to people with infections
  - Monitor self for infection
  - Practice health routines that prevent infection
  - Avoid weight bearing on the affected part

- **Medical complications**
  - Bone necrosis
  - Pathological fractures
  - Sepsis
- **Surgical interventions**
  - Incision and drainage of bone abscess
  - Sequestrectomy
  - Bone graft
  - Bone segment transfer

OSTEOPOROSIS

- **Definition**
  - A metabolic bone dysfunction that results in reduced bone mass and increased porosity
  - Metabolic illnesses or medications that cause osteoporosis increase the risk of skeletal fracture
- **Causes**
  - Lowered estrogen levels
  - Immobility
  - Liver disease
  - Calcium deficiency
  - Vitamin D deficiency
  - Protein deficiency
  - Bone marrow disorders
  - Lack of exercise
  - Increased phosphorus
  - Cushing's syndrome
  - Hyperthyroidism
- **Pathophysiology**
  - Rate of bone resorption exceeds the rate of bone formation
  - Increased phosphate stimulates parathyroid activity, which increases bone resorption
  - Estrogens decrease bone resorption
- **Assessment findings**
  - Dowager's hump (kyphosis)
  - Back pain: thoracic and lumbar
  - Loss of height
  - Unsteady gait
  - Joint pain
  - Weakness
- **Diagnostic test findings**
  - X-ray: thin, porous bone; increased vertebral curvature
  - Dual energy X-ray absorptiometry scan: decreased bone mineral density

Osteoporosis

- A metabolic bone dysfunction that results in reduced bone mass and increased porosity
- Illnesses or medications that cause osteoporosis increase the risk of skeletal fracture

Common signs and symptoms of osteoporosis

- Dowager's hump (kyphosis)
- Back pain: thoracic and lumbar
- Loss of height
- Joint pain

Key diagnostic test findings in osteoporosis

- X-ray: thin, porous bone
- Dual energy X-ray absorptiometry scan: decreased bone mineral density

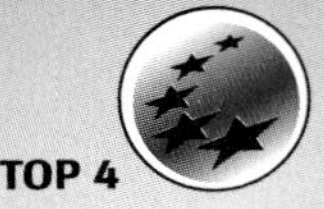

TOP 4

Management options for osteoporosis

1. Estrogen
2. Calcium supplement
3. Vitamin and mineral supplements
4. Exercise program

Key nursing interventions for a patient with osteoporosis

- Maintain the patient's diet.
- Assess musculoskeletal status
- Encourage the patient to express his feelings about changes in his body image.
- Assess pain and administer analgesics, as indicated.

Characteristics of osteogenic sarcoma

- Malignant bone tumor that invades the ends of long bones
- Tumor arises from osteoblasts
- Tumor may spread to the lung

Medical management

- Diet: high in calcium, protein, vitamins, minerals, and boron
- Dietary restrictions: limit caffeine and alcohol
- Activity: as tolerated
- Monitoring: vital signs and I/O
- Laboratory studies: calcium, phosphorus
- Estrogen: estradiol (Estrace)
- Calcium supplement: calcium carbonate (Os-Cal)
- Vitamin and mineral supplements
- Exercise program
- Thiazide diuretic: hydrochlorothiazide (Aldactazide, Dyazide)
- NSAIDs: indomethacin (Indocin), ibuprofen (Motrin), sulindac (Clinoril), piroxicam (Feldene), flurbiprofen (Ansaid), diclofenac (Voltaren), naproxen (Naprosyn), diflunisal (Dolobid)

Nursing interventions

- Maintain the patient's diet
- Assess musculoskeletal status
- Monitor and record vital signs, I/O, and laboratory studies
- Administer medications as prescribed
- Encourage the patient to express his feelings about changes in his body image
- Individualize home care instructions
  - Reinforce the importance of following an exercise program
  - Teach proper body mechanics and posture
  - Provide information about the Osteoporosis Foundation
- Assess pain and administer analgesics, as indicated

Medical complication

- Pathologic fractures

Surgical intervention

- None

OSTEOGENIC SARCOMA (OSTEOSARCOMA)

Definition

- Malignant bone tumor that invades the ends of long bones

Causes

- Osteoblastic activity
- Osteolytic activity

Pathophysiology

- Unregulated cell growth and uncontrolled cell division result in the development of a neoplasm
- Tumor arises from osteoblasts and dissolves the bone and soft tissue
- Tumor may spread to the lung

Assessment findings

- Pain

- Limited movement
- Pathologic fractures
- Soft tissue mass over the tumor site
- Warm tissue over the tumor site
- Elevated body temperature

Diagnostic test findings

- Bone scan: mass
- Biopsy: cytology positive for cancer cells
- Computed tomography scan: mass
- Blood chemistry: increased alkaline phosphatase
- Bone marrow aspiration: cancer cells

Medical management

- Diet: high-protein
- I.V. therapy: saline lock
- Activity: as tolerated
- Monitoring: vital signs and I/O
- Laboratory studies: calcium, phosphorus
- Antiemetics: prochlorperazine (Compazine), ondansetron (Zofran)
- Nutritional support: TPN
- Radiation therapy
- Analgesics: oxycodone (Tylox), meperidine (Demerol)
- Antineoplastics: cyclophosphamide (Cytoxan), vincristine (Oncovin)
- Antidiarrheals: attapulgite (Kaopectate), loperamide (Imodium)

Nursing interventions

- Maintain the patient's diet
- Assess integumentary and musculoskeletal status
- Monitor and record vital signs, I/O, and laboratory studies
- Administer TPN
- Administer medications as prescribed
- Encourage the patient to express his feelings about changes in his body image and a fear of dying
- Provide postchemotherapeutic nursing care
  - Provide prophylactic skin, mouth, and perineal care
  - Monitor dietary intake
  - Administer antiemetics and antidiarrheals as prescribed
  - Monitor for bleeding, infection, and electrolyte imbalance
  - Provide rest periods
- Assess pain
- Individualize home care instructions
  - Provide information about the American Cancer Society
  - Recognize signs and symptoms of a fracture
  - Avoid exposure to people with infections
  - Monitor self for infections
  - Monitor pain control interventions
  - Complete skin care daily

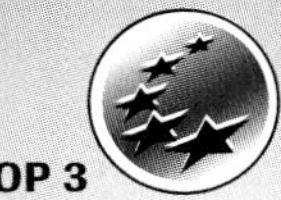

TOP 3

Signs and symptoms of osteogenic sarcoma

1. Pain
2. Pathologic fractures
3. Soft tissue mass over the tumor site

Key diagnostic test findings in osteogenic sarcoma

- Bone scan or CT scan: mass present
- Biopsy: positive for cancer cells
- Bone marrow aspiration: cancer cells present

Key treatment options for osteogenic sarcoma

- Radiation therapy
- Antineoplastics

Key nursing interventions for osteogenic sarcoma

- Assess integumentary and musculoskeletal status.
- Provide postchemotherapeutic nursing care.
- Assess pain.

Carpal tunnel syndrome

- Chronic compression neuropathy of the median nerve at the wrist
- Median nerve supplies motor innervation to the wrist and fingers

Pathophysiology of carpal tunnel syndrome

- Median nerve is compressed in the space between the inelastic transverse carpal ligament and the bones in the wrist.
- Result is pain and numbness in the thumb, index, middle, and half of the ring finger.

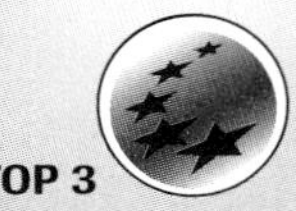

TOP 3

Signs and symptoms of carpal tunnel syndrome

1. Burning and tingling of the hand
2. Impaired sensation in the hand
3. Weakness

Key diagnostic test finding in carpal tunnel syndrome

- Tinel's sign: positive

Medical complications

- Metastasis
- Pathologic fractures

Surgical intervention

- Amputation

CARPAL TUNNEL SYNDROME

Definition

- Chronic compression neuropathy of the median nerve at the wrist

Causes

- Strenuous and repetitive use of the hands
- Fractures and dislocations of the wrist
- Bruising of the wrist
- Menopause
- Genetics
- Pregnancy
- Tenosynovitis
- Rheumatoid arthritis
- Acromegaly
- Hyperparathyroidism
- Obesity
- Gout
- Amyloidosis

Pathophysiology

- Median nerve supplies sensory innervation to the palmar surface of the thumb and the first three fingers (see *The carpal tunnel*)
- Median nerve also supplies motor innervation to the wrist and finger flexion
- Compression of the median nerve in the space between the inelastic transverse carpal ligament and the bones of the wrist (carpal tunnel) leads to pain and numbness in the thumb, index, middle, and half of the ring finger

Assessment findings

- Nocturnal pain and paresthesia in the thumb and first three fingers, relieved by shaking the hand
- Burning and tingling of the hand
- Impaired sensation in the hand
- Pain radiating to forearm, shoulder, neck, and chest
- Thenar atrophy (mound on palm of hand at the base of the thumb)
- Loss of fine motor movement of the hand
- Weakness

Diagnostic test findings

- Tinel's sign: positive (tingling over median nerve on light percussion)

The carpal tunnel

The carpal tunnel is clearly visible in this palmar view and cross section of a right hand. Note the median nerve flexor tendons of fingers, and blood vessels passing through the tunnel on their way from the forearm to the hand.

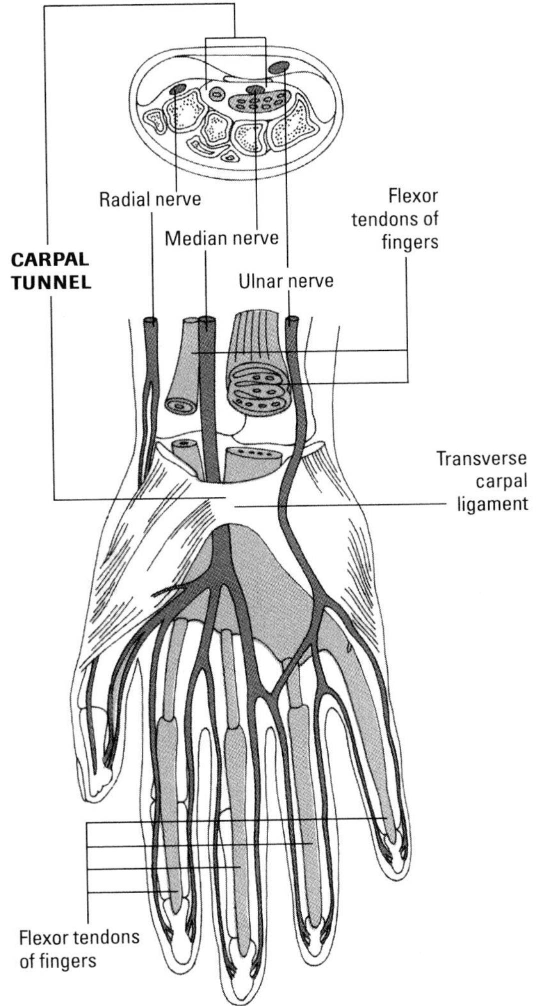

- Motor nerve velocity studies: segmental, distal, median, and motor conduction delay, and conduction block at wrist

Medical management

- Diet: low-sodium
- Dietary restrictions: limit fluids
- Position: avoid flexion of the wrist; elevate the hand
- Activity: avoid using the hand

Parts of the hand and wrist involved in carpal tunnel syndrome

- Carpal tunnel
- Radial nerve
- Median nerve
- Ulnar nerve
- Flexor tendons of fingers
- Transverse carpal ligament

Most common treatments for carpal tunnel syndrome

- Avoid using the hand
- Hand splint
- Glucocorticoids
- NSAIDs

- Monitoring: vital signs, I/O, and neurovascular checks
- Hand splint
- Analgesic: acetaminophen (Tylenol)
- Diuretic: furosemide (Lasix)
- Glucocorticoid: cortisone (Cortone)
- NSAIDs: indomethacin (Indocin), ibuprofen (Motrin), sulindac (Clinoril), piroxicam (Feldene), flurbiprofen (Ansaid), diclofenac (Voltaren), naproxen (Naprosyn), diflunisal (Dolobid)
- Vitamin: pyridoxine (Vitamin B_6)

Nursing interventions

- Maintain the patient's diet
- Assess neurovascular status
- Elevate the patient's hand
- Monitor and record vital signs
- Administer medications as prescribed
- Encourage the patient to express his feelings about inability to use the hand and to perform job requirements
- Provide skin care
- Provide ROM exercises to the splinted hand
- Protect the hand from cold, burns, abrasions, local trauma, and chemical irritations
- **Avoid manual activity that includes dorsiflexion and volar flexion of the wrist**
- Individualize home care instructions
  - Maintain ROM exercises for the hand
  - Avoid activities that increase pain
  - Alternate rest periods with activities involving the hand
  - Protect the hand from trauma
  - Splint the hand
  - Consider vocational retraining, if appropriate
  - Complete skin care daily

Key nursing interventions for a patient with carpal tunnel syndrome

- Assess neurovascular status.
- Encourage the patient to express his feelings about inability to use the hand and to perform job requirements.
- Avoid manual activity that includes dorsiflexion and volar flexion of the wrist

Medical complications

- Contracture
- Loss of thumb abduction and opposition (ape hand)
- Trophic changes of tips of thumbs and index and middle fingers

Surgical intervention

- Carpal tunnel release

HERNIATED NUCLEUS PULPOSA (SLIPPED DISK)

Herniated nucleus pulposa

- Rupture of intervertebral disk
- Two types: lumbrosacral and cervical

Definition

- Rupture of intervertebral disk
- Two types of ruptured disk
  - Lumbrosacral (L4, L5)
  - Cervical (C5, C6, C7)

Causes
- Accidents
- Back or neck strain
- Congenital bone deformity
- Degeneration of disk
- Weakness of ligaments
- Heavy lifting
- Trauma

Pathophysiology
- Protrusion of the nucleus pulposus into the spinal canal compresses the spinal cord or nerve roots
- Compression of the spinal cord or nerve roots causes pain, numbness, and loss of motor function

Assessment findings
- Lumbosacral
  - Acute pain in the lower back radiating across the buttock and down the leg
  - Weakness, numbness, and tingling of the foot and leg
  - Pain on ambulation
- Cervical
  - Neck stiffness
  - Weakness, numbness, and tingling of the hand
  - Neck pain that radiates down the arm to the hand
  - Weakness of affected upper extremities
  - Atrophy of biceps and triceps
  - Straightening of normal lumbar curve with scoliosis away from the affected side

Diagnostic test findings
- Lasègue's sign: positive (pain radiating to the leg when hips and knees are flexed and knee is extended)
- CSF analysis: increased protein
- Myelogram: compression of spinal cord
- EMG: spinal nerve involvement
- X-ray: narrowing of disk space
- Deep tendon reflexes: depressed or absent upper extremity reflexes or Achilles reflex

Medical management
- Diet: calories according to metabolic needs; increase fiber; force fluids
- Keep the patient in semi-Fowler's position
- Activity: bed rest; active and passive ROM and isometric exercises
- Monitoring: vital signs, I/O, neurovascular checks, and laboratory studies
- Heating pad; moist, hot compresses
- Orthopedic devices: back brace, cervical collar
- Analgesic: oxycodone (Tylox)
- Antacids: magnesium and aluminum hydroxide (Maalox), aluminum hydroxide gel (Gelusil)

TOP 3

Causes of herniated nucleus pulposa

1. Accidents
2. Back or neck strain
3. Heavy lifting

Key lumbosacral assessment findings

- Acute pain in the lower back radiating across the buttock and down the leg
- Weakness, numbness, and tingling of the foot and leg
- Pain on ambulation

Key diagnostic test findings

- Lasègue's sign: positive
- Myelogram: compressed spinal cord
- X-ray: narrowing of disk space

Key cervical assessment findings

- Neck stiffness
- Weakness, numbness, and tingling of the hand
- Neck pain that radiates down the arm to the hand
- Weakness of affected upper extremities

Key treatment options for herniated nucleus pulposa

- Neurovascular checks
- Heating pad; moist, hot compresses
- NSAIDs
- Corticosteroids

Key nursing interventions for a patient with herniated nucleus pulposa

- Assess neurovascular status.
- Turn the patient every 2 hours using the logrolling technique.
- Maintain traction, braces, and cervical collar.

Key home care instructions about exercising with a herniated nucleus pulposa

- Exercise regularly with special attention to exercises that strengthen and stretch the muscles.
- Avoid lifting and climbing stairs, as prescribed.
- Avoid flexion, extension, or rotation of the neck.

- Stool softener: docusate (Colace)
- Pelvic traction
- Cervical traction
- Muscle relaxants: diazepam (Valium), cyclobenzaprine (Flexeril)
- Chemonucleolysis using chymopapain (Chymodiactin)
- NSAIDs: indomethacin (Indocin), ibuprofen (Motrin), sulindac (Clinoril), piroxicam (Feldene), flurbiprofen (Ansaid), diclofenac (Voltaren), naproxen (Naprosyn), diflunisal (Dolobid)
- Corticosteroid: cortisone (Cortone)
- Transcutaneous electrical nerve stimulation

Nursing interventions

- Maintain the patient's diet; increase fluid intake
- Assess neurovascular status
- Keep the patient in semi-Fowler's position with moderate hip and knee flexion
- Monitor and record vital signs, I/O, and laboratory studies
- Administer medications as prescribed
- Encourage the patient to express his feelings about changes in his body image and about fears of disability
- Provide skin and back care
- Turn the patient every 2 hours using the logrolling technique
- Maintain bed rest and body alignment
- Maintain traction, braces, and cervical collar
- Promote independence in ADLs
- Apply bed boards
- Individualize home care instructions
  - Exercise regularly with special attention to exercises that strengthen and stretch the muscles
  - Avoid lifting, sleeping in a prone position, climbing stairs, and riding in a car as prescribed
  - Avoid flexion, extension, or rotation of the neck
  - Use one pillow
  - Use a back brace or cervical collar

Medical complications

- Upper respiratory infection
- Urinary tract infection
- Thrombophlebitis
- Chronic pain
- Muscle atrophy
- Progressive paralysis
- Urine retention

Surgical interventions

- Laminectomy
- Spinal fusion
- Microdiskectomy
- Percutaneous lateral diskectomy

FRACTURES

Definition

- Break in the continuity of bone
- Types of fractures (see *Types and causes of fractures,* page 376)
  - Complete
  - Incomplete
  - Comminuted
  - Greenstick
  - Simple
  - Compound
  - Transverse
  - Spiral
  - Oblique
  - Depressed
  - Compression
  - Avulsion
  - Pathologic
- Types of hip fractures
  - Intracapsular
  - Extracapsular
  - Intertrochanteric

Causes

- Trauma
- Osteoporosis
- Multiple myeloma
- Bone tumors
- Immobility
- Malnutrition
- Cushing's syndrome
- Osteomyelitis
- Steroid therapy
- Aging

Pathophysiology

- Fracture occurs when stress placed on the bone is more than the bone can withstand
- Localized tissue injury results in muscle spasm, edema, hemorrhage, compressed nerves, and ecchymosis

Assessment findings

- Pain aggravated by motion
- Tenderness over the fracture site
- Loss of function or motion
- Edema
- Crepitus
- Ecchymosis
- Deformity

Fracture highlights

- Break in the continuity of bone
- Occurs when stress placed on the bone is more than the bone can withstand
- Results in muscle spasm, edema, hemorrhage, compressed nerves, and ecchymosis

Common types of fractures

- Complete
- Incomplete
- Simple
- Compound
- Transverse
- Spiral

Key signs and symptoms of fractures

- Pain aggravated by motion
- Loss of function or motion
- Deformity
- Edema
- Ecchymosis

Fracture descriptions

- Avulsion: pulls bone and tissue from usual attachments
- Closed: skin is closed but bone is fractured
- Compression: bone is squeezed or wedged together at one side
- Greenstick: break in only one cortex of the bone
- Impacted: one end wedged into the opposite end or into the fractured fragment
- Linear: line runs parallel to bone's axis
- Oblique: an oblique angle across both cortices
- Open: skin is open, bone is fractured, and soft tissue trauma may occur
- Pathologic: transverse, oblique, or spiral fracture of a bone weakened by a tumor
- Spiral: fracture curves around both cortices
- Stress: crack in one cortex of a bone
- Transverse: horizontal break through the bone

Diagnostic test findings in fractures

- X-ray: break in continuity of bone
- Hematology: decreased Hb and HCT

Types and causes of fractures

TYPE OF FRACTURE	DESCRIPTION	FORCE CAUSING THE FRACTURE
Avulsion	Fracture that pulls bone and other tissues from their usual attachments	Direct force with resisted extension of the bone and joint
Closed	Skin is closed but bone is fractured	Minor force
Compression	Fracture in which the bone is squeezed or wedged together at one side	Compressive, axial force applied directly above the fracture site
Greenstick	Break in only one cortex of the bone	Minor direct or indirect force
Impacted	Fracture with one end wedged into the opposite end or into the fractured fragment	Compressive, axial force applied directly to the distal fragment
Linear	Fracture line runs parallel to bone's axis	Minor or moderate direct force applied to the bone
Oblique	Fracture at an oblique angle across both cortices	Direct or indirect force with angulation and some compression
Open	Skin is open, bone is fractured, and soft tissue trauma may occur	Moderate to severe force that is continuous and exceeds tissue tolerances
Pathologic	Transverse, oblique, or spiral fracture of a bone weakened by tumor	Minor direct or indirect force
Spiral	Fracture curves around both cortices	Direct or indirect twisting force, with the distal part of the bone held or unable to move
Stress	Crack in one cortex of a bone	Repetitive direct force, as from jogging, running, or osteoporosis
Transverse	Horizontal break through the bone	Direct or indirect force toward the bone

- False motion
- Paresthesia
- Affected leg that appears shorter (fractured hip)

Diagnostic test findings
- X-ray: break in continuity of bone
- Hematology: decreased Hb and HCT

Medical management
- Diet: high-protein, high-vitamin, and low-calcium; increase fluid intake
- Position: elevate a fractured leg; keep the patient flat with the leg abducted for a fractured hip

- Activity: as tolerated for extremity fractures; active and passive ROM exercises for unaffected limbs for fractured hip; isometric exercises
- Monitoring: vital signs, I/O, and neurovascular checks
- Laboratory studies: Hb, HCT, phosphorus, and calcium
- Cast care, pin care, ice packs, incentive spirometry, abductor pillow (fractured hip)
- Analgesic: oxycodone and acetaminophen (Tylox)
- Skin traction: Buck's, Bryant's, or Russell
- Skeletal traction: Thomas splint with Pearson attachment, Steinmann pin, Kirschner wire, or Crutchfield tongs (fractured neck)
- Closed reduction with hip-spica cast (fractured hip)
- Cast or closed reduction (fracture)

Nursing interventions

- Maintain the patient's diet; increase fluid intake
- Assess neurovascular and respiratory status
- Keep the patient in a flat position with the foot of the bed elevated 25 degrees (fractured hip)
- Keep the legs abducted (fractured hip)
- Elevate a fractured extremity
- Monitor and record vital signs, I/O, and laboratory studies
- Administer medications as prescribed
- Allay the patient's anxiety
- Provide skin, pin, and cast care
- Turn the patient to the affected or unaffected side every 2 hours as ordered (fractured hip)
- Keep the hip extended (fractured hip)
- Maintain activity as tolerated (fractures)
- Promote independence in ADLs
- Provide active and passive ROM and isometric exercises for unaffected limbs
- Provide a trapeze
- **Maintain traction to ensure proper body alignment and promote healing** (see *Nursing considerations for a patient in skeletal or skin traction,* page 378)
- Keep side rails up
- Provide appropriate sensory stimulation with frequent reorientation
- Provide turning, coughing, and deep breathing and incentive spirometry
- Prevent constipation as prescribed
- Maintain proper body alignment
- Inspect pin sites for infection
- Provide diversional activities
- Provide heel and elbow protectors and sheepskin
- Apply antiembolism stockings
- Use the logrolling technique to turn the patient
- Individualize home care instructions
  - Complete cast care (fracture)
  - Attend physical therapy sessions

Key ways to manage fractures

- Cast care, pin care, ice packs, incentive spirometry, abductor pillow (fractured hip)
- Analgesic: oxycodone and acetaminophen
- Skin traction: Buck's, Bryant's, or Russell
- Skeletal traction: Thomas splint with Pearson attachment, Steinmann pin, Kirschner wire, or Crutchfield tongs (fractured neck)
- Closed reduction with hip spica cast (fractured hip)
- Cast or closed reduction (fracture)

Key nursing steps for a patient with a fracture

- Assess neurovascular and respiratory status.
- Keep the legs abducted (fractured hip).
- Monitor and record vital signs, I/O, and laboratory studies.
- Provide skin, pin, and cast care.
- Keep the hip extended (fractured hip).
- Provide a trapeze.
- Provide turning, coughing, and deep breathing and incentive spirometry.
- Inspect pin sites for infection.
- Use the logrolling technique to turn the patient.

Key nursing interventions for a patient in skeletal or skin traction

- Check ropes, knots, pulleys, freedom of movement, and intactness.
- Check traction setup.
- Check weights.
- Check all skin surfaces for signs of tolerance or pressure areas
- Provide physical and psychological comfort.
- Answer questions honestly, promptly, and with care.

Possible medical complications of fractures

- Anemia
- Fat embolism
- Pulmonary embolism
- Pneumonia
- Compartment syndrome (fracture)
- Osteomyelitis (fracture)

Nursing considerations for a patient in skeletal or skin traction

NURSING ACTION	RATIONALE
Check ropes, knots, pulleys, freedom of movement, and intactness.	These checks help ensure that the traction is functioning properly.
Check the entire traction setup, pin site, and all suspension apparatus for tightness or signs of loosening.	These actions help ensure that the traction is functioning properly.
Check weights to ensure that they're hanging freely.	These checks help ensure that there's a proper amount of traction.
Make sure the weights aren't "lifted" during care.	This action helps to avoid pain caused by sudden muscle contraction and disrupted fragments of the injured or fractured bone. (Move patients in skeletal traction for position changes without lifting or releasing the weights.)
Take care not to bump the weights or weight holders.	This action helps to avoid pain caused by rope movements, which affect the traction bow and pin.
Check all skin surfaces for signs of tolerance or pressure areas (especially on the occipital area of the head, shoulder blades, elbows, coccyx, and heels).	These checks may uncover signs of pressure that include redness, tenderness or pain, soreness caused by excoriation, and numbness.
Provide physical and psychological comfort. Answer questions honestly, answer the call light promptly, provide prompt and thorough care, encourage patient participation in care, provide diversionary activities, and prepare the patient and family for discharge.	These actions help ensure that the patient participates in and is prepared for self-care.

- Avoid weight bearing on affected limb
- Complete skin and foot care daily

Medical complications

- Deep vein thrombosis
- Anemia
- **Fat embolism**
- **Pulmonary embolism**
- Renal lithiasis
- Pneumonia
- Urinary tract infections
- Compartment syndrome (fracture)
- Hypovolemic shock
- Nonunion
- Osteomyelitis (fracture)
- Avascular necrosis of the femoral head (fractured hip)
- Pressure ulcers

Surgical interventions
- ORIF of the hip
- External fixation for fractures

SYSTEMIC LUPUS ERYTHEMATOSUS (SLE)

Definition
- Chronic connective tissue disease involving multiple organ systems

Causes
- Unknown
- Genetic
- Autoimmune disease
- Viral
- Drug-induced: procainamide (Pronestyl) and hydralazine (Apresoline)

Pathophysiology
- Defect in the body's immunologic mechanism produces serum autoantibodies directed against components of the patient's cell nuclei
- Deposits of antigen or antibody complexes affect connective cells throughout the body, including blood vessels, mucous membranes, joints, skin, kidneys, muscles, brain, and heart

Assessment findings
- Oral and nasopharyngeal ulcerations
- Alopecia
- Photosensitivity
- Early-morning joint stiffness
- Low-grade fever
- Butterfly erythema on face
- Erythema on palms
- Muscle pain
- Abdominal pain
- Malaise and weakness
- Weight loss
- Lymphadenopathy
- Anorexia

Diagnostic test findings
- Hematology: decreased Hb, HCT, WBCs, platelets; increased ESR
- Rheumatoid factor: positive
- LE cell preparation test: positive
- Urine chemistry: proteinuria, hematuria
- Blood chemistry: decreased complement fixation
- ANA test: positive

Medical management
- Diet: high in iron, protein, and vitamins (especially vitamin C)
- I.V. therapy: saline lock
- Activity: as tolerated

SLE defined
- Chronic connective tissue disease involving multiple organ systems
- Deposits of antigen or antibody complexes affect the connective cells throughout the body

Key signs and symptoms of SLE
- Early-morning joint stiffness
- Butterfly erythema on face
- Malaise and weakness

Key test findings for SLE
- LE cell preparation test: positive
- Urine chemistry: proteinuria, hematuria
- ANA test: positive

Key medication options for SLE

- Corticosteroids
- NSAIDs
- Immunosuppressants

Key nursing interventions for a patient with SLE

- Assess musculoskeletal and renal status.
- Encourage the patient to express his feelings about changes in his body image and the chronicity of the disease.
- Maintain seizure precautions.
- Maintain a quiet environment.

Key steps in providing care after chemotherapy for a patient with SLE

- Provide prophylactic skin, mouth, and perineal care.
- Monitor for bleeding, infection, and electrolyte imbalance.

- Monitoring: vital signs and I/O
- Laboratory studies: Hb, HCT, WBCs, platelets, ESR, BUN, and creatinine
- Plasmapheresis
- Precautions: seizure
- Analgesic: acetaminophen (Tylenol)
- Antacids: magnesium and aluminum hydroxide (Maalox), aluminum hydroxide gel (Gelusil)
- Corticosteroid: prednisone (Deltasone)
- Antimalarial: hydroxychloroquine (Plaquenil)
- Antipyretic: aspirin
- NSAIDs: indomethacin (Indocin), ibuprofen (Motrin), sulindac (Clinoril), piroxicam (Feldene), flurbiprofen (Ansaid), diclofenac (Voltaren), naproxen (Naprosyn), diflunisal (Dolobid)
- Antianemics: ferrous sulfate (Feosol), ferrous gluconate (Fergon)
- Immunosuppressants: azathioprine (Imuran), cyclophosphamide (Cytoxan)
- Vitamins and minerals
- Surgical placement of shunt for dialysis if needed

Nursing interventions

- Avoid foods high in L-canavanine
- Assess musculoskeletal and renal status
- Monitor and record vital signs, I/O, laboratory studies, and daily weight
- Administer medications as prescribed
- Encourage the patient to express his feelings about changes in his body image and the chronicity of the disease
- Avoid exposing the patient to sunlight
- Minimize environmental stress
- Maintain seizure precautions
- Provide rest periods
- Prevent infection
- Maintain a quiet environment
- Don't use dusting powder on the patient
- Promote independence in ADLs
- Provide postchemotherapeutic nursing care
  - Provide prophylactic skin, mouth, and perineal care
  - Monitor dietary intake
  - Administer antiemetics and antidiarrheals as prescribed
  - Monitor for bleeding, infection, and electrolyte imbalance
- Individualize home care instructions
  - Provide information about the Lupus Foundation
  - Stop smoking
  - Identify ways to reduce stress
  - Recognize the signs and symptoms of renal failure
  - Avoid exposure to people with infections
  - Monitor self for infection
  - Monitor self for fatigue and joint pain

- Complete mouth care daily
- Avoid over-the-counter medications
- Avoid exposure to sunlight
- Don't use hair spray or hair coloring
- Don't take hormonal contraceptives
- Use liquid cosmetics to cover rashes
- Maintain a quiet environment

Medical complications

- Necrosis of glomerular capillaries
- Inflammation of cerebral and ocular blood vessels
- Necrosis of lymph nodes
- Vasculitis of GI tract and pleura
- Degeneration of the skin's basal layer
- Heart failure
- Seizures
- Depression
- Infection
- Peripheral neuropathy

Surgical interventions

- None

NCLEX CHECKS

It's never too soon to begin your NCLEX preparation. Now that you've reviewed this chapter, carefully read each of the following questions and choose the best answer. Then compare your responses to the correct answers.

1. The nurse notes a positive Tinel's sign in a patient. Presence of this sign might indicate:

☐ **A.** thrombophlebitis.
☐ **B.** osteoporosis.
☐ **C.** rheumatoid arthritis.
☐ **D.** carpal tunnel syndrome.

2. A patient received a hip prosthesis for a right hip fracture sustained after a fall. In the immediate postoperative period, the nurse should maintain the leg:

☐ **A.** in an abducted position.
☐ **B.** in an adducted position.
☐ **C.** in a neutral position.
☐ **D.** with the hip flexed more than 90 degrees.

3. A 78-year-old patient has a history of osteoarthritis. Which signs and symptoms would the nurse expect to find on physical assessment?

☐ **A.** Joint pain, crepitus, Heberden's nodes
☐ **B.** Hot, inflamed joints; crepitus; joint pain
☐ **C.** Tophi, enlarged joints, Bouchard's nodes
☐ **D.** Swelling, joint pain, tenderness on palpation

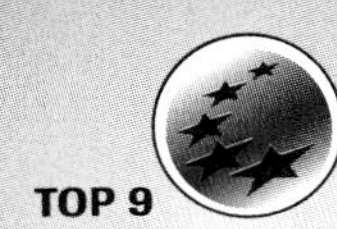

TOP 9

Items to study for your next test on the musculoskeletal system

1. Structures and functions of the musculoskeletal system
2. Nursing interventions after arthroscopy and arthrocentesis
3. Patient care after total hip replacement
4. Preoperative and postoperative care for amputation
5. Assessment findings in rheumatoid arthritis and osteoarthritis
6. What happens in osteoarthritis
7. Nursing interventions for carpal tunnel syndrome
8. Types of fractures
9. Nursing care for a patient in skin or skeletal traction

4. When teaching an elderly female patient who has osteoporosis, the nurse should include information about which major complication?

☐ **A.** Loss of estrogen
☐ **B.** Bone fracture
☐ **C.** Negative calcium balance
☐ **D.** Dowager's hump

5. A patient with a sports injury undergoes a diagnostic arthroscopy of his left knee. After the procedure, the nurse assesses the patient's leg. What are the priority nursing assessment factors?

☐ **A.** Wound and skin
☐ **B.** Mobility and sensation
☐ **C.** Vascular and integumentary
☐ **D.** Circulatory and neurologic

6. A patient develops L5-S1 herniated nucleus pulposus, which impinges on the left nerve root. Most likely, the patient would experience pain that radiates:

☐ **A.** up the spinal column.
☐ **B.** to the lower abdomen.
☐ **C.** down the left leg.
☐ **D.** across to the right pelvis.

7. A patient is undergoing rehabilitation following a fracture. As part of his regimen, the patient performs isometric exercises. Which of the following provides the best evidence that the patient understands the proper technique?

☐ **A.** Exercising bilateral extremities simultaneously
☐ **B.** Periodic monitoring of his heart rate
☐ **C.** Forced resistance against stable objects
☐ **D.** Swinging of limbs through full ROM

8. A patient in balanced suspension traction for a fractured femur needs to be repositioned toward the head of the bed. During repositioning, the nurse should:

☐ **A.** place slight additional tension on the traction cords.
☐ **B.** release the weights and replace immediately after positioning.
☐ **C.** lift the traction and the patient during repositioning.
☐ **D.** maintain the same degree of traction tension.

9. While assessing a patient with osteoarthritis, you palpate a grating sensation as the patient bends her fingers. This assessment finding is called:

______________.

ANSWERS AND RATIONALES

1. CORRECT ANSWER: D
You may observe a positive Tinel's sign — tingling over the median nerve on light percussion — in a patient with carpal tunnel syndrome. A positive Tinel's sign isn't associated with thrombophlebitis, osteoporosis, or rheumatoid arthritis.

2. Correct answer: A

After receiving a hip prosthesis, the patient should keep the affected leg abducted. Adduction may dislocate the hip. Keep the hip in a neutral position if an internal fixation device was used. The hip must not be flexed more than 90 degrees for the first 2 months and even less than that for the first 10 days.

3. Correct answer: A

Signs and symptoms of osteoarthritis include joint pain, crepitus, Heberden's nodes, Bouchard's nodes, and enlarged joints. Hot, inflamed joints rarely occur with osteoarthritis. Tophi are deposits of sodium urate crystals that occur with chronic gout, not osteoarthritis. Swelling, joint pain, and tenderness on palpation occur with a sprain injury.

4. Correct answer: B

Bone fracture is a major complication of osteoporosis that results when loss of calcium and phosphate increases the fragility of bones. Estrogen deficiencies result from menopause, not osteoporosis. Calcium and vitamin D supplements may be used to support bone metabolism, but a negative calcium balance isn't a complication of osteoporosis. Dowager's hump results from bone fractures; it develops when repeated vertebral fractures increase spinal curvature.

5. Correct answer: D

Following a procedure on an extremity, focus assessments on neurovascular status of the extremity. Swelling of the extremity can impair both neurologic and circulatory function of the leg. After establishing the neurovascular stability of the extremity, the nurse can address the other concerns of skin, mobility, and pain.

6. Correct answer: C

The pain associated with herniated nucleus pulposus of L5-S1 primarily affects the lower back with radiation down the leg. Pain that radiates up the spinal column, to the lower abdomen, or across to the right pelvis isn't associated with a lumbar herniation.

7. Correct answer: C

Isometric exercises involve applying pressure against a stable object, such as pressing the hands together or pushing an arm against a wall. Exercising extremities simultaneously isn't characteristic of isometrics. Heart rate monitoring is associated with aerobic exercising. Limb swinging isn't isometric.

8. Correct answer: D

Traction is used to reduce the fracture and must be maintained at all times, including during repositioning. It isn't appropriate to increase traction tension or release or lift the traction during repositioning.

9. Correct answer: Crepitation

Crepitation is the grating sensation that can be felt or heard that's associated with degenerative joint diseases such as osteoarthritis.

9

Integumentary system

LEARNING OBJECTIVES

After studying this chapter, you should be able to:

- Describe the psychosocial impact of integumentary disorders.
- Differentiate between modifiable and nonmodifiable risk factors in the development of an integumentary disorder.
- List three probable and three possible nursing diagnoses for a patient with an integumentary disorder.
- Identify nursing interventions for a patient with an integumentary disorder.
- Identify three teaching topics for a patient with an integumentary disorder.

CHAPTER OVERVIEW

Caring for the patient with an integumentary disorder requires a sound understanding of integumentary anatomy and physiology as well as the management of modifiable risk factors. A thorough assessment is essential to planning and implementing appropriate patient care. The assessment includes a complete history, physical examination, diagnostic testing, identification of modifiable and nonmodifiable risk factors, and information related to the psychosocial impact of the disorder on the patient.

Nursing diagnoses focus primarily on impaired skin integrity and body image disturbance. Nursing interventions are designed to support healing of the skin, prevent further injury to the affected area, and help the patient adjust to the

What's in your skin

This cross section of the skin illustrates major skin structures.

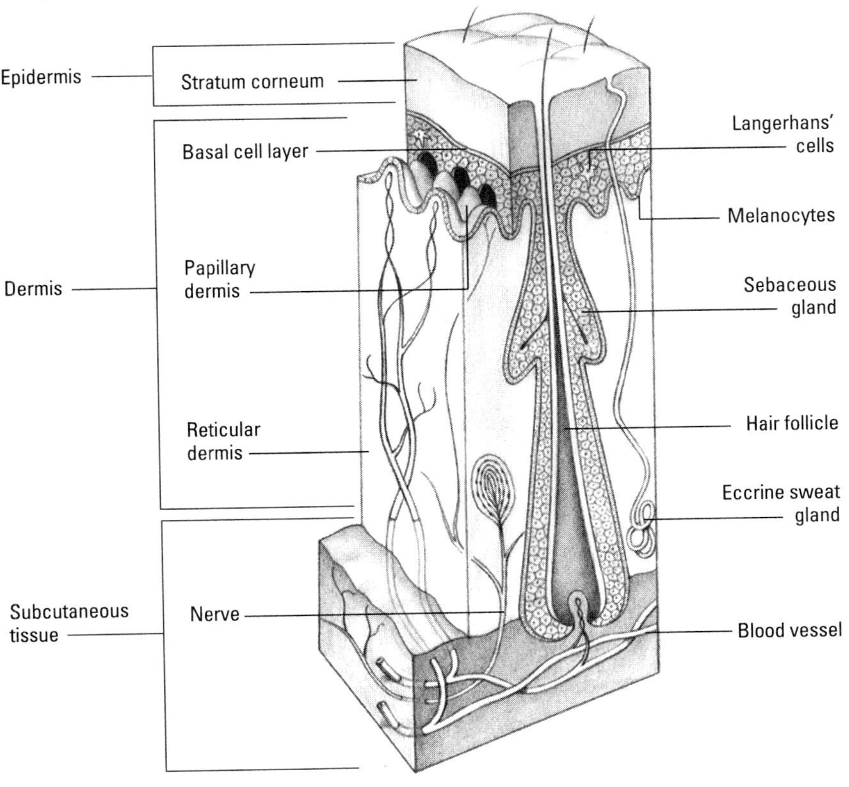

change in his body image. Patient teaching—a crucial nursing activity—involves providing information about medical follow-up, medication regimens, signs and symptoms of possible complications, and reducing modifiable risk factors by preventing skin damage and infection.

ANATOMY AND PHYSIOLOGY REVIEW

Skin

- First line of defense against microorganisms
- Composed of three layers (see *What's in your skin*)
  - Epidermis
    - Outer avascular layer composed of dense squamous cells that shed constantly
    - Keratinocytes and melanocytes are found in this layer
  - Dermis
    - Origin of hair, nails, sebaceous glands, eccrine sweat glands, and apocrine sweat glands

Parts of the skin

- Stratum corneum
- Basal cell layer
- Langerhans' cells
- Melanocytes
- Papillary dermis
- Sebaceous gland
- Hair follicle
- Reticular dermis
- Eccrine sweat gland
- Nerve
- Blood vessel

3 layers of skin

- Epidermis: outer layer; composed of dense squamous cells
- Dermis: origin of hair, nails, sebaceous glands, eccrine sweat glands, and apocrine sweat glands
- Subcutaneous tissue: third layer of skin; provides heat, insulation, shock absorption, and a reserve of calories

- Collagen layer that supports the epidermis and contains nerves and blood vessels
- Subcutaneous tissue (hypodermis)
  - Third layer of skin is composed of loose connective tissue filled with fatty cells
  - Provides heat, insulation, shock absorption, and a reserve of calories

Functions of the hair and nails

- Hair: protects and covers the body
- Nails: protect the tips of the fingers and toes

Hair
- Protects and covers the body, except for the palms, lips, soles of the feet, nipples, and external genitalia
- Hormones stimulate differential growth

Nails
- Composed of dead cells filled with keratin
- Protect the tips of the fingers and toes

Glandular appendages
- Three types: sebaceous, eccrine, and apocrine
- Sebaceous glands (oil), which lubricate hair and epidermis, are stimulated by sex hormones
- Eccrine sweat glands regulate body temperature through water secretion
- Apocrine sweat glands are located in the axilla, nipple, anal, and pubic areas and secrete odorless fluid; decomposition of this fluid by bacteria causes odor

Functions of the glandular appendages

- Sebaceous glands lubricate hair and epidermis
- Eccrine sweat glands regulate body temperature
- Apocrine sweat glands secrete odorless fluid

ASSESSMENT FINDINGS

History
- Change in skin color, texture, and temperature
- Perspiration or dryness
- Itching
- Brittle, thick, or soft nails
- Fever
- Hair loss
- Rash

Key assessment findings in a disorder of the integumentary system

- Change in skin color, texture, and temperature
- Perspiration or dryness
- Itching

Physical examination
- Pattern of pigmentation and hair distribution
- Skin texture, turgor, color, and temperature (see *Evaluating skin turgor*)
- Peripheral edema
- Trophic changes: skin, hair, and nails
- Skin lesions: type, shape, and character
- Pruritus
- Nevi and scars
- Elevated body temperature
- Erythema
- Petechiae and ecchymosis

Evaluating skin turgor

To assess skin turgor in an adult, gently squeeze the skin on the forearm or sternal area between your thumb and forefinger, as shown. In an infant, roll a fold of loosely adherent abdominal skin between your thumb and forefinger, then release the skin.

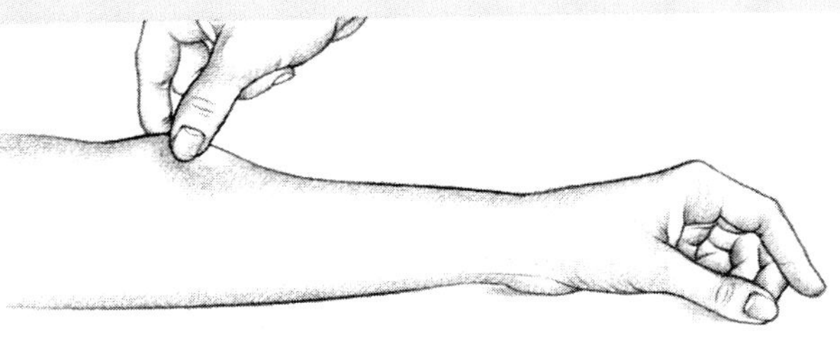

If the skin quickly returns to its original shape, the patient has normal turgor. If the skin doesn't return to its original shape within 30 seconds or if it maintains a tented position as shown, it has poor turgor.

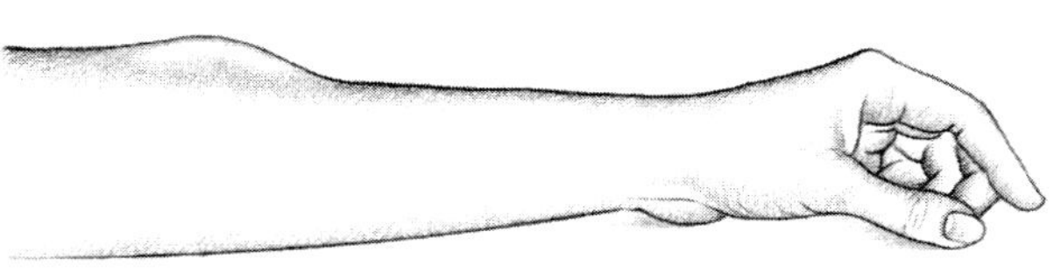

Assessing skin turgor

- Squeeze the skin on the forearm or sternal area.
- If the skin returns to normal shape, the skin has normal turgor.
- If the skin doesn't return to original shape in 30 seconds or if it maintains a tented position, it has poor turgor.

DIAGNOSTIC TESTS AND PROCEDURES

Blood chemistry

- Definition and purpose
  - Laboratory test of a blood sample
  - Analysis for potassium, sodium, calcium, phosphorus, ketones, glucose, osmolality, chloride, blood urea nitrogen (BUN), and creatinine
- Nursing interventions
  - Withhold food and fluids before the procedure as directed
  - Check the site for bleeding after the procedure

Blood chemistry

- Blood test
- Analysis for potassium, sodium, calcium, phosphorus and other factors
- Intervention: check the site for bleeding after the procedure

Hematologic studies

- Definition and purpose
  - Laboratory test of a blood sample
  - Analysis for red blood cell (RBC) count, white blood cell (WBC) count, erythrocyte sedimentation rate, platelets, prothrombin time, partial thromboplastin time, hemoglobin (Hb), and hematocrit (HCT)
- Nursing intervention: check the site for bleeding

Hematologic studies

- Blood test
- Analysis for RBCs, WBCs, platelets, Hb, and other factors
- Intervention: check the site for bleeding

Skin biopsy (punch biopsy)

- Definition and purpose
  - Procedure using a circular punch instrument to remove a small amount of skin tissue
  - Histologic evaluation
- Nursing intervention: check the site for bleeding and infection

Skin testing

- Definition and purpose
  - Procedure using a patch, scratch, or intradermal technique
  - Administration of an allergen to the skin's surface or into the dermis
- Nursing interventions
  - Keep the area dry
  - Record the site, date, and time of test
  - Inspect the site for erythema, papules, vesicles, edema, and induration
  - Record the date and time for follow-up site reading

Skin scrapings

- Definition and purpose
  - Procedure calling for cells scraped by a scalpel and covered with potassium hydroxide
  - Microscopic examination of scales, nails, and hair
- Nursing intervention: check the scraping site for bleeding and infection

Skin studies

- Definition and purpose
  - Laboratory test
  - Microscopic examination of skin, including Gram stain, culture and sensitivity, cytology, and immunofluorescence
- Nursing interventions
  - Follow laboratory procedure guidelines
  - Note current antibiotic therapy

Wood's light

- Definition and purpose
  - Procedure using ultraviolet (UV) light
  - Direct examination of skin
- Nursing interventions
  - Explain the procedure
  - Allay the patient's anxiety

Skin biopsy

- Procedure to remove a small amount of skin
- Histologic evaluation
- Intervention: check the site for bleeding and infection

Skin testing

- Procedure using a patch, scratch, or intradermal technique
- Administers allergens to the skin
- Intervention: keep the area dry

Skin scraping

- Procedure in which cells are scraped and covered with potassium hydroxide
- Examines scales, nails, and hair
- Intervention: check the site for bleeding and infection

Skin studies

- Test in which the skin is microscopically examined
- Intervention: note current antibiotic therapy

Wood's light

- Procedure using a UV light
- Examines the skin
- Intervention: explain the procedure to the patient

PSYCHOSOCIAL IMPACT OF INTEGUMENTARY DISORDERS

Developmental impact

- Changes in body image
- Fear of rejection
- Changes in role performance
- Decreased self-esteem

Economic impact
- Cost of cosmetics
- Disruption or loss of employment
- Cost of hospitalizations and follow-up care
- Cost of medications

Occupational and recreational impact
- Restrictions in physical activity
- Changes in leisure activity

Social impact
- Social isolation
- Sexual dysfunction

Possible psychosocial impact of integumentary disorders
- Changes in body image
- Costs of cosmetics, hospitalizations, and medications
- Restrictions in activities

RISK FACTORS

Modifiable risk factors
- Infection
- Occupation
- Exposure to chemical and environmental pollutants
- Exposure to radiation
- Exposure to the sun
- Personal hygiene habits
- Climate
- Use of cosmetics and soaps
- Stress
- Nutritional deficiencies
- Medications
- Crowded living conditions
- Skin moles

Nonmodifiable risk factors
- Aging
- History of endocrine, vascular, or immune disorders
- Family history of skin disease or allergies
- History of allergies
- Exposure to communicable disease
- Pregnancy
- Menopause

Key modifiable risk factors for integumentary disorders
- Infection
- Occupation
- Exposure to pollutants and radiation
- Exposure to the sun

Key nonmodifiable risk factors for integumentary disorders
- Aging
- History of endocrine, vascular, or immune disorders
- Family history of skin disease or allergies

NURSING DIAGNOSES

Probable nursing diagnoses
- Impaired skin integrity
- Disturbed body image
- Situational low self-esteem
- Acute pain
- Disturbed sensory perception: tactile

Probable nursing diagnoses for a patient with an integumentary disorder
- Impaired skin integrity
- Disturbed body image
- Disturbed sensory perception: tactile

Possible nursing diagnoses

- Ineffective breathing pattern
- Ineffective coping
- Risk for deficient fluid volume
- Risk for infection
- Anxiety
- Social isolation

SKIN GRAFT

Characteristics of a skin graft

- Replacement of damaged skin with healthy skin to protect underlying structures or reconstruct areas
- Three types: split-thickness graft, full-thickness graft, and pinch graft

Description

- Replacement of damaged skin with healthy skin to protect underlying structures or to reconstruct areas for cosmetic or functional purposes
- Split-thickness graft: graft of half of the epidermis, which is removed by a dermatome
- Full-thickness graft: graft of the entire epidermis
- Pinch graft: graft of a small piece of skin, obtained by elevating the skin with a needle and removing it with scissors

Key nursing interventions before a skin graft

- Demonstrate postoperative turning, coughing, deep breathing, splinting, and ROM exercises.
- Complete a preoperative checklist.
- Prepare the donor and graft sites.

Preoperative nursing interventions

- Complete patient and family preoperative teaching
  - Determine the patient's understanding of the procedure
  - Describe the operating room, postanesthesia care unit, and preoperative and postoperative routines
  - Demonstrate postoperative turning, coughing, deep breathing, splinting, and range-of-motion (ROM) exercises
  - Explain the postoperative need for drainage tubes, surgical dressings, oxygen therapy, I.V. therapy, and pain control
- Complete a preoperative checklist
- Administer preoperative medications as prescribed
- Allay the patient's and family's anxiety about surgery
- Document the patient's history and physical assessment data
- Prepare the donor and graft sites

Key nursing interventions after a skin graft

- Avoid weight bearing on the extremity with the graft site.
- Elevate and immobilize the graft site.
- Administer antibiotics as prescribed.
- Assess the graft site for infection, hematoma, and fluid accumulation under the graft.
- Keep the donor site dry and open to air.

Postoperative nursing interventions

- Assess pain and administer analgesics as prescribed
- Assess for return of peristalsis; provide solid foods and liquids as tolerated
- Administer I.V. fluids
- Allay the patient's anxiety
- Provide hydrotherapy as directed
- Reinforce turning, coughing, and deep breathing
- Provide incentive spirometry
- Maintain activity as tolerated; active and passive ROM and isometric exercises
- Avoid weight bearing on the extremity with the graft site
- Monitor and record vital signs, intake and output (I/O), and neurovascular checks distal to the recipient site
- Elevate and immobilize the graft site

- Encourage the patient to express his feelings about changes in his body image
- Administer antibiotics as prescribed
- Assess the graft site for infection, hematoma, and fluid accumulation under the graft; keep the graft and donor sites free from pressure
- Keep the donor site dry and open to air
- Prevent scratching
- Apply a heat lamp to the donor site
- Apply sterile saline or antibiotic solution to the graft site, as ordered
- Change graft site dressing, as ordered
- Individualize home care instructions
  - Continue physical therapy
  - Apply lubricating lotion to the graft site
  - Protect the graft site from direct sunlight
  - Demonstrate cosmetic camouflage techniques

Possible surgical complications

- Infection of the graft and donor sites
- Graft rejection or failure
- Hematoma under the graft
- Fluid accumulation under the graft

Common complications for a skin graft

- Infection of the graft and donor sites
- Graft rejection or failure

CONTACT DERMATITIS

Definition

- Inflammatory response of the skin after contact with a specific antigen

Causes

- Mechanical, biological, and chemical irritants
- Cosmetics and hair dyes
- Detergents, cleaning agents, and soaps
- Insecticides
- Poison ivy
- Wool

Pathophysiology

- Contact with an antigen triggers a localized inflammatory response
- Inflammatory response produces skin changes

Assessment findings

- Pruritus and burning
- Erythema at point of contact
- Localized edema
- Vesicles and papules
- Lichenification
- Pigmentation changes
- Eczema
- Scaling

Contact dermatitis defined

- Inflammatory response of the skin
- Occurs after contact with a specific antigen
- Produces skin change

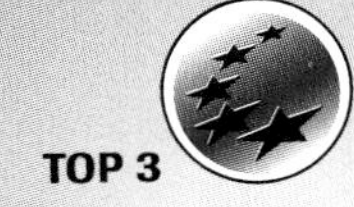

TOP 3

Signs and symptoms of contact dermatitis

1. Pruritus and burning
2. Erythema at point of contact
3. Vesicles and papules

Key diagnostic test finding for contact dermatitis

- Skin test: positive

Key treatments for contact dermatitis

- Cool, wet dressings with aluminum acetate solution, tepid baths, and bed cradle
- Antipruritics or antihistamines
- Corticosteroids

Key nursing interventions for a patient with contact dermatitis

- Provide tepid baths, bed cradle, and cool, wet dressings.
- Prevent scratching and rubbing of affected areas.
- Maintain a cool environment.

Psoriasis defined

- Chronic, noninfectious skin inflammation that occurs in patches
- Papules coalesce to form plaques

Diagnostic test findings

- Skin test (patch): positive to specific antigen
- Visual examination: area of dermatitis correlates with area of antigen contact

Medical management

- Position: elevation of extremity
- Activity: as tolerated
- Monitoring: vital signs and neurovascular checks
- Treatments: cool, wet dressings with aluminum acetate solution (Burow's solution), tepid baths, and bed cradle
- Antibiotic: ampicillin (Omnipen)
- Antipruritic/antihistamine: diphenhydramine (Benadryl)
- Corticosteroid: hydrocortisone (Cort-Dome)
- Antianxiety agents: diazepam (Valium), oxazepam (Serax)

Nursing interventions

- Assess and record neurovascular status
- Maintain elevation of affected extremity
- Monitor and record vital signs
- Administer medications as prescribed
- Encourage the patient to express his feelings about changes in his physical appearance
- Provide tepid baths, bed cradle, and cool, wet dressings
- Avoid soaps
- Avoid using heating pads or blankets
- Avoid temperature extremes
- Prevent scratching and rubbing of affected area; increases risk of further irritation, inflammation, and possible infection
- Maintain a cool environment
- Provide diversional activities
- Individualize home care instructions: avoid causative agent (for teaching tips, see *Patients with integumentary disorders*)

Medical complications

- Infection

Surgical interventions

- None

PSORIASIS

Definition

- Chronic, noninfectious skin inflammation that occurs in patches

Causes

- Stress
- Epidermal trauma
- Streptococcal infection
- Changes in climate

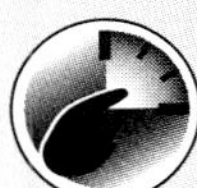

TIME-OUT FOR TEACHING

Patients with integumentary disorders

Be sure to include the following topic areas in your teaching plan when caring for patients with integumentary disorders.

- Follow-up appointments
- Smoking cessation
- Optimal body weight maintenance
- Medication therapy, including the action, adverse effects, and scheduling
- Prevention of skin damage and irritation, including:
  - extreme temperatures
  - skin dryness
  - cool environment
  - sunlight and wind
  - scratching and rubbing
  - trauma
  - detergents and soaps
- Dressing changes as directed
- Infection control measures
- Avoidance of over-the-counter skin medications
- Daily skin care
- Signs and symptoms of skin infection
- Community agencies and resources for supportive services
- Fluid intake

- Genetics
- Anxiety
- Alcoholism
- Rheumatoid arthritis
- Drug induced: lithium, propranolol
- Hormones
- Obesity

Pathophysiology

- Loss of normal regulatory mechanisms of cell division leads to rapid multiplication of epidermal cells that interferes with formation of normal protective layer of skin
- Papules coalesce to form plaques

Assessment findings

- Pruritus
- Shedding, scaling plaques
- Yellow discoloration and thickening of nails
- Erythema
- Papules on sacrum, nails, palms
- Plaques, on visual examination

Diagnostic test finding

- Skin biopsy: positive
- Serum uric acid level: increased

Medical management

- Monitoring: vital signs and neurovascular checks
- Treatments: bed cradle, daily soaks, and tepid, wet compresses
- Corticosteroids: triamcinolone (Kenalog) covered with occlusive dressing, betamethasone (Valisone)

Key teaching topics for a patient with an integumentary disorder

- Medication therapy
- Prevention of skin damage and irritation
- Dressing changes
- Infection control measures

Key symptoms of psoriasis

- Pruritus
- Shedding, scaling plaques
- Papules on sacrum, nails, palms

Diagnostic test findings for psoriasis

- Skin biopsy: positive
- Serum uric acid level: increased

Medications available to treat psoriasis

- Corticosteroids
- Antipsoriatics
- Antimetabolites
- Photochemotherapy
- Keratolytics
- Antimicrobials

- Antipsoriatics: anthralin (Anthra-Derm), coal tar (Estar), followed by exposure to UV light, etretinate (Tegison)
- Antimetabolite: methotrexate (Amethopterin)
- Photochemotherapy (PUVA therapy): methoxsalen (Oxsoralen) followed by exposure to black light
- Keratolytics: benzoyl peroxide (Benzagel), salicylic acid (Keratex gel, Sal-Acid)
- Antimicrobial: sulfasalazine (Azulfidine)
- Diet: high-protein, high-calorie, frequent feedings

Key nursing interventions for a patient with psoriasis

- Encourage the patient to express his feelings about changes in his body image.
- Administer UV light and PUVA therapy.
- Prevent scratching.
- Provide information about the National Psoriasis Foundation.

Nursing interventions

- Assess and record neurovascular status
- Monitor and record vital signs
- Administer medications as prescribed
- Encourage the patient to express his feelings about changes in his body image
- Administer UV light and PUVA therapy
- Apply occlusive dressings
- Prevent scratching
- Help the patient to remove scales during soaks
- Provide information about the National Psoriasis Foundation
- Maintain the patient's diet
- Individualize home care instructions
  - Identify ways to reduce stress
  - Wear light cotton clothing over affected areas

Medical complications

- Depression
- Infection
- Rheumatoid arthritis

Surgical interventions

- None

HERPES ZOSTER (SHINGLES)

Facts about herpes zoster

- Acute viral infection of nerve structure
- Caused by varicella zoster
- Affects spinal and cranial sensory ganglia and posterior gray matter of the spinal cord

Definition

- Acute viral infection of nerve structure caused by varicella zoster

Causes

- Cytotoxic drug-induced immunosuppression
- Hodgkin's lymphoma
- Exposure to varicella zoster
- Debilitating disease

Pathophysiology

- Activation of dormant varicella zoster virus causes an inflammatory reaction
- Affected areas include spinal and cranial sensory ganglia and posterior gray matter of the spinal cord

Assessment findings

- Neuralgia
- Malaise
- Pruritus
- Burning
- Unilaterally clustered skin vesicles along peripheral sensory nerves on trunk, thorax, or face
- Erythema
- Fever
- Anorexia
- Headache
- Paresthesia
- Edematous skin

Diagnostic test findings

- Antinuclear antibody: positive
- Skin cultures and stains: identification of organism

Medical management

- Activity: as tolerated
- Monitoring: vital signs, seventh cranial nerve function, and neurovascular checks
- Treatments: air mattress, acetic acid compresses, tepid baths, and bed cradle
- Analgesics: acetaminophen (Tylenol), oxycodone (Tylox)
- Antianxiety agents: diazepam (Valium), hydroxyzine (Vistaril)
- Antipruritic: diphenhydramine (Benadryl)
- Corticosteroids: hydrocortisone (Cortef), triamcinolone (Kenalog)
- Nerve block using lidocaine (Xylocaine)
- Antiviral agents: acyclovir (Zovirax), vidarabine (Vira-A), interferon (Roferon-A)
- Laboratory studies: culture and sensitivity

Nursing interventions

- Assess pain
- Monitor and record vital signs, laboratory results, and neurologic status
- Administer medications as directed
- Encourage the patient to express his feelings about changes in his physical appearance and the recurrent nature of the illness
- Provide acetic acid compresses, tepid baths, bed cradle, and air mattress
- Prevent scratching and rubbing of affected areas
- Allay the patient's anxiety
- Individualize home care instructions
  - Recognize the signs and symptoms of hearing loss
  - Avoid wool and synthetic clothing
  - Wear lightweight, loose cotton clothing
  - Keep blisters intact

Medical complications

- Infection

Key symptoms of herpes zoster

- Neuralgia
- Unilaterally clustered skin vesicles along peripheral sensory nerves on trunk, thorax, or face

Diagnostic test findings

- Antinuclear antibody: positive
- Skin culture: positive

Key medications available to treat herpes zoster

- Analgesics
- Antianxiety agents
- Antipruritic
- Corticosteroids
- Nerve blocking agents
- Antiviral agents

Key nursing interventions for a patient with herpes zoster

- Encourage the patient to express his feelings about changes in his physical appearance and the recurrent nature of the illness.
- Provide acetic acid compresses, tepid baths, bed cradle, and air mattress.
- Prevent scratching and rubbing of affected areas.

Characteristics of burns

- Destruction of epidermis, dermis, and subcutaneous layers of skin
- Amount of cell destruction is related to the extent and degree of burn
- Three types: first-degree, second-degree, and third-degree

First-degree burn assessment findings

- Erythema
- Edema
- Pain
- Blanching

Second-degree burn assessment findings

- Pain
- Oozing, fluid-filled vesicles
- Erythema
- Shiny, wet subcutaneous layer after vesicles rupture

Third-degree burn assessment findings

- Eschar
- Edema
- Little or no pain

- Posttherapeutic neuralgia
- Ophthalmic herpes zoster
- Facial paralysis
- Vertigo
- Tinnitus
- Hearing loss
- Visceral dissemination

Surgical interventions

- None

BURNS

Definition

- Destruction of epidermis, dermis, and subcutaneous layers of skin

Causes

- Radiation: X-ray, sun, nuclear reactors
- Mechanical: friction
- Chemical: acids, alkalies, vesicants
- Electrical: lightning, electrical wires
- Thermal: flame, frostbite, scald

Pathophysiology

- Cell destruction causes loss of intracellular fluid and electrolytes
- Amount of cell destruction is directly related to the extent (area) and degree (depth) of burn
- First-degree (superficial partial thickness) involves epidermal layer (see *Burn classification*)
- Second-degree (dermal partial thickness) involves epidermal and dermal layers
- Third-degree (full thickness) involves epidermal, dermal, subcutaneous layers, and nerve endings

Assessment findings

- **Visual examination: extent of burn determined by Rule of Nines, Lund and Browder chart**
- First-degree
  - Erythema
  - Edema
  - Pain
  - Blanching
- Second-degree
  - Pain
  - Oozing, fluid-filled vesicles
  - Erythema
  - Shiny, wet subcutaneous layer after vesicles rupture
- Third-degree
  - Eschar

Burn classification

CHARACTERISTIC	FIRST-DEGREE BURN	SECOND-DEGREE BURN	THIRD-DEGREE BURN
Thickness	Superficial, partial-thickness	Deep, partial-thickness	Full-thickness
Appearance	Dry with no blisters	Weeping, edematous blisters	Dry, leathery, and possibly edematous
Color	Pink	White to pink or red	White to charred
Comfort	Painful	Very painful	Little or no pain
Depth	Epidermis only	Epidermis, dermis, and possibly some subcutaneous tissue	Subcutaneous tissue and possibly fascia, muscle, and bone

- Edema
- Little or no pain

Diagnostic test findings

- Blood chemistry: increased potassium; decreased sodium, albumin, complement fixation, immunoglobulins
- Arterial blood gas (ABG) analysis: metabolic acidosis
- 24-hour urine collection: decreased creatinine clearance, negative nitrogen balance
- Hematology: increased Hb, HCT; decreased fibrinogen, platelets, WBCs
- Urine chemistry: hematuria, myoglobinuria

Medical management

- Withhold oral food and fluids until allowed by the physician
- Diet: high in protein, fat, calories, carbohydrates; small, frequent feedings
- I.V. therapy: hydration and electrolyte replacement using Evan, Brooke, Parkland, or Massachusetts General Hospital protocols; saline lock
- Oxygen therapy
- Intubation and mechanical ventilation
- GI decompression: nasogastric (NG) tube, Miller-Abbott tube
- Position: semi-Fowler's
- Activity: bed rest
- Monitoring: vital signs, electrocardiogram, hemodynamic variables, I/O, neurovital signs, neurovascular checks, and stool for occult blood
- Laboratory studies: potassium, sodium, glucose, osmolality, creatinine, BUN, Hb, HCT, platelets, WBCs, ABG levels, culture and sensitivity
- Nutritional support: total parental nutrition (TPN), NG feedings
- Treatments: indwelling urinary catheter, postural drainage, chest physiotherapy, incentive spirometry, bed cradle, intermittent positive pressure breathing, suction, Jobst clothing, and Hubbard tank bath

Depth and burn classification

- First-degree: epidermis only
- Second-degree: epidermis, dermis, and possibly some subcutaneous tissue
- Third-degree: subcutaneous tissue and possibly fascia, muscle, and bone

Key diagnostic test findings in burns

- Blood chemistry: increased potassium; decreased sodium and albumin
- 24-hour urine collection: decreased creatinine clearance
- Urine chemistry: hematuria, myoglobinuria

Key ways to treat burns

- I.V. therapy: hydration and electrolyte replacement
- Oxygen therapy
- Intubation and mechanical ventilation
- GI decompression

Most common medications used to treat burns

- Antibiotics
- Anti-infectives
- Antitetanus
- Analgesics
- Colloids
- Mucosal barrier fortifiers

Key nursing interventions for a patient with burns

- Administer I.V. fluids to prevent hypovolemia.
- Administer oxygen.
- Assess respiratory status and fluid balance.
- Assess pain and administer analgesics, as indicated.
- Administer TPN.
- Maintain protective and standard precautions.

- Precaution: protective; standard
- Transfusion therapy: fresh frozen plasma, platelets, packed RBCs, plasma
- Antibiotic: gentamicin sulfate (Garamycin)
- Anti-infectives: mafenide (Sulfamylon), silver sulfadiazine (Silvadene), silver nitrate, povidone-iodine (Betadine)
- Antianxiety: diazepam (Valium)
- Antitetanus: tetanus toxoid
- Analgesic: morphine (Roxanol)
- Antacids: magnesium and aluminum hydroxide (Maalox), aluminum hydroxide gel (AlternaGEL)
- Histamine antagonists: cimetidine (Tagamet), ranitidine (Zantac)
- Vitamins: phytonadione (AquaMEPHYTON), cyanocobalamin (vitamin B_{12})
- Colloid: 5% albumin (Albuminar-5)
- Diuretic: mannitol (Osmitrol)
- Sedative: oxazepam (Serax)
- Cardiac glycoside: digoxin (Lanoxin)
- Escharotomy
- Biological dressings
- Early excisional therapy
- Specialized bed: air fluidized (Clinitron, Skytron, Fluid Air)
- Pulse oximetry
- Mucosal barrier fortifier: sucralfate (Carafate)

Nursing interventions

- Maintain the patient's diet; withhold food and fluids, as ordered
- Administer I.V. fluids to prevent hypovolemia
- Administer oxygen
- Provide suction; turning, coughing, and deep breathing; intermittent positive pressure breathing; chest physiotherapy; and postural drainage
- Assess respiratory status and fluid balance
- Assess pain and administer analgesics, as indicated
- Maintain position, patency, and low suction of NG tube
- Keep the patient in semi-Fowler's position
- Monitor and record vital signs, I/O, laboratory studies, hemodynamic variables, neurovital signs, stool for occult blood, specific gravity, calorie count, daily weight, neurovascular checks, and pulse oximetry
- Provide tracheostomy care or endotracheal care
- Administer TPN
- Administer medications as prescribed
- **Encourage the patient to express his feelings about disfigurement, immobility from scarring, and a fear of dying**
- Allay the patient's anxiety
- Provide treatments: ROM exercises, tanking, bed cradle, splints, and Jobst clothing
- Elevate affected extremities
- Maintain a warm environment during acute period
- Maintain protective and standard precautions
- Provide skin and mouth care

- Assess bowel sounds
- Individualize home care instructions
  - Follow dietary recommendations and restrictions
  - Avoid wearing restrictive clothing
  - Lubricate healing skin with cocoa butter
  - Use splints and Jobst clothing
  - Seek help from community agencies and resources

Medical complications

- Paralytic ileus
- Curling's ulcer
- Acute renal failure
- Pneumonia
- Heart failure
- Septicemia
- Pulmonary edema
- Hypovolemic shock

Surgical intervention

- Skin grafting

SKIN CANCER

Definition

- Malignant primary tumor of the epidermal layer of the skin
- Three types of skin cancer
  - Basal cell epithelioma
  - Melanoma
  - Squamous cell carcinoma

Causes

- Heredity
- Chemical irritants
- Ultraviolet rays
- Radiation
- Friction or chronic irritation
- Immunosuppressive drugs
- Precancerous lesions: leukoplakia, nevi, senile keratoses
- Infrared heat or light

Pathophysiology

- Unregulated cell growth and uncontrolled cell division result in the development of a neoplasm
- Basal cell epithelioma: basal cell keratinization causes tumor growth in basal layer of the epidermis
- Melanoma: tumor arises from melanocytes of the epidermis
- Squamous cell carcinoma: tumor arises from keratinocytes

Assessment findings

- Basal cell epithelioma: waxy nodule with telangiectasis

Key home care instructions for a patient with burns

- Avoid wearing restrictive clothing.
- Lubricate healing skin with cocoa butter.
- Use splints and Jobst clothing.

Facts about skin cancer

- Malignant primary tumor of the epidermal layer of the skin
- Three types: basal cell epithelioma, melanoma, and squamous cell carcinoma

Skin cancer pathophysiology

- Unregulated cell growth and uncontrolled cell division cause a neoplasm
- Tumor growth occurs
- Tumor arises from melanocytes or keratinocytes

Key signs and symptoms of skin cancer

- Basal cell epithelioma: waxy nodule with telangiectasis
- Melanoma: irregular, circular bordered lesion with hues of tan, black, or blue
- Squamous cell carcinoma: small, red, nodular lesion that begins as an erythematous macule or plaque with indistinct margins
- Change in color, size, or shape of preexisting lesion

Diagnostic test finding

- Skin biopsy: positive for cancer cells

Key treatment options for skin cancer

- Cryosurgery with liquid nitrogen
- Chemosurgery with zinc chloride
- Curettage and electrodesiccation
- Antimetabolites

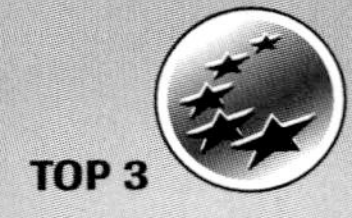
TOP 3

Home care instructions for a patient with skin cancer

1. Avoid contact with chemical irritants.
2. Use sun-screen lotions and wear layered clothing when outdoors.
3. Monitor for lesions and moles that don't heal or that change characteristics.

- Melanoma: irregular, circular bordered lesion with hues of tan, black, or blue
- Squamous cell carcinoma: small, red, nodular lesion that begins as an erythematous macule or plaque with indistinct margins
- Pruritus
- Local soreness
- Change in color, size, or shape of preexisting lesion
- Oozing, bleeding, crusting lesion

Diagnostic test findings

- Skin biopsy: cytology positive for cancer cells

Medical management

- I.V. therapy: saline lock
- Monitoring: vital signs, graft viability (with dressing changes)
- Radiation therapy
- Cryosurgery with liquid nitrogen
- Chemosurgery with zinc chloride
- Curettage and electrodesiccation
- Immunotherapy for melanoma: bacille Calmette-Guérin (BCG) vaccine
- Alkylating agents: carmustine (BiCNU), dacarbazine (DTIC-Dome)
- Antineoplastics: hydroxyurea (Hydrea), vincristine (Oncovin)
- Antimetabolite: fluorouracil (Adrucil)
- Antiemetics: prochlorperazine (Compazine), ondansetron (Zofran)

Nursing interventions

- Monitor and record vital signs
- Administer medications as prescribed
- Encourage the patient to express his feelings about changes in his body image and a fear of dying
- Provide postchemotherapeutic and postradiation nursing care
  - Provide prophylactic skin, mouth, and perineal care
  - Monitor dietary intake
  - Administer antiemetics and antidiarrheals as prescribed
  - Monitor for bleeding, infection, and electrolyte imbalance
  - Provide rest periods
- Assess lesions
- Individualize home care instructions
  - Avoid contact with chemical irritants
  - Use sun-screen lotions and wear layered clothing when outdoors
  - Monitor self for lesions and moles that don't heal or that change characteristics
  - Have moles that are subject to chronic irritation removed
  - Provide information about the Skin Cancer Foundation
  - Seek help from community agencies and resources

Medical complication

- Metastasis (melanoma)

Surgical interventions
- Surgical excision of tumor
- Melanoma: bone marrow transplant

PRESSURE ULCERS

Definition
- Localized areas of cellular necrosis in the skin and subcutaneous tissue over bony prominences

Causes
- Pressure, particularly over bony prominences
- Shearing forces

Pathophysiology
- Pressure interrupts circulation, producing tissue ischemia and increased capillary pressure (see *Pressure points: Common sites of pressure ulcers,* page 402)
- As capillaries collapse, thrombosis occurs, leading to edema and tissue necrosis
- Necrotic tissue predisposes to bacterial invasion and infection

Assessment findings
- Visual inspection reveals pressure ulcer
- Stage I
  - Nonblanchable erythema of intact skin
  - Skin discoloration
  - Warmth and hardness
- Stage II
  - Abrasion
  - Blister
  - Partial-thickness skin loss involving the epidermis and dermis
  - Shallow crater
- Stage III
  - Deep-crater with or without undermining of adjacent tissue
  - Full-thickness skin loss involving damage or necrosis of subcutaneous tissue that may extend down to, but not through, underlying fascia
- Stage IV
  - Damage to muscle, bone, tendon, or joint
  - Full-thickness skin loss with extensive destruction
  - Tissue necrosis

Diagnostic test finding
- Wound culture and sensitivity: identifies infecting organism

Medical management
- Diet: high-protein, high-calorie diet in small frequent feedings; nutritional supplements, such as vitamin C and zinc
- I.V. therapy: saline lock, hydration
- Position: reposition every 2 hours keeping weight off ulcer site

Characteristics of pressure ulcers
- Localized areas of cellular necrosis in the skin and subcutaneous tissue over bony prominences
- Necrotic tissue predisposes to bacterial invasion and infection
- Caused by pressure and shearing forces

Key assessment findings in the four stages of pressure ulcers
- Stage I: nonblanchable erythema of intact skin
- Stage II: partial-thickness skin loss involving the epidermis and dermis
- Stage III: full-thickness skin loss involving damage or necrosis of subcutaneous tissue
- Stage IV: damage to muscle, bone, tendon, or joint; full-thickness skin loss with extensive destruction

Diagnostic test finding
- Wound culture: positive

16 sites of pressure points

- Shoulder blade
- Sacrum
- Ischial tuberosity
- Posterior knee
- Foot
- Heel
- Occiput
- Rim of ear
- Dorsal thoracic area
- Elbow
- Side of head
- Shoulder
- Iliac crest
- Trochanter
- Anterior knee
- Malleolus

Pressure points: Common sites of pressure ulcers

Pressure ulcers may develop in any of these 16 pressure points. To prevent ulcers, reposition the patient frequently, and check carefully for any change in the patients skin tone.

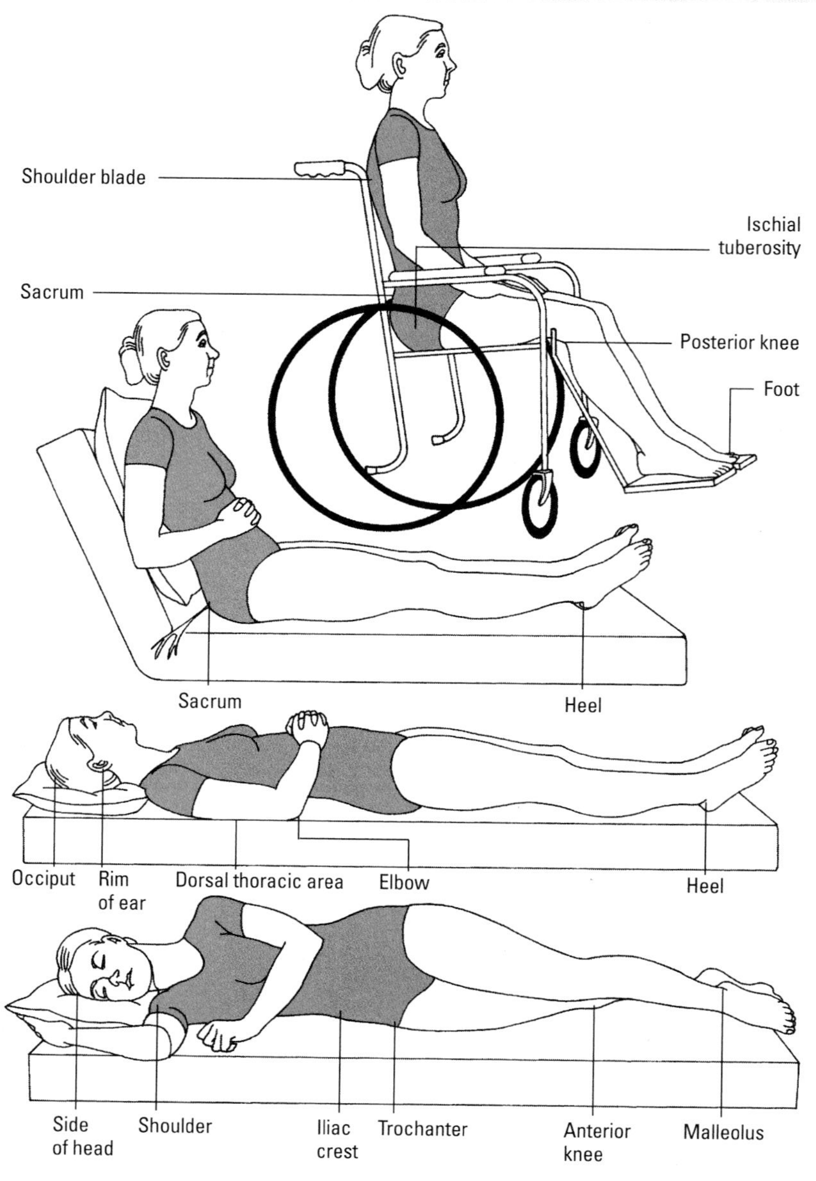

- Treatments: foam, gel, or air mattress, dressing changes, debridement
- Activity: as tolerated, active or passive ROM exercises
- Monitoring: vital signs and I/O

- Laboratory studies: electrolytes, Hb, RBC, WBC, platelet, complete blood count, serum albumin, serum protein
- Nutritional support: parenteral or enteral feedings if the patient can't or won't take adequate nourishment orally

Nursing interventions

- Maintain the patient's diet and encourage oral intake
- Reposition the patient every 2 hours
- Monitor and record vital signs, I/O, laboratory studies, and daily weight
- Provide meticulous skin care
- Assess skin integrity and watch for signs of infection
- Assess and document pressure ulcer
- Provide wound care and dressing changes, as ordered
- Encourage fluid intake
- Use special mattress on bed
- Individualize home care instructions
  - Change positions frequently
  - Perform meticulous skin care
  - Recognize signs and symptoms of skin breakdown
  - Eat a nutritious diet

Complications

- Progression of ulcer to more severe stage
- Sepsis
- Loss of limb from bone involvement

Surgical interventions

- Debridement
- Tissue flap

NCLEX CHECKS

It's never too soon to begin your NCLEX preparation. Now that you've reviewed this chapter, carefully read each of the following questions and choose the best answer. Then compare your responses to the correct answers.

1. What key symptom would a second-degree burn wound show?

☐ **A.** Edema
☐ **B.** Blanching
☐ **C.** Eschar
☐ **D.** Fluid-filled vesicles

2. What's the best method for preventing hypovolemic shock in a patient admitted with severe burns?

☐ **A.** Administering dopamine
☐ **B.** Applying medical antishock trousers
☐ **C.** Infusing I.V. fluids
☐ **D.** Infusing fresh frozen plasma

Treatment options for pressure ulcers

- High-protein, high-calorie diet in small frequent feedings
- Nutritional supplements, such as vitamin C and zinc
- Foam, gel, or air mattress
- Dressing changes
- Debridement

Key nursing interventions for a patient with pressure ulcers

- Maintain the patient's diet and encourage oral intake.
- Reposition the patient every 2 hours.
- Assess skin integrity and watch for signs of infection.
- Provide wound care and dressing changes, as ordered.
- Use special mattress on bed.

3. A patient undergoes a biopsy to confirm a diagnosis of skin cancer. Immediately following the procedure, the nurse should observe the site for:

- ☐ **A.** skin color changes.
- ☐ **B.** dehiscence.
- ☐ **C.** hemorrhage.
- ☐ **D.** swelling.

4. The skin lesions evident in herpes zoster are similar to those seen in:

- ☐ **A.** impetigo.
- ☐ **B.** syphilis.
- ☐ **C.** varicella.
- ☐ **D.** rubella.

5. A patient experiences problems in body temperature regulation associated with a skin impairment. Which gland is most likely involved?

- ☐ **A.** Eccrine
- ☐ **B.** Sebaceous
- ☐ **C.** Apocrine
- ☐ **D.** Endocrine

6. The nurse is caring for a patient with a new skin donor site that was harvested to treat a burn. The nurse should position the patient to: (Select all that apply.)

- ☐ **A.** allow ventilation of the site.
- ☐ **B.** make the site dependent.
- ☐ **C.** avoid pressure on the site.
- ☐ **D.** keep the site elevated.
- ☐ **E.** keep the donor site dry and open to air.
- ☐ **F.** be lying on the site.

7. A patient is admitted with a suspected malignant melanoma on his left shoulder. When performing the physical assessment, the nurse would expect to find which of the following?

- ☐ **A.** A brown birthmark that has lightened in color
- ☐ **B.** An area of petechiae
- ☐ **C.** A brown or black mole with areas of blue and irregular borders
- ☐ **D.** A red birthmark that has recently become darker

8. When assessing the skin of a patient, the nurse notes reddened, intact skin over the sacrum that doesn't blanch. The nurse determines that this patient has which stage pressure ulcer?

- ☐ **A.** Stage I
- ☐ **B.** Stage II
- ☐ **C.** Stage III
- ☐ **D.** Stage IV

TOP 6

Items to study for your next test on the integumentary system

1. Layers of the skin
2. Nursing interventions after a skin graft
3. What causes herpes zoster
4. Classification of burns
5. Types of skin cancer
6. Four stages of pressure ulcers

ANSWERS AND RATIONALES

1. Correct answer: D
Second-degree burn wounds show fluid-filled vesicles. Edema and blanching on pressure are characteristics of first-degree burns. Eschar is seen in third-degree burns.

2. Correct answer: C
During the early postburn period, large amounts of plasma fluid extravasates into interstitial spaces. Restoring the fluid loss is necessary to prevent hypovolemic shock. Fresh frozen plasma is expensive and carries a slight risk of disease transmission. Apply medical antishock trousers to treat—not prevent—shock. Dopamine causes vasoconstriction and elevates blood pressure but it doesn't prevent hypovolemia in burn patients.

3. Correct answer: C
The nurse's main concern following a skin biopsy procedure is bleeding. Infection is a later possible consequence of a biopsy. Dehiscence is more likely in larger wounds such as surgical wounds of the abdomen or thorax. Skin color change and swelling are normal reactions associated with any event that traumatizes the skin.

4. Correct answer: C
Varicella (chickenpox) characteristically has vesicles as the hallmark lesion. Impetigo has pustules. In syphilis the primary lesion is the chancre, and in rubella the lesion is a maculopapular rash.

5. Correct answer: A
Eccrine glands are associated with body temperature regulation, sebaceous glands lubricate the skin and hair, and apocrine glands are involved in bacteria decomposition. Endocrine glands are a group of glands that secrete hormones responsible for the regulation of body processes, such as metabolism and glucose regulation.

6. Correct answer: A, C, D, E
Allowing ventilation of the site, avoiding pressure on the site, elevating the site, and keeping the donor site dry and open to air are all appropriate interventions for this patient. Elevating the site, rather than keeping dependent, may reduce edema. If the patient lies on the site, it will be exposed to pressure, which the patient should avoid.

7. Correct answer: C
Melanomas have an irregular shape and lack uniformity in color. They may appear brown or black with red, white, or blue areas. The other assessment findings don't describe melanomas.

8. Correct answer: A
In a stage I pressure ulcer, the skin is intact with nonblanchable erythema. Intact, nonblanchable skin isn't characteristic of stage II, III, or IV ulcers.

10 Hematologic and lymphatic systems

LEARNING OBJECTIVES

After studying this chapter, you should be able to:

- Describe the psychosocial impact of hematologic or lymphatic disorders.
- Differentiate between modifiable and nonmodifiable risk factors in the development of a hematologic or lymphatic disorder.
- List three probable and three possible nursing diagnoses for a patient with any hematologic or lymphatic disorder.
- Identify nursing interventions for a patient with a hematologic or lymphatic disorder.
- Identify three teaching topics for a patient with a hematologic or lymphatic disorder.

CHAPTER OVERVIEW

Caring for the patient with a hematologic or lymphatic disorder requires a sound understanding of cardiovascular and lymphatic anatomy and physiology, hemodynamics, and fluid balance. A thorough assessment is essential to planning and implementing appropriate care. The assessment includes a complete history, a physical examination, diagnostic testing, identification of modifiable and nonmodifiable risk factors, and information related to the psychosocial impact of the disorder on the patient.

Nursing diagnoses focus primarily on activity intolerance, risk for infection, and anxiety. Nursing interventions are designed to monitor bleeding, prevent infection, and assist the patient to adjust to the effects of chronic illness. Patient teaching — a crucial nursing activity — involves providing the patient information about medical follow-up, medication regimens, signs and symptoms of possible complications, and reducing modifiable risk factors by adhering to infection control measures and by changing behaviors that lead to increased bleeding.

ANATOMY AND PHYSIOLOGY REVIEW

- **Lymphatic vessels**
  - Consist of capillary-like structures that are permeable to large molecules
  - Prevent edema by moving fluid and proteins from interstitial spaces to venous circulation
  - Reabsorb fats from the small intestine
- **Lymph nodes**
  - Tissue that filters out bacteria and other foreign cells
  - Regional grouping of lymph nodes: cervicofacial, supraclavicular, axillary, epitrochlear, inguinal, and femoral
- **Lymph**
  - Fluid found in interstitial spaces
  - Composition of lymph: water and end products of cell metabolism
- **Spleen**
  - The largest lymphatic organ
  - Filters blood
  - Traps formed particles
  - Destroys bacteria
  - Serves as blood reservoir
  - Forms lymphocytes and monocytes
- **Erythrocytes: red blood cells (RBCs)**
  - RBCs are formed in the bone marrow
  - RBCs contain hemoglobin (Hb)
  - Oxygen binds with Hb to form oxyhemoglobin
- **Thrombocytes (platelets)**
  - Formed in the bone marrow
  - Function in the coagulation of blood
- **Leukocytes: white blood cells (WBCs)**
  - WBCs are formed in the bone marrow and lymphatic tissue (see *WBC types and functions,* page 408)
  - WBCs include granulocytes and agranulocytes
  - Provide immunity and protection from infection by phagocytosis
- **Plasma**
  - Liquid portion of the blood
  - Composition of plasma: water, protein (albumin and globulin), glucose, and electrolytes

Lymphatic vessel characteristics

- Consists of capillary-like structures
- Prevents edema
- Reabsorbs fats

Facts about the spleen

- Largest lymphatic organ
- Filters blood
- Traps particles
- Destroys bacteria
- Acts as blood reservoir
- Forms lymphocytes and monocytes

Blood cells

- RBCs: formed in bone marrow; contain Hb
- WBCs: formed in bone marrow and lymphatic tissue; include granulocytes and agranulocytes; provide immunity and protection from infection

Plasma

- Liquid portion of blood
- Contains water, protein, glucose, and electrolytes

Types of WBCs

- Neutrophils: predominant form; help devour invading organisms
- Eosinophils: minor granulocytes; defend against parasites and infections
- Basophils: minor granulocytes; participate in delayed hypersensitivity reactions
- Monocytes: help devour invading organisms; help process antigens
- Lymphocytes: occur as B cells and T cells
- Plasma cells: reside in tissue; produce antibodies

ABO blood groups

- Antigens that determine blood type
- Blood types: A antigen, B antigen, AB antigens, O antigens
- Blood type O: universal donor; blood type AB: universal recipient

Bone marrow characteristics

- Red: source of lymphocytes and macrophages; carries out hematopoiesis
- Yellow: red bone marrow that has changed to fat

WBC types and functions

White blood cells (WBCs), or leukocytes, protect the body against harmful bacteria and infection. WBCs are classified as granular leukocytes (basophils, neutrophils, and eosinophils) or nongranular leukocytes (lymphocytes, monocytes, and plasma cells). WBCs are usually produced in bone marrow; lymphocytes and plasma cells are produced in lymphoid tissue as well. Neutrophils have a circulating half-life of less than 6 hours, while some lymphocytes may survive for weeks or months. Normally, WBCs number between 5,000 and 10,000 µl. There are six types of WBCs:

- Neutrophils – The predominant form of granulocyte, neutrophils make up about 60% of WBCs and help devour invading organisms by phagocytosis.
- Eosinophils – Minor granulocytes, eosinophils may defend against parasites and lung and skin infections, and may act in allergic reactions. They account for 1% to 5% of the total WBC count.
- Basophils – Minor granulocytes, basophils may release heparin and histamine into the blood and participate in delayed hypersensitivity reactions. They account for up to 1% of the total WBC count.
- Monocytes – Along with neutrophils, monocytes help devour invading organisms by phagocytosis. Monocytes help process antigens for lymphocytes and form macrophages in the tissues. They account for 1% to 6% of total WBC count.
- Lymphocytes – These occur as B cells and T cells: B cells form lymphoid follicles, produce humoral antibodies, and help T-cell mediated delayed hypersensitivity reactions and the rejection of foreign cells or cell products. Lymphocytes account for 20% to 40% of the total WBC count.
- Plasma cells – Residing in tissue, plasma cells develop from lymphoblasts and produce antibodies.

ABO blood groups

- System of antigens located on the surface of RBCs that determines blood type
- Blood types: A antigen, B antigen, AB antigens, O (zero) antigens
- Universal donor: blood type O
- Universal recipient: blood type AB

Coagulation

- Blood clotting
- Series of reactions involving the conversion of prothrombin to thrombin to fibrinogen to fibrin to form a clot

Bone marrow

- Two types exist: red and yellow
- Hematopoiesis is carried out by red marrow
- Hematopoiesis produces erythrocytes, leukocytes, and thrombocytes
- Red bone marrow is a source of lymphocytes and macrophages
- Yellow bone marrow is red bone marrow that has changed to fat

Liver

- The largest organ in the body
- Produces bile (main function), which emulsifies fats and stimulates peristalsis
- Conveys bile to the duodenum at the sphincter of Oddi through the common bile duct
- Metabolizes carbohydrates, fats, and proteins
- Synthesizes coagulation factors VII, IX, X, and prothrombin
- Stores vitamins A, D, B_{12}, and iron
- Detoxifies chemicals
- Excretes bilirubin
- Receives dual blood supply from portal vein and hepatic artery
- Produces and stores glycogen
- Promotes erythropoiesis when bone marrow production is insufficient

Key functions of the liver

- Produces and conveys bile
- Metabolizes carbohydrates, fats, and proteins
- Stores vitamins
- Detoxifies chemicals
- Excretes bilirubin
- Produces and stores glycogen

ASSESSMENT FINDINGS

History

- Enlarged glands
- Pain
- Fatigue and weakness
- Bleeding
- Pallor
- Lassitude
- Shortness of breath
- Fainting
- Vertigo
- Jaundice
- Night sweats
- Fever
- Weight loss
- Tachycardia
- Activity intolerance
- Frequent infections
- Melena
- Headache

Key history findings in hematologic and lymphatic disorders

- Enlarged glands
- Pain
- Fatigue and weakness
- Bleeding
- Activity intolerance

Physical examination

- Lymph node enlargement
- Anemia
- Ecchymosis
- Skin: pallor, cyanosis, jaundice, and petechiae
- Gingivitis
- Ophthalmoscopic examination: bleeding fundi
- Sclera: jaundice, capillary hemorrhage
- Hepatomegaly
- Sternal tenderness

Key physical assessment findings

- Lymph node enlargement
- Anemia
- Ecchymosis
- Skin: pallor, cyanosis, jaundice, and petechiae

- Splenomegaly
- Myocardial hypertrophy
- Epistaxis
- Dyspnea on exertion

DIAGNOSTIC TESTS AND PROCEDURES

Blood chemistry

- Definition and purpose
  - Laboratory test of a blood sample
  - Analysis for potassium, calcium, blood urea nitrogen (BUN), creatinine, protein, albumin, and bilirubin
- Nursing interventions
  - Withhold food and fluids, as directed, before the procedure
  - Check the site for bleeding after the procedure

Hematologic studies

- Definition and purpose
  - Laboratory test of a blood sample
  - Analysis for WBCs, RBCs, erythrocyte sedimentation rate (ESR), Hb, and hematocrit (HCT)
- Nursing interventions
  - Note current drug therapy before the procedure
  - Check the site for bleeding after the procedure

Lymphangiography

- Definition and purpose
  - Procedure involving an injection of contrast media through a catheter into lymphatic vessels in the hands and feet
  - Radiographic picture of lymphatic system and dissection of lymph vessel taken at intervals after injection
- Nursing interventions before the procedure
  - **Note the patient's allergies to iodine, seafood, and radiopaque dyes**
  - Inform the patient of possible throat irritation and flushing of the face after injection of the dye
  - Place obtained written informed consent in the patient's chart
  - Withhold food and fluids, as directed
- Nursing interventions after the procedure
  - Assess vital signs and peripheral pulses
  - Check catheter insertion site for bleeding
  - Encourage fluids
  - Advise the patient that skin, stool, and urine will have a blue discoloration

Bone marrow examination (aspiration or biopsy)

- Definition and purpose
  - Procedure involving the percutaneous removal of bone marrow

Blood chemistry

- Laboratory test of a blood sample
- Analysis for potassium, calcium, BUN, creatinine, protein, albumin, and bilirubin
- Intervention: check the site for bleeding after the procedure

Hematologic studies

- Laboratory test of a blood sample
- Analysis for WBCs, RBCs, ESR, Hb, and HCT
- Intervention: note current drug therapy before the procedure

Lymphangiography

- Procedure involving an injection of contrast media into lymphatic vessels in the hands and feet
- Intervention: after injection, radiographic pictures of the lymphatic system and lymph vessel are taken

Bone marrow examination

- Procedure that involves the percutaneous removal of bone marrow
- Examines erythrocytes, leukocytes, thrombocytes, and precursor cells
- Intervention: administer analgesics or anxiolytics, as ordered

- Examination of erythrocytes, leukocytes, thrombocytes, and precursor cells
- Nursing interventions before the procedure
  - Place obtained written informed consent in the patient's chart
  - Administer analgesics or anxiolytics, as ordered
  - Determine the patient's ability to lie still during aspiration
- Nursing interventions after the procedure
  - Maintain pressure dressing
  - Check the aspiration site for bleeding and infection

Schilling test

- Definition and purpose
  - Procedure involving administration of oral radioactive cyanocobalamin and I.M. cyanocobalamin
  - Microscopic examination of a 24-hour urine sample for cyanocobalamin (vitamin B_{12})
- Nursing interventions before the procedure
  - Withhold food and fluids after midnight
  - Place obtained written informed consent in the patient's chart
- Nursing interventions after the procedure
  - Instruct the patient to save all voided urine for 24 hours
  - Keep urine at room temperature

Shilling test

- Administration of oral radioactive cyanocobalamin and I.M. cyanocobalamin
- Microscopic examination of 24-hour urine sample for cyanocobalamin
- Intervention: withhold food and fluids after midnight

Gastric analysis

- Definition and purpose
  - Procedure involving the aspiration of stomach contents through a nasogastric (NG) tube
  - Fasting analysis of gastric secretions to measure acidity and diagnose pernicious anemia
- Nursing interventions before the procedure
  - Withhold food and fluids
  - Instruct the patient not to smoke for 8 to 12 hours before the test
  - Withhold medications that can affect gastric secretions
- Nursing interventions after the procedure
  - Obtain vital signs
  - Assess for reactions to gastric acid stimulant, if used

Gastric analysis

- Procedure involving aspiration of stomach contents through an NG tube
- Measures acidity and helps diagnose pernicious anemia
- Intervention: withhold medications that can affect gastric secretions

Urine urobilinogen

- Definition and purpose
  - Laboratory test of a 2-hour or a 24-hour urine sample
  - Microscopic examination to diagnose hemolytic jaundice
- Nursing interventions
  - Use a bottle with a preservative and refrigerate specimen
  - Note salicylate use
  - Start urine collection in the afternoon when food is being digested for a 2-hour specimen
  - Begin the 24-hour collection after the first voided specimen in the morning

Urine urobilinogen

- Laboratory test of a 2-hour or 24-hour urine sample
- Helps diagnose hemolytic jaundice
- Intervention: begin the 24-hour collection after the first voided specimen in the morning

Erythrocyte life span determination

- Definition and purpose
  - Procedure involving reinjection of the patient's blood that has been tagged with chromium 51
  - Measurement of the life span of circulating RBCs
- Nursing interventions
  - Inform the patient that frequent blood samples will be drawn over a 2-week period
  - Check the venipuncture site for bleeding
  - Apply a pressure dressing after the procedure

Erythrocyte life span determination

- Procedure involving reinjection of the patient's blood that has been tagged with chromium 51
- Measures life span of RBCs
- Intervention: inform the patient that frequent blood samples will be drawn over a 2-week period

Bence Jones protein assay

- Definition and purpose
  - Procedure involving a 24-hour urine sample
  - Microscopic examination for the Bence Jones protein to help diagnose multiple myeloma
- Nursing interventions
  - Withhold all medications for 48 hours before the test
  - Instruct the patient to void and note the time (collection of urine starts with the next voiding)
  - Place urine container on ice
  - Measure each voided urine
  - Instruct the patient to void at the end of the 24-hour period
  - Note any medications that might interfere with the test

Bence Jones protein assay

- Involves 24-hour urine sample
- Examines for Bence Jones protein
- Helps diagnose multiple myeloma
- Intervention: instruct the patient to void and note the time

Romberg's test

- Definition and purpose
  - Physical test
  - Examination to assess loss of balance in pernicious anemia
- Nursing interventions
  - Explain the procedure
  - Monitor for imbalance
  - Prevent the patient from falling

Romberg's test

- Physical test
- Helps assess loss of balance
- Intervention: prevent the patient from falling

Erythrocyte fragility test

- Definition and purpose
  - Laboratory test of a blood sample
  - Analysis to measure the rate at which RBCs burst in varied hypotonic solutions
- Nursing interventions
  - Explain the procedure
  - Send the specimen to the laboratory

Erythrocyte fragility test

- Laboratory test of blood sample
- Measures the rate at which RBCs burst in hypotonic solutions
- Intervention: send the specimen to the laboratory

Rumpel-Leede capillary fragility tourniquet test

- Definition and purpose
  - Crude physical test
  - Examination of vascular resistance, platelet count, and function
- Nursing interventions
  - Explain that a blood pressure cuff will be placed on the arm for 5 minutes, followed by counting of petechiae

Rumpel-Leede test

- Physical test
- Examines vascular resistance, platelet count, and function
- Intervention: explain that the blood pressure cuff will be placed on the arm for 5 minutes

Bone scan
- Definition and purpose
  - Procedure using an I.V. injection of radioisotope
  - Visual imaging of bone metabolism
- Nursing interventions before the procedure
  - Determine the patient's ability to lie still

Coagulation studies
- Definition and purpose
  - Laboratory tests of a blood sample
  - Analysis for platelet function, platelet count, prothrombin time (PT), partial thromboplastin time (PTT), coagulation time, and bleeding time
- Nursing interventions
  - Note current drug therapy before procedure
  - Check the site for bleeding after the procedure

PSYCHOSOCIAL IMPACT OF HEMATOLOGIC AND LYMPHATIC DISORDERS

Developmental impact
- Fear of dying
- Decreased self-esteem
- Fear of rejection

Economic impact
- Disruption or loss of employment
- Cost of hospitalization
- Cost of medications

Occupational and recreational impact
- Restrictions in work activity
- Changes in leisure activity

Social impact
- Changes in role performance
- Social isolation

RISK FACTORS

Modifiable risk factors
- Exposure to chemical and environmental pollutants
- Sexual activity patterns
- Aspirin use
- Alcohol consumption
- Drug toxicity
- Diet
- Exposure to occupational radiation or radiation therapy

Bone scan
- Procedure involving injection of radioisotope
- Visual imaging of bone metabolism
- Intervention: determine the patient's ability to lie still

Coagulation studies
- Laboratory test of blood sample
- Analysis for platelet function, platelet count, PT, PTT, coagulation time, and bleeding time
- Intervention: check the site for bleeding after the procedure

Major impacts of hematologic and lymphatic system disorders
- Costs of loss of employment, hospitalizations, and medications
- Restrictions in activity
- Changes in role performance

Key modifiable risk factors
- Exposure to pollutants
- Sexual activity patterns
- Aspirin use

Probable nursing diagnoses

- Risk for activity intolerance
- Ineffective breathing pattern
- Chronic pain
- Impaired gas exchange

Splenectomy defined

- Surgical removal of the spleen

Key nursing steps before splenectomy

- Monitor PT, PTT, HCT, Hb, and platelet count.
- Administer vitamin K.
- Verify inoculation with polyvalent pneumococcal vaccine 2 weeks before the procedure.

- **Nonmodifiable risk factors**
  - Ethnic background
  - Age
  - Malabsorption syndromes
  - History of liver disease
  - History of malignancy

NURSING DIAGNOSES

- **Probable nursing diagnoses**
  - Risk for activity intolerance
  - Ineffective breathing pattern
  - Chronic pain
  - Impaired gas exchange
- **Possible nursing diagnoses**
  - Risk for infection
  - Imbalanced nutrition: Less than body requirements
  - Impaired oral mucous membrane
  - Disturbed body image
  - Situational low self-esteem
  - Anxiety
  - Social isolation
  - Risk for impaired skin integrity

SPLENECTOMY

- **Description**
  - Surgical removal of the spleen
- **Preoperative nursing interventions**
  - Complete patient and family preoperative teaching
    - Determine the patient's understanding of the procedure
    - Describe the operating room, postanesthesia care unit (PACU), and preoperative and postoperative routines
    - Demonstrate postoperative turning, coughing, deep breathing, splinting, and range-of-motion (ROM) exercises
    - Explain the postoperative need for drainage tubes, surgical dressings, oxygen therapy, I.V. therapy, and pain control
  - Complete a preoperative checklist
  - Administer preoperative medications, as prescribed
  - Allay the patient's and his family's anxiety about surgery
  - Document the patient's history and physical assessment database
  - Monitor PT, PTT, HCT, Hb, and platelet count
  - Administer vitamin K
  - Verify inoculation with polyvalent pneumococcal vaccine 2 weeks before the procedure
  - Administer antibiotics, as prescribed

Postoperative nursing interventions
- Assess cardiac, respiratory, and neurologic status
- Assess pain and administer postoperative analgesics, as prescribed
- Assess for return of peristalsis; provide solid foods and liquids, as tolerated
- Administer I.V. fluids, total parenteral nutrition (TPN), and transfusion therapy, as prescribed
- Allay the patient's anxiety
- Inspect the surgical dressing and change, as directed
- Reinforce turning, coughing, and deep breathing, and splinting of incision
- Keep the patient in semi-Fowler's position
- Provide incentive spirometry
- Increase activity as tolerated
- Monitor and record vital signs, intake and output (I/O), laboratory studies, and pulse oximetry
- Monitor and maintain position and patency of drainage tubes
- Apply abdominal binder
- Monitor for abdominal distention
- Individualize home care instructions
  - Complete incision care daily
  - State the need for prophylactic use of antibiotics
  - Avoid contact sports

Surgical complications
- Pneumococcal pneumonia
- Infection
- Hemorrhage
- Sepsis
- Disseminated intravascular coagulation (DIC)
- Atelectasis
- Subphrenic abscess
- Thrombophlebitis

Key nursing steps after splenectomy
- Assess cardiac, respiratory, and neurologic status.
- Monitor and record vital signs, I/O, laboratory studies, and pulse oximetry.
- Monitor and maintain position and patency of drainage tubes.
- Monitor for abdominal distention.

BONE MARROW TRANSPLANT

Description
- Bone marrow is aspirated from multiple sites along the iliac crest of the donor
- Donor bone marrow is infused intravenously into the recipient

Preoperative nursing interventions
- Complete patient and family preoperative teaching
  - Determine the patient's understanding of the procedure
  - Describe the operating room, PACU, and preoperative and postoperative routines
  - Demonstrate postoperative turning, coughing, deep breathing, splinting, and ROM exercises
  - Explain the postoperative need for drainage tubes, surgical dressings, oxygen therapy, I.V. therapy, and pain control

Bone marrow transplant
- Bone marrow is aspirated from multiple sites along the iliac crest of the donor.
- Donor bone marrow is infused intravenously into the recipient.

Key nursing steps before bone marrow transplant

- Verify bone marrow compatibility.
- Administer chemotherapy for 3 days before the transplant.
- Maintain the radiation treatment schedule.
- Maintain protective isolation or the use of a laminar airflow room.
- Monitor for infection.

Key nursing steps after bone marrow transplant

- Maintain protective precautions.
- Administer antibiotics, as prescribed.
- Provide postchemotherapeutic and postradiation nursing care.
- Inspect for bruising and petechiae.
- Administer immunosuppressants, as prescribed.

Agranulocytosis defined

- Profound decrease in the number of granulocytes
- Reduced number of granulocytes diminishes resistance to disease

- Complete a preoperative checklist
- Administer preoperative medications, as prescribed
- Allay the patient's and his family's anxiety about surgery
- Document the patient's history and physical assessment database
- Verify bone marrow compatibility
- Administer chemotherapy for 3 days before the transplant
- Maintain the radiation treatment schedule
- Maintain protective isolation or the use of a laminar airflow room
- Monitor for infection

Postoperative nursing interventions

- Assess cardiac and respiratory status
- Administer I.V. fluids
- Allay the patient's anxiety
- Keep the patient in semi-Fowler's position
- Maintain activity, as tolerated
- Monitor and record vital signs; I/O; central venous pressure (CVP); laboratory studies; urine, stool, and emesis for occult blood; daily weight; specific gravity; urine glucose, ketones, and protein; and pulse oximetry values
- Precautions: protective
- Encourage the patient to express feelings about a fear of dying
- Administer antibiotics, as prescribed
- Provide postchemotherapeutic and postradiation nursing care
  - Provide prophylactic skin, mouth, and perineal care
  - Monitor dietary intake
  - Administer antiemetics and antidiarrheals, as prescribed
  - Monitor for bleeding, infection, and electrolyte imbalance
  - Provide rest periods
- Inspect for bruising and petechiae
- Administer immunosuppressants, as prescribed
- Individualize home care instructions
  - Recognize the signs and symptoms of infection and bleeding
  - Identify changes in vision

Surgical complications

- Marrow graft rejection
- Graft versus host disease
- Cataracts
- Stomatitis
- Hemorrhage

AGRANULOCYTOSIS (GRANULOCYTOPENIA)

Definition

- Profound decrease in the number of granulocytes

Causes

- Idiopathic
- Exposure to chemicals

- Drug induced: chloramphenicol (Chloromycetin), chlorpromazine (Thorazine), or phenytoin (Dilantin)
- Chemotherapy
- Radiation
- Radioisotopes
- Hemodialysis
- Viral infection

Pathophysiology

- Number of granulocytes is reduced because of increased utilization, lack of maturation, or shortened life span
- The reduced number of granulocytes diminishes resistance to disease

Assessment findings

- Fatigue
- Malaise
- Elevated temperature
- Chills
- Sore throat
- Multiple infections
- Weakness
- Dysphagia
- Enlarged cervical lymph nodes
- Tachycardia
- Ulcerations of oral mucosa and throat

Diagnostic test findings

- Hematology: decreased WBCs, granulocytes; increased ESR
- Bone marrow biopsy: absence of polymorphonuclear leukocytes
- Culture and sensitivity: positive identification of organisms

Medical management

- Diet: high-protein, high-vitamin, high-calorie, bland, and soft
- I.V. therapy: saline lock
- Position: semi-Fowler's
- Activity: bed rest and active and passive ROM exercises
- Monitoring: vital signs and I/O
- Laboratory studies: WBCs, granulocytes, and urine and blood for culture and sensitivity
- Treatment: saline gargles
- Precautions: protective
- Transfusion therapy: packed WBCs and whole blood
- Antibiotics: ticarcillin (Ticar), tobramycin (Nebcin)
- Antipyretic: acetaminophen (Tylenol)
- Sedative: oxazepam (Serax)
- Stool softener: docusate (Colace)
- Analgesic: ibuprofen (Motrin)
- Antifungal: fluconazole (Diflucan)
- Hematopoietic growth factor: epoetin alfa (Epogen)

Key assessment findings in agranulocytosis

- Fatigue
- Elevated temperature
- Chills
- Weakness

Key diagnostic test findings in agranulocytosis

- Hematology: decreased WBCs, granulocytes; increased ESR
- Bone marrow biopsy: absence of polymorphonuclear leukocytes
- Culture and sensitivity: positive identification of organisms

Key management options for a patient with agranulocytosis

- Laboratory studies: WBCs, granulocytes, and urine and blood for culture and sensitivity
- Precautions: protective
- Antibiotics

Key teaching topics for a patient with a hematologic or lymphatic disorder

- Infection control measures
- Signs and symptoms of infection and bleeding
- Medication therapy
- Daily skin, mouth, and foot care
- Medical identification jewelry

Key nursing interventions for a patient with agranulocytosis

- Provide tepid baths and saline gargles.
- Maintain protective precautions.
- Monitor for infection.
- Tell the patient to avoid raw fruits and vegetables and exposure to flowers and plants in the room.

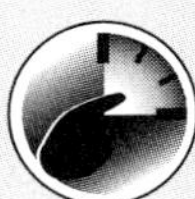

TIME-OUT FOR TEACHING

Patients with hematologic or lymphatic disorders

Be sure to include the following topics in your teaching plan when caring for patients with hematologic or lymphatic disorders.

- Follow-up appointments
- Smoking cessation
- Optimal body weight maintenance
- Medication therapy, including the action, adverse effects, and scheduling of medications
- Infection control measures
- Signs and symptoms of infection and bleeding
- Daily skin, mouth, and foot care
- Dietary recommendations and restrictions
- Avoidance of over-the-counter medications
- Prevention of constipation
- Medical identification jewelry
- Safe environment
- Independence in activities of daily living (ADLs)
- Reactions to limitation on lifestyle and ADLs
- Rest and activity patterns, including any limitations or restrictions
- Community agencies and resources for supportive services

Nursing interventions

- Maintain the patient's diet
- Encourage fluids
- Promote turning, coughing, and deep breathing
- Assess respiratory status
- Keep the patient in semi-Fowler's position
- Monitor and record: vital signs, I/O, laboratory studies, and stool count
- Administer medications, as prescribed
- Encourage the patient to express feelings about imposed isolation
- Maintain bed rest
- Provide tepid baths and saline gargles
- Maintain protective precautions
- Administer transfusion therapy, as prescribed
- Provide gentle mouth and skin care
- Monitor for infection
- Instruct the patient to avoid enemas and rectal temperatures
- **Instruct the patient to avoid raw fruits and vegetables**
- **Tell the patient to avoid exposure to flowers and plants in the room**
- Individualize home care instructions (for teaching tips, see *Patients with hematologic or lymphatic disorders*)
  - Avoid using over-the-counter medications
  - Prevent constipation

Complications

- Sepsis
- Rectal abscess

- Pneumonia
- Hemorrhagic necrosis of mucous membranes
- Parenchymal liver damage

Possible surgical intervention
- Splenectomy

LEUKEMIA

Definition
- Unregulated proliferation or accumulation of WBCs in the bone marrow
- Three types
  - Acute myelogenous
  - Chronic lymphocytic
  - Chronic myelocytic

Causes
- Unknown
- Genetic influence
- Viral pathogenesis
- Exposure to chemicals
- Radiation
- Altered immune system
- Chemotherapy
- Polycythemia vera

Pathophysiology
- Normal hemopoietic cells are replaced by leukemic cells in bone marrow
- Immature forms of WBCs circulate in the blood, infiltrating the liver, spleen, and lymph nodes, and invading nonhematologic organs, such as the meninges, GI tract, kidneys, and skin

Assessment findings
- Petechiae
- Ecchymosis
- Frequent infections
- Elevated temperature
- Enlarged lymph nodes, spleen, and liver
- Weakness and fatigue
- Joint, abdominal, and bone pain
- Gingivitis
- Night sweats
- Stomatitis
- Prolonged menses
- Hematemesis
- Melena
- Jaundice
- Tachycardia
- Hypotension

Key facts about leukemia

- Unregulated proliferation or accumulation of WBCs in the bone marrow
- Three types: acute myelogenous, chronic lymphocytic, and chronic myelocytic

Key causes of leukemia

- Genetic influence
- Viral pathogenesis
- Exposure to chemicals

Pathophysiology of leukemia

- Leukemic cells replace normal hemopoietic cells in bone marrow.
- Immature forms of WBCs circulate in the blood, infiltrating and invading organs.

TOP 3

Leukemia assessment findings

1. Frequent infections
2. Enlarged lymph nodes, spleen, and liver
3. Weakness and fatigue

- Epistaxis
- Generalized pain

Diagnostic test findings

- Hematology: decreased HCT, Hb, RBCs, and platelets; increased ESR, immature WBCs, and bleeding time
- Bone marrow biopsy: large number of immature leukocytes

Diagnostic test findings in leukemia

- Hematology: decreased HCT, Hb, RBCs, and platelets; increased ESR, immature WBCs, and bleeding time
- Bone marrow biopsy: large number of immature leukocytes

Medical management

- Diet: high-protein, high-vitamin and mineral, high-calorie, low-roughage, bland and soft in small, frequent feedings
- I.V. therapy: hydration and saline lock
- Oxygen therapy
- Position: semi-Fowler's
- Activity: bed rest and active and passive ROM and isometric exercises
- Monitoring: vital signs and I/O
- Laboratory studies: Hb, HCT, WBCs, platelets, BUN, creatinine, and surveillance cultures
- Nutritional support: TPN
- Radiation therapy
- Chemotherapy
- Treatments: sitz baths, bed cradle, and tepid baths
- Precautions: protective or laminar airflow room
- Transfusion therapy: platelets, packed RBCs, and whole blood
- Antibiotics: doxorubicin (Adriamycin), plicamycin (Mithracin)
- Antipyretic: acetaminophen (Tylenol)
- Stool softener: docusate (Colace)
- Analgesic: ibuprofen (Motrin)
- Antigout: allopurinol (Zyloprim)
- Tranquilizer: oxazepam (Serax)
- Systemic alkalinizer: sodium bicarbonate
- Antimetabolites: fluorouracil (Adrucil), methotrexate (MTX)
- Alkylating agents: busulfan (Myleran), chlorambucil (Leukeran)
- Antineoplastics: vinblastine (Velban), vincristine (Oncovin)
- Enzyme: Asparaginase (Elspar)
- Estrogen: diethylstilbestrol (DES)
- Progestin: medroxyprogesterone (Provera)
- Immune globulin G (IgG) antibody: immune globulin I.V. (Gammagard)
- Antiemetic: prochlorperazine (Compazine)
- Leukopheresis
- Antifungal: fluconazole (Mycostatin)
- Hematopoietic growth factor: epoetin alfa (Epogen)

Key medication options for leukemia

- Antibiotics
- Antimetabolites
- Alkylating agents
- Antineoplastics
- Hematopoietic growth factor

Nursing interventions

- Maintain the patient's diet
- Encourage fluids
- Administer I.V. fluids
- Administer oxygen

- Promote turning, coughing, and deep breathing
- Assess cardiovascular, neurologic, respiratory, and renal status and fluid balance
- Keep the patient in semi-Fowler's position
- Monitor and record vital signs, I/O, laboratory studies, daily weight, and urine, stool, and emesis for occult blood
- Administer TPN
- Administer transfusion therapy, as prescribed
- Administer medications, as prescribed
- Encourage the patient to express feelings about changes in body image and a fear of dying
- Maintain bed rest
- Provide treatments: sitz baths, bed cradle, and tepid baths
- Allay the patient's anxiety
- **Monitor for bleeding and infection**
- Maintain protective precautions
- Provide gentle mouth and skin care
- **Avoid giving the patient I.M. injections and enemas and taking his temperature rectally**
- Avoid using straight razors on the patient
- Provide postchemotherapeutic and postradiation nursing care
  - Provide prophylactic skin, mouth, and perineal care
  - Monitor dietary intake
  - Administer antiemetics and antidiarrheals, as prescribed
  - Monitor for bleeding, infection, and electrolyte imbalance
  - Provide rest periods
- Individualize home care instructions
  - Provide information about the American Cancer Society
  - Recognize the signs and symptoms of occult blood
  - Prevent constipation
  - Use an electric razor
  - Avoid using over-the-counter medications
  - Monitor stool for occult blood
  - Increase fluid intake

Complications

- Gross systemic hemorrhage
- Acute renal failure
- Stroke
- Thrombocytopenia
- Perirectal abscess
- GI bleeding
- Fungal and bacterial infection
- Meningitis

Possible surgical intervention

- Bone marrow transplant

Key nursing interventions for a patient with leukemia

- Monitor and record vital signs, I/O, laboratory studies, daily weight, and urine, stool, and emesis for occult blood.
- Administer transfusion therapy, as prescribed.
- Monitor for bleeding and infection.
- Maintain protective precautions.
- Provide gentle mouth and skin care.
- Avoid giving the patient I.M. injections and enemas and taking his temperature rectally.
- Provide postchemotherapeutic and postradiation nursing care.

Key nursing interventions after chemotherapy and radiation for leukemia

- Provide prophylactic skin, mouth, and perineal care.
- Administer antiemetics and antidiarrheals, as prescribed.
- Monitor for bleeding, infection, and electrolyte imbalance.

Description and types of lymphomas

- Neoplastic cells of lymphoid origin
- Hodgkin's disease: proliferation of malignant Reed-Sternberg cells within lymph nodes
- Malignant lymphoma: malignant tumors of lymph nodes and lymphatic tissues that can't be classified as Hodgkin's disease
- Classes of malignant lymphoma: B-lymphocyte malignancies, T-lymphocyte malignancies, and histiocyte malignancies

Most common assessment finding in Hodgkin's disease

- Enlarged, nontender, firm, and movable lymph nodes in lower cervical regions

Most common assessment finding in malignant lymphoma

- Prominent, painless, generalized lymphadenopathy

LYMPHOMAS

Definition

- Neoplastic cells of lymphoid origin
- Hodgkin's disease: proliferation of malignant Reed-Sternberg cells within lymph nodes
- Malignant lymphoma: malignant tumors of lymph nodes and lymphatic tissues that can't be classified as Hodgkin's disease
- Classes of malignant lymphoma: B-lymphocyte malignancies, T-lymphocyte malignancies, and histiocyte malignancies

Causes

- Unknown
- Viral
- Genetic (Hodgkin's disease)
- Environmental (Hodgkin's disease)
- Immunologic

Pathophysiology

- Reed-Sternberg cells proliferate in a single lymph node and travel contiguously through the lymphatic system to other lymphatic nodes and organs (Hodgkin's disease)
- Immune system cell tumors occur throughout lymph nodes and lymphatic organs in unpredictable patterns (malignant lymphoma)

Assessment findings

- Enlarged, nontender, firm, and movable lymph nodes in lower cervical regions (Hodgkin's disease)
- Recurrent, intermittent fever
- Night sweats
- Weight loss
- Malaise
- Lethargy
- Severe pruritus
- Dyspnea (Hodgkin's disease)
- Anorexia
- Bone pain (Hodgkin's disease)
- Cough
- Recurrent infection
- Hepatomegaly
- Splenomegaly
- Dysphagia (Hodgkin's disease)
- Edema and cyanosis of face and neck (Hodgkin's disease)
- Prominent, painless, generalized lymphadenopathy (malignant lymphoma)

Diagnostic test findings

- Bone marrow aspiration and biopsy: small, diffuse lymphocytic or large, follicular-type cells (malignant lymphoma)

- Hematology: decreased Hb, HCT, and platelets (malignant lymphoma and Hodgkin's disease); increased ESR (Hodgkin's disease and malignant lymphoma); increased leukocytes and gamma globulin (Hodgkin's disease)
- Lymphangiogram: positive lymph node involvement (Hodgkin's disease)
- Lymph node biopsy: positive for Reed-Sternberg cells (Hodgkin's disease)
- Chest X-ray: lymphadenopathy (Hodgkin's disease)
- Blood chemistry: increased alkaline phosphatase and copper (Hodgkin's disease)
- Stage I: asymptomatic; malignant cells found in a single lymph node
- Stage II: symptomatic; malignant cells found in two or three adjacent lymph nodes on the same side of the diaphragm
- Stage III: symptomatic; malignant cells widely disseminated to lymph nodes on both sides of the diaphragm and to organs
- Stage IV: symptomatic; malignant cells found in one or more extralymphatic organs or tissues with or without lymphatic involvement

Medical management

- Diet: high-protein, high-calorie, high-vitamin and mineral, high-iron, high-calcium, bland, and soft
- I.V. therapy: saline lock
- Oxygen therapy
- Position: semi-Fowler's
- Activity: bed rest and active and passive ROM exercises
- Monitoring: vital signs and I/O
- Laboratory studies: Hb, HCT, WBCs, and platelets
- Radiation therapy
- Precautions: protective
- Transfusion therapy: packed RBCs
- Combined chemotherapy
  - MOPP chemotherapy protocol (Hodgkin's disease): mechlorethamine (Mustargen), vincristine (Oncovin), procarbazine (Matulane), and prednisone (Deltasone)
  - ABVD chemotherapy protocol (Hodgkin's disease): doxorubicin (Adriamycin), bleomycin (Blenoxane), vinblastine (Velban), and dacarbazine (DTIC-Dome)
  - CVP chemotherapy protocol (malignant lymphoma): cyclophosphamide (Cytoxan), vincristine (Oncovin), and prednisone (Deltasone)
  - CHOP chemotherapy protocol (malignant lymphoma): cyclophosphamide (Cytoxan), hydroxydaunorubicin (Adriamycin), vincristine (Oncovin), and prednisone (Deltasone)
- Analgesic: meperidine (Demerol)
- Sedative: oxazepam (Serax)
- Stool softener: docusate (Colace)
- Antipruritic: diphenhydramine (Benadryl)
- Antiemetic: prochlorperazine (Compazine)

Nursing interventions

- Maintain the patient's diet

Key diagnostic test findings in lymphomas

- Bone marrow aspiration and biopsy: small, diffuse lymphocytic or large, follicular-type cells (malignant lymphoma)
- Lymph node biopsy: positive for Reed-Sternberg cells (Hodgkin's disease)

Key management options for lymphomas

- Radiation therapy
- Transfusion therapy: packed RBCs
- MOPP chemotherapy protocol (Hodgkin's disease): mechlorethamine, Oncovin, procarbazine, and prednisone
- CHOP chemotherapy protocol (malignant lymphoma): cyclophosphamide, hydroxydaunorubicin, Oncovin, and prednisone

Key nursing interventions for a patient with lymphoma

- Encourage fluids.
- Administer transfusion therapy, as prescribed.
- Avoid giving aspirin to the patient.
- Provide postchemotherapeutic and postradiation nursing care.
- Maintain protective precautions.

Key nursing steps after chemotherapy and radiation

- Provide prophylactic skin, mouth, and perineal care.
- Administer antiemetics and antidiarrheals, as prescribed.
- Monitor for bleeding, infection, and electrolyte imbalance.

Common complications of lymphomas

- Metastasis
- Pleural effusion
- Paraplegia
- Infections
- Leukemia

- Encourage fluids
- Administer I.V. fluids
- Administer oxygen
- Promote turning, coughing, and deep breathing
- Assess respiratory, cardiovascular, and neurologic status and fluid balance
- Keep the patient in semi-Fowler's position
- Monitor and record vital signs, I/O, laboratory studies, and specific gravity
- Administer medications, as prescribed
- Encourage the patient to express feelings about changes in body image and a fear of dying
- Maintain bed rest
- Give frequent baths with mild soap
- Provide mouth and skin care
- Administer transfusion therapy, as prescribed
- Allay the patient's anxiety
- **Avoid giving aspirin to the patient**
- Avoid using straight razors on the patient
- Provide postchemotherapeutic and postradiation nursing care
  - Provide prophylactic skin, mouth, and perineal care
  - Monitor dietary intake
  - Administer antiemetics and antidiarrheals, as prescribed
  - Monitor for bleeding, infection, and electrolyte imbalance
  - Provide rest periods
- Monitor for jaundice and infection
- Maintain protective precautions
- Individualize home care instructions
  - Provide information about the American Cancer Society
  - Recognize the signs and symptoms of motor and sensory deficits
  - Increase fluid intake
  - Use electric razors
  - Avoid using over-the-counter medications
  - Avoid taking aspirin

Complications

- Metastasis (Hodgkin's disease)
- Hypersplenism
- Pleural effusion (Hodgkin's disease)
- Herpes zoster (Hodgkin's disease)
- Depression
- Pancytopenia (Hodgkin's disease)
- Pneumonitis (Hodgkin's disease)
- Paraplegia
- Pericarditis (Hodgkin's disease)
- Nephritis (Hodgkin's disease)
- Hypothyroidism (Hodgkin's disease)
- Neuralgia (Hodgkin's disease)
- Obstructive jaundice (Hodgkin's disease)
- Infections: viral, bacterial, fungal (malignant lymphoma)

- Intestinal obstruction (malignant lymphoma)
- Leukemia (malignant lymphoma)
- Superior vena cava obstruction (malignant lymphoma)

Possible surgical interventions

- Splenectomy

ACQUIRED IMMUNODEFICIENCY SYNDROME (AIDS)

Definition

- Defect in T-cell mediated immunity that allows the development of fatal opportunistic infections
- Caused by human immunodeficiency virus (HIV)
- An illness characterized by laboratory evidence of HIV infection coexisting with one or more indicator diseases, such as herpes simplex virus, cytomegalovirus, mycobacteria, candidal infection, *Pneumocystis carinii,* Kaposi's sarcoma, wasting syndrome, or dementia

Causes

- Exposure to blood containing HIV: transfusions, contaminated needles, handling of blood, or in utero
- Exposure to semen and vaginal secretions containing HIV: sexual intercourse or handling of semen and vaginal secretions

Pathophysiology

- HIV is transmitted by contact with infected blood or body fluids
  - HIV-infected lymphocytes are carried in semen, vaginal secretions, and blood
  - Infected lymphocytes in semen and vaginal secretions are transferred through minute breaks in the skin and mucosa
  - Infected lymphocytes in blood are transferred via transfusion, fetal circulation, and minute breaks in the skin and mucosa
- HIV, a retrovirus, selectively infects human cells containing $CD4^+$ antigen on their surface, the majority of which are T4 lymphocytes
- HIV virus reproduces within the T4 lymphocytes and destroys them
- The destruction of the T4 lymphocytes diminishes resistance to disease

Assessment findings

- Fatigue
- Weakness
- Anorexia
- Weight loss
- Recurrent diarrhea
- Fever
- Lymphadenopathy
- Pallor
- Night sweats
- Malnutrition
- Disorientation, confusion, dementia

AIDS definition and cause

- Defect in T-cell mediated immunity that allows the development of fatal opportunistic infections
- Caused by HIV

Key signs and symptoms of AIDS

- Anorexia
- Weight loss
- Recurrent diarrhea
- Night sweats
- Disorientation, confusion, dementia
- Opportunistic infections

- Opportunistic infections

Diagnostic test findings

- Hematology: decreased WBCs, RBCs, platelets
- Blood chemistry: increased transaminase, alkaline phosphatase, and gamma globulin; decreased albumin
- Enzyme linked immunosorbent assay (ELISA): positive HIV antibody titer
- Western blot: positive
- $CD4^+$ level: less than 200

Key diagnostic test findings for AIDS

- ELISA: positive HIV antibody titer
- Western blot: positive
- $CD4^+$ level: less than 200

Medical management

- Diet: high-calorie, high-protein in small, frequent feedings
- I.V. therapy: hydration, electrolyte replacement, and saline lock
- Oxygen therapy
- Position: semi-Fowler's
- Activity: as tolerated, active and passive ROM exercises
- Monitoring: vital signs, I/O, and neurovital signs
- Laboratory studies: WBCs, RBCs, platelets, and albumin
- Nutritional support: TPN
- Treatments: chest physiotherapy, postural drainage, and incentive spirometry
- Precautions: standard
- Transfusion therapy: fresh frozen plasma, platelets, and packed RBCs
- Antibiotics: aerosolized pentamidine (NebuPent), co-trimoxazole (Bactrim)
- Antivirals: dapsone, didanosine (Videx), ganciclovir (Cytovene), zidovudine (Retrovir, AZT), acyclovir (Zovirax), and pentamidine (Pentam)
- Antiretrovirals in various combinations
  - Nucleoside reverse transcriptase inhibitors: zidovudine (Retrovir, AZT), didanosine (Videx), zalcitabine (Dideoxycytidine, ddC), lamivudine (Epivir), abacavir (Ziagen), and stavudine (Zerit)
  - Protease inhibitors: ritonavir (Norvir), indinavir (Crixivan), nelfinavir (Viracept), amprenavir (Agenerase), and saquinavir (Invirase)
  - Nonnucleoside reverse transcriptase inhibitors: nevirapine (Viramune), efavirenz (Sustiva), and delavirdine (Rescriptor)
- Plasmapheresis
- Interferon
- Interleukin II
- Specialized bed: active or static, low air loss (Kin Air, Biodyne)
- Antifungals: fluconazole (Diflucan) and amphotericin B (Fungizone)
- Pulse oximetry
- Antiemetic: prochlorperazine (Compazine)

Main therapies for a patient with AIDS

- Transfusion therapy: fresh frozen plasma, platelets, and packed RBCs
- Antibiotics
- Antivirals
- Antiretrovirals in various combinations

Combinations of antiretrovirals to treat AIDS

- Nucleoside reverse transcriptase inhibitors
- Protease inhibitors
- Nonnucleoside reverse transcriptase inhibitors

Nursing interventions

- Maintain the patient's diet
- Encourage fluids
- Administer I.V. fluids
- Administer oxygen
- Provide incentive spirometry

- Promote turning, coughing, and deep breathing
- Assess respiratory and neurologic status and fluid balance
- Keep the patient in semi-Fowler's position
- Monitor and record vital signs, I/O, laboratory studies, daily weight, specific gravity, and pulse oximetry
- Administer TPN
- Administer medications, as prescribed
- Encourage the patient to express feelings about changes in body image, a fear of dying, and social isolation
- Maintain activity, as tolerated
- Allay the patient's anxiety
- Provide rest periods
- Provide skin and mouth care
- **Maintain standard precautions**
- Monitor for opportunistic infections
- Caution the patient to avoid anal sex
- Caution an I.V. drug user to clean drug paraphernalia with bleach
- Make referrals to community agencies for support
- Individualize home care instructions
  - Refrain from donating blood
  - Avoid using alcohol and recreational drugs
  - Use condoms during sexual intercourse

Complications

- *Pneumocystis carinii* pneumonia
- Cryptococcal meningitis
- Burkitt's lymphoma
- Encephalopathy
- Depression
- Herpes simplex virus
- Cytomegalovirus infection
- Epstein-Barr virus
- Oral and esophageal candidiasis
- Kaposi's sarcoma
- Toxoplasmosis
- *Mycobacterium avium* intracellular infection
- Neuropathies
- Myopathies

Possible surgical intervention

- Bone marrow transplant

IRON DEFICIENCY ANEMIA

Definition

- Chronic, slowly progressive decrease in circulating RBCs

Causes

- Acute and chronic bleeding

Key nursing interventions for a patient with AIDS

- Monitor and record vital signs, I/O, laboratory studies, daily weight, specific gravity, and pulse oximetry.
- Encourage the patient to express his feelings about changes in his body image, a fear of dying, and social isolation.
- Provide skin and mouth care.
- Maintain standard precautions
- Monitor for opportunistic infections.
- Make referrals to community agencies for support.

Key home care instructions for a patient with AIDS

- Refrain from donating blood.
- Avoid using alcohol and recreational drugs.
- Use condoms during sexual intercourse.

Iron deficiency anemia defined

- Chronic, slowly progressive decrease in circulating RBCs
- Iron deficiency caused by inadequate absorption or excessive loss of iron
- Decreased iron affects formation of Hb and RBCs

- Inadequate intake of iron-rich foods
- Gastrectomy
- Malabsorption syndrome
- Vitamin B_6 deficiency
- Pregnancy
- Menstruation
- Alcohol abuse
- Drug induced

Key causes of iron deficiency anemia
- Acute and chronic bleeding
- Gastrectomy
- Malabsorption syndrome
- Vitamin B_6 deficiency

Pathophysiology
- Iron deficiency is caused by inadequate absorption or excessive loss of iron
- Decreased iron affects formation of Hb and RBCs
- Decreased Hb and RBCs reduce the capacity of the blood to transport oxygen to cells

Assessment findings
- Palpitations
- Dizziness
- Sensitivity to cold
- Stomatitis
- Dyspnea
- Weakness and fatigue
- Pale, dry mucous membranes
- Papillae atrophy of the tongue
- Cheilosis
- Pallor
- Koilonychia

Chief assessment findings in iron deficiency anemia
- Sensitivity to cold
- Weakness and fatigue
- Pallor

Diagnostic test findings
- Hematology: decreased Hb, HCT, iron, ferritin, reticulocytes, red cell indices, transferrin saturation; absent hemosiderin; increased iron-binding capacity
- Peripheral blood smear: microcytic and hypochromic RBCs

Hematology test findings
- Decreased Hb, HCT, and iron levels
- Increased iron-binding capacity

Medical management
- Diet: high-iron, high-roughage, high-protein, high-ascorbic acid, high-vitamin with increased fluids; avoid teas
- Oxygen therapy
- Position: semi-Fowler's
- Activity: bed rest
- Monitoring: vital signs and I/O
- Laboratory studies: arterial blood gas (ABG) analysis, Hb, HCT, iron, iron-binding capacity
- Transfusion therapy: packed RBCs
- Antianemics: ferrous sulfate (Feosol), iron dextran (DexFerrum)
- Vitamins: pyridoxine (vitamin B_6), ascorbic acid (vitamin C)

Key management options for iron deficiency anemia
- High-iron, high-roughage, high-protein, high-ascorbic acid, high-vitamin diet with increased fluids; avoid teas
- Antianemics
- Vitamins

Nursing interventions
- Maintain the patient's diet

How to inject iron solutions

For deep I.M. injections of iron solutions, use the Z-track technique to avoid subcutaneous irritation and discoloration from leaking medication.

Choose a 19G to 20G, 2″ to 3″ (5- to 7.5-cm) needle. After drawing up the solution, change to a fresh needle to avoid tracking the solution through the subcutaneous tissue. Draw 0.5 cc of air into the syringe as an "air lock."

Displace the skin and fat at the injection site (in the upper outer quadrant of buttocks or the ventro-gluteal site only) firmly to one side. Clean the area, and insert the needle. Aspirate to check for entry into a blood vessel. Inject the solution slowly, followed by the 0.5 cc of air in the syringe. Wait 10 seconds then pull the needle straight out, and release tissues.

Apply direct pressure to the site, but don't massage it. Caution the patient against vigorous exercise for 15 to 30 minutes.

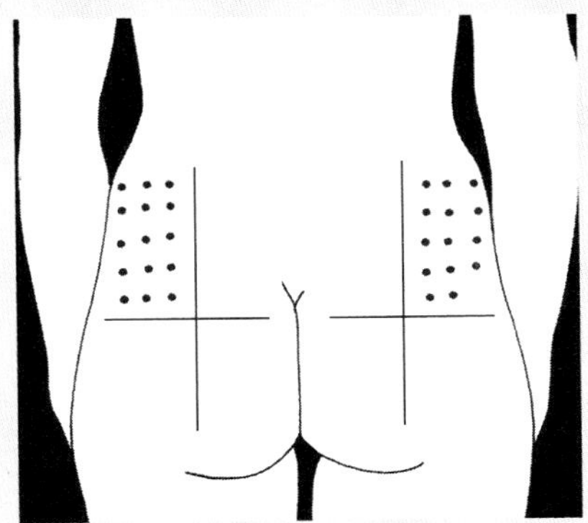

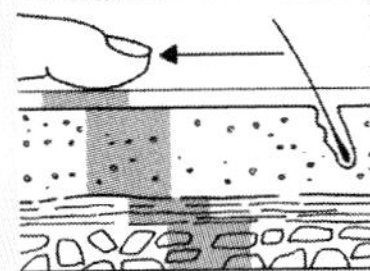

1. Displace tissues.

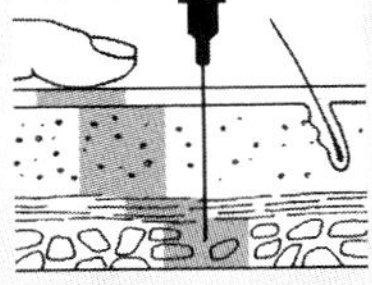

2. Inject solution.

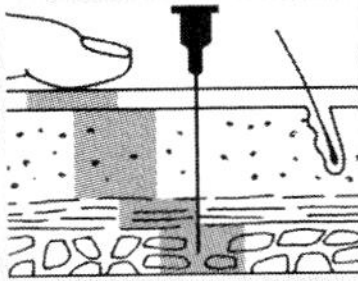

3. Wait 10 seconds.

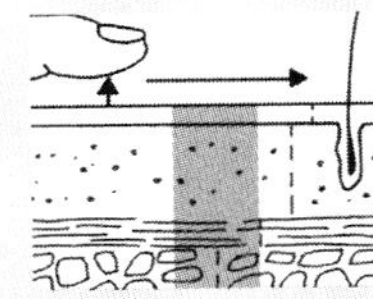

4. Release tissues.

- Encourage fluids
- Administer oxygen, as needed
- Assess cardiovascular and respiratory status
- Keep the patient in semi-Fowler's position
- Monitor and record vital signs, I/O, and laboratory studies
- Administer medications, as prescribed (see *How to inject iron solutions*)
- Allay the patient's anxiety
- Monitor stool, urine, and emesis for occult blood
- Provide rest periods
- Provide mouth, skin, and foot care
- Protect the patient from falls
- Keep the patient warm
- Individualize home care instructions
  - Recognize the signs and symptoms of bleeding
  - Monitor stools for occult blood
  - Avoid using hot pads and hot water bottles

Complications

- Plummer-Vinson syndrome

How to inject iron solutions

- Choose a 19G to 20G needle.
- After drawing up the solution, change to a fresh needle to avoid tracking the solution through the subcutaneous tissue.
- Draw 0.5 cc of air into the syringe as air lock.
- Displace the skin and fat at the injection site firmly to one side.
- Clean the area and insert the needle.
- Aspirate to check for entry into a blood vessel.
- Inject the solution and 0.5 cc of air slowly.
- Wait 10 seconds and draw the needle out, releasing tissues.
- Apply pressure to the site.
- Caution the patient against vigorous exercise for 15 to 30 minutes.

Key nursing interventions for a patient with iron deficiency anemia

- Assess cardiovascular and respiratory status.
- Monitor stool, urine, and emesis for occult blood.
- Provide mouth, skin, and foot care.
- Provide rest periods.

- Angina pectoris
- Heart failure

Possible surgical interventions
- None

Pernicious anemia highlights
- Chronic, progressive macrocytic anemia
- Caused by a deficiency of intrinsic factor

PERNICIOUS ANEMIA

Definition
- Chronic, progressive macrocytic anemia caused by a deficiency of intrinsic factor

Causes
- Deficiency of intrinsic factor
- Gastric mucosal atrophy
- Genetics
- Prolonged iron deficiency
- Autoimmune disease
- Lack of administration of vitamin B_{12} after small-bowel resection or total gastrectomy
- Malabsorption
- Bacterial or parasitic infections

Common causes of pernicious anemia
- Deficiency of intrinsic factor
- Gastric mucosal atrophy
- Genetics
- Prolonged iron deficiency

Pathophysiology
- Without intrinsic factor, dietary vitamin B_{12} can't be absorbed by the ileum
- Normal deoxyribonucleic acid synthesis is inhibited, resulting in defective maturation of cells

Assessment findings
- Weakness
- Pallor
- Dyspnea
- Palpitations
- Fatigue
- Sore mouth
- Glossitis
- Weight loss and anorexia
- Dyspepsia
- Constipation or diarrhea
- Mild jaundice of sclera
- Tingling and paresthesia of hands and feet
- Paralysis
- Depression
- Delirium
- Gait disturbances
- Tachycardia

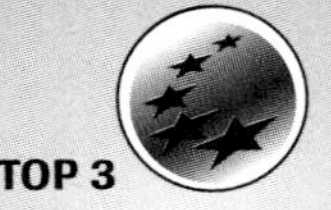

TOP 3

Assessment findings in pernicious anemia
1. Weight loss and anorexia
2. Dyspepsia
3. Tingling and paresthesia of hands and feet

Diagnostic test findings
- Schilling test: positive

Foods high in folic acid

Below is a list of foods high in folic acid.

FOOD	MCG/100 G
Asparagus spears	109
Beef liver	294
Broccoli spears	54
Collards (cooked)	102
Mushrooms	24
Oatmeal	33
Peanut butter	57
Red beans	180
Wheat germ	305

- Romberg test: positive
- Gastric analysis: hypochlorhydria
- Peripheral blood smear: oval, macrocytic, hyperchromic erythrocytes
- Bone marrow: increased megaloblasts; few maturing erythrocytes; defective leukocyte maturation
- Blood chemistry: increased bilirubin and lactate dehydrogenase (LD)
- Hematology: decreased HCT and Hb
- Upper GI series: atrophy of gastric mucosa

Medical management

- Diet: high in iron and protein, with increased intake of vitamin B_{12} and folic acid; restrict highly seasoned, coarse, or extremely hot foods (see *Foods high in folic acid*)
- Position: semi-Fowler's
- Activity: as tolerated
- Monitoring: vital signs and neurovital signs
- Laboratory studies: Hb, HCT, and bilirubin
- Treatment: bed cradle
- Transfusion therapy: packed RBCs
- Antianemics: ferrous sulfate (Feosol) and iron dextran (DexFerrum)
- Vitamins: pyridoxine (vitamin B_6), ascorbic acid (vitamin C), cyanocobalamin (vitamin B_{12}), folic acid (Folvite)

Nursing interventions

- Maintain the patient's diet
- Assess neurologic, cardiovascular, and respiratory status
- Keep the patient in semi-Fowler's position
- Monitor and record vital signs, laboratory studies, and neurovital signs

Foods high in folic acid

- Asparagus spears
- Beef liver
- Broccoli spears
- Collards
- Mushrooms
- Oatmeal
- Peanut butter
- Red beans
- Wheat germ

Key diagnostic test findings in pernicious anemia

- Peripheral blood smear results: oval, macrocytic, hyperchromic erythrocytes
- Bone marrow: increased megaloblasts; few maturing erythrocytes; defective leukocyte maturation

Key management option for pernicious anemia

- Vitamins:
  - Pyridoxine (vitamin B_6)
  - Ascorbic acid (vitamin C)
  - Cyanocobalamin (vitamin B_{12})
  - Folic acid (Folvite)

Key nursing interventions for a patient with pernicious anemia

- Assess neurologic, cardiovascular, and respiratory status.
- Provide mouth care before and after meals.
- Use soft toothbrushes when brushing the patient's teeth.
- Prevent the patient from falling.

Common complications of pernicious anemia

- Chronic renal failure
- Arrhythmias
- Gastric cancer
- GI bleeding

Aplastic anemia defined

- Failure of bone marrow to produce adequate amounts of erythrocytes, leukocytes, and platelets
- Primarily idiopathic cause

- Administer medications, as prescribed
- Allay the patient's anxiety
- Maintain activity, as tolerated
- Provide treatments: bed cradle
- Monitor and record amount, consistency, and color of stools
- Provide mouth care before and after meals
- Use soft toothbrushes when brushing the patient's teeth
- Maintain warm environment
- Provide foot and skin care
- Prevent the patient from falling
- Individualize home care instructions
  - Recognize the signs and symptoms of skin breakdown
  - Alter activities of daily living (ADLs) to compensate for paresthesia
  - Comply with lifelong, monthly injections of vitamin B_{12}
  - Avoid using heating pads and electric blankets

Complications
- Chronic renal failure
- Arrhythmias
- Gastric cancer
- GI bleeding
- Heart failure
- Angina
- Neurogenic bladder
- Stroke

Possible surgical interventions
- None

APLASTIC ANEMIA (PANCYTOPENIA)

Definition
- Failure of bone marrow to produce adequate amounts of erythrocytes, leukocytes, and platelets

Causes
- Idiopathic
- Exposure to chemicals
- Drug induced: chloramphenicol (Chloromycetin), phenylbutazone (Butazolidin), phenytoin (Dilantin)
- Chemotherapy
- Radiation
- Viral hepatitis

Pathophysiology
- Bone marrow suppression, destruction, or aplasia results in failure of bone marrow to produce an adequate number of stem cells
- Without an adequate number of stem cells, sufficient amounts of erythrocytes, leukocytes, and platelets can't be produced
- Pancytopenia includes leukopenia, thrombocytopenia, and anemia

Assessment findings

- Fatigue
- Dyspnea
- Multiple infections
- Elevated temperature
- Headache
- Weakness
- Anorexia
- Gingivitis
- Epistaxis
- Purpura
- Petechiae
- Ecchymosis
- Pallor
- Palpitations
- Tachycardia
- Tachypnea
- Melena

Diagnostic test findings

- Peripheral blood smear: pancytopenia
- Hematology: decreased granulocytes, thrombocytes, RBCs
- Fecal occult blood: positive
- Urine chemistry: hematuria
- Bone marrow biopsy: fatty marrow with reduction of stem cells

Medical management

- Diet: high-protein, high-calorie, high-vitamin
- I.V. therapy: hydration and saline lock
- Oxygen therapy
- Position: semi-Fowler's
- Activity: as tolerated
- Monitoring: vital signs and I/O
- Laboratory studies: RBCs, WBCs, platelets, and stool for occult blood
- Treatments: tepid sponge baths and cooling blankets
- Precautions: protective
- Transfusion therapy: platelets and packed RBCs
- Antibiotics: penicillin G (Pentids), ticarcillin (Ticar), and tobramycin (Nebcin)
- Analgesics: ibuprofen (Motrin) and acetaminophen (Tylenol)
- Antithymocyte globulin (ATG)
- Androgenic steroids: fluoxymesterone (Halotestin) and oxymethalone (Anadrol)
- Recombinant human granulocyte-macrophage colony stimulating factor (GM-CSF)
- Hematopoietic growth factor: epoetin alfa (Epogen)

Nursing interventions

- Maintain the patient's diet

Key assessment findings in aplastic anemia

- Dyspnea
- Multiple infections
- Epistaxis
- Purpura
- Petechiae
- Ecchymosis
- Pallor
- Palpitations
- Tachycardia
- Tachypnea
- Melena

Key test findings in aplastic anemia

- Hematology: decreased granulocytes, thrombocytes, RBCs
- Bone marrow biopsy: fatty marrow with reduction of stem cells

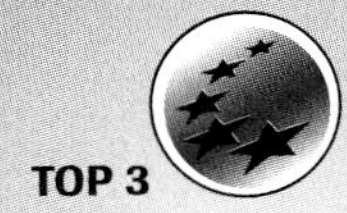

TOP 3

Therapy options for aplastic anemia

1. Transfusion therapy: platelets and packed RBCs
2. ATG
3. Hematopoietic growth factor

Key nursing interventions for a patient with aplastic anemia

- Administer oxygen.
- Monitor and record vital signs; I/O; laboratory studies; stool, urine, and emesis for occult blood; and specific gravity.
- Administer transfusion therapy, as prescribed.
- Maintain protective precautions.
- Avoid giving the patient I.M. injections.
- Monitor for infection, bleeding, and bruising.

Key home care instructions for a patient with aplastic anemia

- Recognize the signs and symptoms of bleeding.
- Avoid taking aspirin.

ITP defined

- Increased premature destruction of platelets
- Decreased number of circulating platelets causes bleeding

- Encourage fluids
- Administer I.V. fluids
- Administer oxygen
- Promote turning, coughing, and deep breathing
- Assess cardiovascular and respiratory status and fluid balance
- Keep the patient in semi-Fowler's position
- Monitor and record vital signs; I/O; laboratory studies; stool, urine, and emesis for occult blood; and specific gravity
- Administer transfusion therapy, as prescribed
- Administer medications, as prescribed
- Allay the patient's anxiety
- Alternate rest periods with activity
- Provide cooling blankets and tepid sponge baths
- Maintain protective precautions
- Provide mouth care before and after meals
- Provide skin care
- Protect the patient from falls
- **Avoid giving the patient I.M. injections**
- Avoid using hard toothbrushes and straight razors on the patient
- Monitor for infection, bleeding, and bruising
- Individualize home care instructions
  - Recognize the signs and symptoms of bleeding
  - Avoid contact sports
  - Wear medical identification jewelry
  - Avoid using over-the-counter medications
  - Monitor stool for occult blood
  - Use an electric razor
  - Avoid taking aspirin

Complications

- Hemorrhage
- Infection
- Septicemia
- Stroke
- GI bleeding

Possible surgical interventions

- Bone marrow transplant
- Splenectomy

IDIOPATHIC THROMBOCYTOPENIC PURPURA (ITP)

Definition

- Increased premature destruction of platelets

Causes

- Unknown
- Autoimmune disease

- Viral infection

Pathophysiology

- Antibody-coated platelets are removed from circulation by reticuloendothelial cells of the spleen and liver
- Decreased number of circulating platelets causes bleeding

Assessment findings

- Petechiae
- Ecchymosis
- Epistaxis
- Gingivitis
- Vision disturbances
- Dizziness
- Menorrhagia
- Hematomas
- Increased bleeding after dental extraction
- GI bleeding

Diagnostic test findings

- Hematology: decreased Hb, HCT, and platelets; normal PT and PTT; prolonged bleeding time
- Urine chemistry: hematuria
- Fecal occult blood: positive
- Blood chemistry: increased immunoglobulins, complement fixation
- Bone marrow biopsy: increased and abnormal megakaryocytes
- Rumpel-Leede capillary fragility tourniquet test: positive with increased capillary fragility

Medical management

- Diet: soft and bland
- I.V. therapy: saline lock
- Activity: bed rest
- Monitoring: vital signs, daily weight, and stool for occult blood
- Laboratory studies: Hb, HCT, and platelets
- Precautions: protective
- Transfusion therapy: fresh frozen plasma, platelets, packed RBCs, and plasma
- IgG antibody: immune globulin I.V. (Gammagard)
- Stool softener: docusate (Colace)
- Immunosuppressants: azathioprine (Imuran), cyclophosphamide (Cytoxan), vincristine (Oncovin)
- Anabolic steroid: danazol (Cyclomen)
- Corticosteroid: prednisone (Deltasone)

Nursing interventions

- Maintain the patient's diet
- Encourage fluids
- Administer I.V. fluids and transfusion therapy
- Assess for bruising, bleeding, and infection

Key assessment findings in ITP

- Petechiae
- Ecchymosis
- Epistaxis

Key diagnostic test findings in ITP

- Hematology: decreased Hb, HCT, and platelets; normal PT and PTT; prolonged bleeding time
- Bone marrow biopsy: increased and abnormal megakaryocytes

Key medications for treating ITP

- IgG antibody: immune globulin I.V.
- Corticosteroids

Key steps in monitoring a patient with ITP

- Assess for bruising, bleeding, and infection.
- Monitor and record vital signs; I/O; laboratory studies; daily weight; stool, urine, and emesis for occult blood; neurovital signs; pad count; and blood loss.
- Protect the patient from falls.
- Rotate extremities for blood pressure monitoring.

Key home care instructions for a patient with aplastic anemia

- Recognize the signs and symptoms of bleeding.
- Wear medical identification jewelry.
- Use electric razors and soft toothbrushes.

Characteristics of polycythemia vera

- Myeloproliferative disorder
- Results in the increased production of erythrocytes, Hb, myelocytes, and thrombocytes
- Overproduction causes increased blood viscosity, increased total blood volume, and severe congestion of all tissues and organs

- Monitor and record vital signs; I/O; laboratory studies; daily weight; stool, urine, and emesis for occult blood; neurovital signs; pad count; and blood loss
- Administer medications, as prescribed
- Allay the patient's anxiety
- Provide gentle mouth care
- Protect the patient from falls
- Avoid giving the patient I.M. injections, aspirin, enemas, and rectal temperatures
- Avoid using straight razors, tape, and tourniquets on the patient
- Alternate rest periods with activity
- **Rotate extremities for blood pressure monitoring**
- Individualize home care instructions
  - Recognize the signs and symptoms of bleeding
  - Avoid contact sports
  - Wear medical identification jewelry
  - Use electric razors and soft toothbrushes
  - Avoid sneezing, coughing, nose blowing, straining while defecating, and heavy lifting
  - Avoid using over-the-counter medications

Complications

- Hypersplenism
- Stroke
- Shock
- Hemothorax
- Peripheral paralysis and paresthesia
- Bleeding into diaphragm

Possible surgical intervention

- Splenectomy

POLYCYTHEMIA VERA

Definition

- Myeloproliferative disorder that results in the increased production of erythrocytes, Hb, myelocytes, and thrombocytes

Causes

- Unknown
- Hypernephroma
- Hepatoma
- Uterine fibroids
- Pheochromocytoma
- Lung tumors
- Adrenal cancer
- Cerebral hemangioblastoma

Pathophysiology

- Hyperplasia of bone marrow results in increased production of erythrocytes, Hb, granulocytes, and platelets
- Overproduction results in increased blood viscosity, increased total blood volume, and severe congestion of all tissues and organs

Assessment findings

- Ruddy complexion
- Dusky mucosa
- Vertigo
- Headaches
- Dizziness
- Dyspnea and orthopnea
- Tachycardia
- Ecchymosis
- Hepatomegaly and splenomegaly
- Increased gastric secretions
- Weakness and fatigue
- Pruritus
- Epistaxis
- GI bleeding
- Angina

Diagnostic test findings

- Blood chemistry: increased uric acid, unconjugated bilirubin, vitamin B_{12}, alkaline phosphatase, serum aspartate aminotransferase (AST), serum alanine aminotransferase (ALT), and LD
- Hematology: increased RBCs, WBCs, platelets, HCT, and Hb
- Bone marrow biopsy: increased number of immature cell forms and decreased iron in marrow
- Urine chemistry: hematuria
- Stool specimen: positive for blood
- ABG analysis: normal partial pressure of arterial oxygen

Medical management

- Diet: soft foods, low-iron
- I.V. therapy: saline lock
- Activity: as tolerated
- Monitoring: vital signs, CVP, I/O, and neurovital signs
- Laboratory studies: Hb, HCT, WBCs, RBCs, platelets, and unconjugated bilirubin
- Treatment: tepid sponge baths
- Analgesic: acetaminophen (Tylenol)
- Antacids: magnesium and aluminum hydroxide (Maalox) and aluminum hydroxide gel (AlternaGEL)
- Histamine antagonists: cimetidine (Tagamet) and ranitidine (Zantac)
- Antihistamine: diphenhydramine (Benadryl)
- Antigouts: colchicine (Colchicine) and allopurinol (Zyloprim)
- Radioactive phosphorus

Key signs and symptoms of polycythemia vera

- Ruddy complexion
- Headaches
- Dizziness
- Dyspnea and orthopnea

Key diagnostic test findings in polycythemia vera

- Blood chemistry: increased uric acid, unconjugated bilirubin, vitamin B_{12}, alkaline phosphatase, serum AST, serum ALT, and LD
- Hematology: increased RBCs, WBCs, platelets, HCT, and Hb
- Bone marrow biopsy: increased number of immature cell forms and decreased iron in marrow

Key therapies to treat polycythemia vera

- Antigout agents
- Phlebotomy
- Myelosuppressants

- Phlebotomy
- Myelosuppressants: busulfan (Myleran), chlorambucil (Leukeran), and cyclophosphamide (Cytoxan)
- Mucosal barrier fortifier: sucralfate (Carafate)

Nursing interventions
- Maintain the patient's diet
- Encourage fluids
- Assess cardiovascular and respiratory status
- Keep the patient in semi-Fowler's position
- Monitor and record vital signs, I/O, laboratory studies, CVP, neurovital signs, and fecal occult blood
- Administer medications, as prescribed
- Allay the patient's anxiety
- Protect the patient from falls
- Provide treatments: tepid baths and ROM exercises
- Provide postchemotherapeutic and postradiation nursing care
  - Provide prophylactic skin, mouth, and perineal care
  - Monitor dietary intake
  - Administer antiemetics and antidiarrheals, as prescribed
  - Monitor for bleeding, infection, and electrolyte imbalance
  - Provide rest periods
- Individualize home care instructions
  - Recognize the signs and symptoms of heart failure and thrombophlebitis
  - Avoid taking hot showers

Complications
- Hypertension
- Heart failure
- Stroke
- Myocardial infarction
- Deep vein thrombosis
- Hemorrhage
- Peptic ulcer
- Gout
- Acute leukemia

Possible surgical interventions
- None

DISSEMINATED INTRAVASCULAR COAGULATION (DIC)

Definition
- Body's response to injury or disease in which widespread clotting in small vessels obstructs blood supply of organs, causing clotting factors and platelets to be used up and hemorrhage to occur throughout the body

Key nursing steps for a patient with polycythemia vera

- Encourage fluids.
- Assess cardiovascular and respiratory status.
- Monitor and record vital signs, I/O, laboratory studies, CVP, neurovital signs, and fecal occult blood.

Key steps after chemotherapy and radiation

- Provide prophylactic skin, mouth, and perineal care.
- Monitor for bleeding, infection, and electrolyte imbalance.

DIC defined

- Body's response to injury or disease in which widespread clotting in small vessels obstructs blood supply of organs
- Causes clotting factors and platelets to be used up and hemorrhage to occur throughout the body

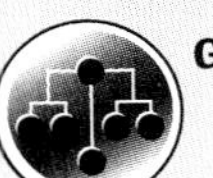

GO WITH THE FLOW

Understanding DIC

This simplified illustration shows the pathophysiology of disseminated intravascular coagulation (DIC). Circulating thrombin activates coagulation and fibrinolysis, leading to paradoxical bleeding and clotting.

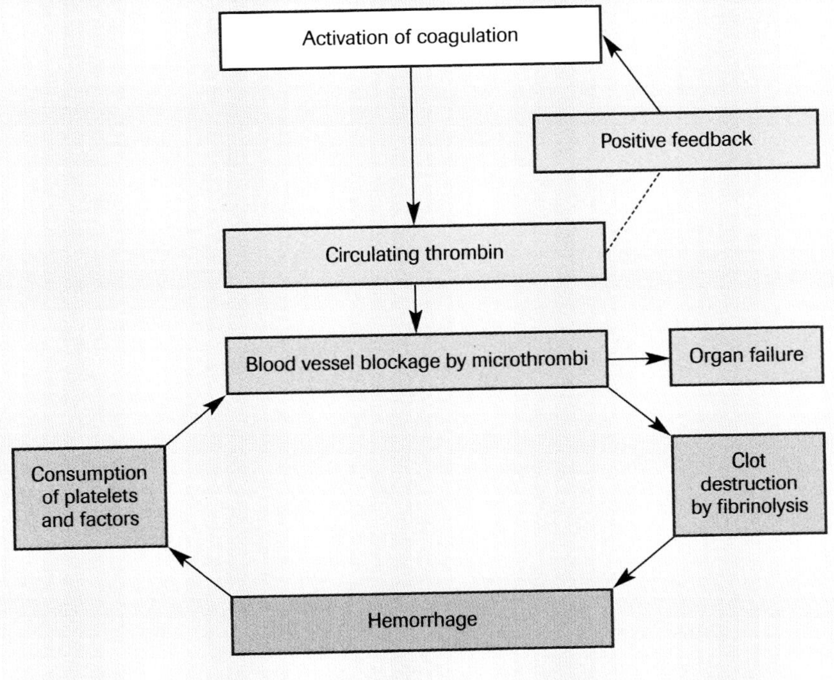

Causes

- Unknown
- Frequent, rapid transfusions
- Gram-negative sepsis
- Neoplastic disease
- Massive burns
- Massive trauma
- Anaphylaxis
- Chronic disease

Pathophysiology

- Underlying disease causes release of thromboplastic substances that promote the deposition of fibrin throughout the microcirculation (see *Understanding DIC*)
- RBCs are trapped in fibrin strands and are hemolyzed
- Platelets, prothrombin, and other clotting factors are destroyed, leading to bleeding

Pathophysiology of DIC

- Activation of coagulation
- Circulating thrombin
- Blood vessel blockage by microthrombi
- Organ failure
- Clot destruction by fibrinolysis
- Hemorrhage
- Consumption of platelets and factors

Most common causes of DIC

- Unknown cause
- Frequent, rapid transfusions
- Gram-negative sepsis

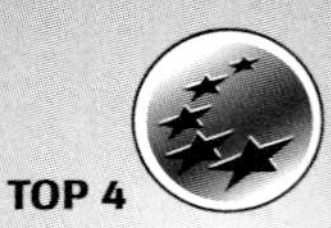

TOP 4
DIC assessment findings

1. Petechiae
2. Ecchymosis
3. Hemorrhage
4. Oliguria

Key test findings for DIC

- Hematology: decreased platelets, RBCs, fibrinogen, and factor assay (II, V, VII); increased fibrin split products, thrombin, PT, and PTT; positive protamine sulfate test
- Urine chemistry: hematuria

Key treatment options for DIC

- Transfusion therapy: platelets, packed RBCs, fresh frozen plasma, whole blood, volume expanders, and cryoprecipitates
- Anticoagulants

- Excessive clotting activates the fibrinolytic system that inhibits platelet function, causing further bleeding
- Acute activation of clotting mechanism results in consumption of plasma-clotting factors that the liver can't replenish quickly enough
- Activation of the thrombin and fibrinolytic system results in simultaneous bleeding and thrombosis

Assessment findings

- Petechiae
- Ecchymosis
- Prolonged bleeding after venipuncture
- Hemorrhage
- Oliguria
- Anxiety
- Restlessness
- Purpura
- Acrocyanosis
- Joint pain
- Dyspnea
- Hemoptysis
- Crackles

Diagnostic test findings

- Hematology: decreased platelets, RBCs, fibrinogen, and factor assay (II, V, VII); increased fibrin split products, thrombin, PT, and PTT; positive protamine sulfate test
- Urine chemistry: hematuria
- ABG analysis: metabolic acidosis
- Ophthalmoscopic exam: retinal hemorrhage
- Fecal occult blood: positive

Medical management

- Diet: withhold food and fluids
- I.V. therapy: hydration, electrolyte replacement, and saline lock
- Oxygen therapy
- Intubation and mechanical ventilation
- GI decompression: NG tube
- Position: semi-Fowler's
- Activity: bed rest and active and passive ROM exercises
- Monitoring: vital signs, I/O, electrocardiogram, and hemodynamic variables
- Laboratory studies: PT, PTT, platelets, fibrinogen, and fibrin split products
- Nutritional support: TPN
- Treatment: indwelling urinary catheter
- Transfusion therapy: platelets, packed RBCs, fresh frozen plasma, whole blood, volume expanders, and cryoprecipitates
- Glucocorticoids: prednisone (Deltasone) and hydrocortisone (Cortef)
- Analgesics: ibuprofen (Motrin) and acetaminophen (Tylenol)
- Antacids: magnesium and aluminum hydroxide (Maalox) and aluminum hydroxide gel (AlternaGEL)

- Stool softener: docusate (Colace)
- Anticoagulant: heparin
- Hemodialysis
- Precautions: seizure
- Pulse oximetry

Nursing interventions

- Withhold food and fluids
- Administer I.V. fluids
- Administer oxygen
- Provide suction, as necessary
- Promote turning, coughing, and deep breathing
- Assess cardiovascular and respiratory status and fluid balance
- Maintain position, patency, and low suction of NG tube
- Irrigate NG tube gently
- Keep the patient in semi-Fowler's position
- Monitor and record vital signs, I/O, laboratory studies, hemodynamic variables, neurovital signs, fecal occult blood, and pulse oximetry
- Administer TPN
- Administer medications, as prescribed
- Allay the patient's anxiety
- Maintain bed rest
- Provide gentle mouth and skin care
- Avoid giving the patient I.M. injections, enemas, and rectal temperatures
- Avoid using straight razors and tape on the patient
- **Rotate extremities for blood pressure monitoring**
- Maintain seizure precautions
- Administer transfusion therapy, as prescribed
- Maintain endotracheal tube to mechanical ventilator
- Individualize home care instructions
  - Recognize the signs and symptoms of occult bleeding
  - Wear medical identification jewelry
  - Avoid straining while defecating
  - Avoid using enemas
  - Avoid using over-the-counter medications, especially aspirin
  - Monitor stool for occult blood
  - Use an electric razor

Complications

- Acute renal failure
- Shock
- Stroke
- Convulsions
- Hemothorax
- Hemorrhage
- Coma

Possible surgical interventions

- None

Key nursing interventions for a patient with DIC

- Assess cardiovascular and respiratory status and fluid balance.
- Monitor and record vital signs, I/O, laboratory studies, hemodynamic variables, neurovital signs, fecal occult blood, and pulse oximetry.
- Maintain bed rest.
- Provide gentle mouth and skin care.
- Rotate extremities for blood pressure monitoring.
- Administer transfusion therapy, as prescribed.
- Avoid giving the patient I.M. injections, enemas, and rectal temperatures.

Key home care instructions for a patient with DIC

- Recognize the signs and symptoms of occult bleeding.
- Monitor stool for occult blood.
- Avoid using over-the-counter medications, especially aspirin.
- Use an electric razor.

MULTIPLE MYELOMA

Definition
- Abnormal proliferation of plasma cells in the bone marrow

Causes
- Unknown
- Genetic
- Environmental

Pathophysiology
- Single tumor in bone marrow disseminates into lymph nodes, liver, spleen, kidneys, and bone
- Plasma cell tumors produce abnormal amounts of immunoglobulins
- Tumor cells trigger osteoblastic activity, leading to bone destruction throughout the body

Assessment findings
- Headaches
- Constant, severe bone pain
- Pathologic fractures
- Skeletal deformities of sternum and ribs
- Renal calculi
- Multiple infections
- Hepatomegaly
- Splenomegaly
- Loss of height
- Hemorrhage

Diagnostic test findings
- X-ray: diffuse, round, punched out bone lesions; osteoporosis; osteolytic lesions of the skull; and widespread demineralization
- Bone scan: increased uptake
- Bone marrow biopsy: increased number of immature plasma cells
- Hematology: decreased HCT, WBCs, and platelets; increased ESR
- Blood chemistry: increased calcium, uric acid, BUN, creatinine, globulins, and protein; decreased albumin-globulin ratio
- Urine chemistry: increased calcium and uric acid
- Immunoelectrophoresis: monoclonal spike
- Bence Jones protein assay: positive

Medical management
- Diet: high-protein, high-carbohydrate, high-vitamin and mineral in small, frequent feedings
- I.V. therapy: hydration, electrolyte replacement, and saline lock
- Activity: as tolerated
- Monitoring: vital signs, I/O, and neurovital signs
- Laboratory studies: HCT, calcium, BUN, creatinine, uric acid, WBCs, protein, platelets, and surveillance cultures
- Radiation therapy

Multiple myeloma

- Abnormal proliferation of plasma cells in the bone marrow
- Plasma cells produce abnormal amounts of immunoglobulins, which triggers osteoblastic activity

Key assessment findings in multiple myeloma

- Constant, severe bone pain
- Pathologic fractures
- Hemorrhage
- Multiple infections

X-ray findings in multiple myeloma

- Diffuse, round, punched out bone lesions
- Osteoporosis
- Osteolytic lesions of the skull
- Widespread demineralization

- Chemotherapy
- Precautions: seizure
- Transfusion therapy: packed RBCs
- Antibiotics: doxorubicin (Adriamycin) and plicamycin (Mithracin)
- Antigout: allopurinol (Zyloprim)
- Alkylating agents: melphalan (Alkeran) and cyclophosphamide (Cytoxan)
- Antineoplastics: vinblastine (Velban) and vincristine (Oncovin)
- Analgesic: meperidine (Demerol)
- Diuretic: furosemide (Lasix)
- Glucocorticoid: prednisone (Deltasone)
- Antacids: magnesium and aluminum hydroxide (Maalox) and aluminum hydroxide gel (AlternaGEL)
- Androgen: fluoxymesterone (Halotestin)
- Orthopedic devices: braces, splints, and casts
- Peritoneal and hemodialysis
- Antiemetic: prochlorperazine (Compazine)

Nursing interventions

- Maintain the patient's diet
- Encourage fluids
- Administer I.V. fluids
- Promote turning, coughing, and deep breathing
- Assess renal, cardiovascular, and respiratory status and fluid balance
- Monitor and record vital signs, I/O, laboratory studies, specific gravity, daily weight, urine and stool for occult blood, and neurovital signs
- Administer transfusion therapy, as prescribed
- Administer medications, as prescribed
- Allay the patient's anxiety
- Maintain seizure precautions
- Provide skin and mouth care
- Alternate rest periods with activity
- Monitor for infection and bruising
- Prevent the patient from falling
- Provide postchemotherapeutic and postradiation nursing care
  - Provide prophylactic skin, mouth, and perineal care
  - Monitor dietary intake
  - Administer antiemetics and antidiarrheals, as prescribed
  - Monitor for bleeding, infection, and electrolyte imbalance
  - Provide rest periods
- Assess bone pain
- Move the patient gently
- Apply and maintain braces, splints, and casts
- Individualize home care instructions
  - Provide information about the American Cancer Society
  - Exercise regularly, with particular attention to muscle-strengthening exercises
  - Recognize the signs and symptoms of renal calculi, fractures, and seizures

Key treatment options for a patient with multiple myeloma

- Antibiotics
- Antigout agents
- Alkylating agents
- Antineoplastics
- Glucocorticoid
- Androgen

Key nursing interventions for a patient with multiple myeloma

- Administer I.V. fluids.
- Assess renal, cardiovascular, and respiratory status and fluid balance.
- Monitor for infection and bruising.
- Provide postchemotherapeutic and postradiation nursing care.
- Assess bone pain.
- Move the patient gently.

Key nursing interventions after chemotherapy and radiation

- Provide prophylactic skin, mouth, and perineal care.
- Administer antiemetics and antidiarrheals, as prescribed.
- Monitor for bleeding, infection, and electrolyte imbalance.

- Limit activities, such as avoiding lifting
- Take measures to avoid constipation
- Avoid over-the-counter medications
- Monitor urine, stool, and emesis for occult blood
- Use braces, splints, and casts

Key home care instructions for a patient with multiple myeloma

- Exercise regularly, with particular attention to muscle-strengthening exercises.
- Recognize the signs and symptoms of renal calculi, fractures, and seizures.

Complications

- Paraplegia
- Acute renal failure
- Hemorrhage
- Infection
- Urolithiasis
- Pathologic fractures
- Seizures
- Gout

Possible surgical interventions

- None

HEMOPHILIA

Hemophilia highlights

- Hereditary bleeding disorder
- Two types: hemophilia A and hemophilia B

Definition

- Hereditary bleeding disorder
- Two types
  - Hemophilia A — most common type caused by deficiency of factor VIII
  - Hemophilia B — deficiency of factor IX

Causes

- Inherited as X-linked traits, primarily by males
- Asymptomatic mothers and sisters as carriers

Pathophysiology

- Hemophilia A: deficiency of factor VIII causes extended clotting time
- Hemophilia B: deficiency of factor IX causes extended clotting time

Common signs and symptoms of hemophilia

- Bleeding into muscles, joints, and soft tissues after minimal trauma
- Pain in joints
- Joint swelling
- Spontaneous hematuria

Assessment findings

- Large spreading bruises
- Bleeding into muscles, joints, and soft tissues after minimal trauma
- Pain in joints
- Joint swelling and limited ROM
- Recurrent joint hemorrhages
- Spontaneous hematuria
- Spontaneous GI bleeding

Diagnostic test findings

- HCT and Hb: decreased
- Coagulation time: prolonged
- Bleeding time: normal
- PT and PTT: normal
- Platelet function and count: normal
- Factor VIII: missing (Hemophilia A)

- Factor IX: missing (Hemophilia B)

Medical management

- Activity: as tolerated
- Monitoring: vital signs and I/O
- Laboratory studies: HCT, Hb, and coagulation time
- I.V. therapy: saline lock, whole blood, blood components, and I.V. fluids
- Nonsteroidal anti-inflammatory drug (NSAID): ibuprofen (Motrin)
- Stool softener: docusate (Colace)
- Treatment: cold compresses
- Hemostatic: factor VIII concentrate (Hemophilia A) or factor IX concentrate (Hemophilia B)
- Hemostatic: aminocaproic acid (Amicar)
- Corticosteroid: hydrocortisone (Solu-Cortef)
- Vasopressor: desmopressin (DDAVP)

Nursing interventions

- Assess the patient for internal bleeding, hematuria, melena, hematemesis, joint space hemorrhages, and muscle hematomas
- Assess cardiac, renal, and respiratory status
- Monitor and record vital signs, I/O, and laboratory studies
- Administer medications, as prescribed
- Allay the patient's anxiety
- Provide skin and mouth care
- Administer I.V. fluids, blood, and blood components, as prescribed
- Turn the patient every 2 hours if on bed rest
- Use padded side rails
- Assess the location and intensity of pain, and medicate, as necessary
- **Avoid aspirin and I.M. injections**
- **Apply gentle pressure to external bleeding sites**
- Apply cold compresses, as prescribed
- Individualize home care instructions
  - Make the patient aware that there's a potential for hemorrhage with dental extractions and surgery
  - Administer factor VIII or factor IX at first sign of bleeding
  - Avoid nose blowing, coughing, straining while defecating, and lifting
  - Maintain regular dental hygiene appointments
  - Wear joint and muscle splints and orthopedics, as prescribed
  - Use soft toothbrush
  - Use cane or crutches, as directed
  - Use electric razor
  - Prevent stress on joints
  - Take warm baths for joint pain unless there's active bleeding
  - Avoid contact sports

Complications

- Ankylosis
- Hypovolemia
- Shock

TOP 4

Therapy options for hemophilia

1. Factor VIII concentrate for hemophilia A
2. Factor IX concentrate for hemophilia B
3. Aminocaproic acid
4. Desmopressin

Key nursing interventions for a patient with hemophilia

- Assess the patient for internal bleeding, hematuria, melena, hematemesis, joint space hemorrhages, and muscle hematomas.
- Assess cardiac, renal, and respiratory status.
- Administer I.V. fluids, blood, and blood components, as prescribed.
- Avoid aspirin and I.M. injections.
- Apply gentle pressure to external bleeding sites.
- Apply cold compresses, as prescribed.

- Hematuria
- GI bleeding
- Hematemesis
- Melena
- Sensitization to antihemolytic factor

Possible surgical interventions

- None

SICKLE CELL ANEMIA

Sickle cell anemia defined

- Congenital hemolytic anemia resulting from a defective Hb molecule (Hb S)
- Causes RBCs to roughen and become sickle-shaped

Definition

- Congenital hemolytic anemia resulting from a defective Hb molecule (Hb S) that causes RBCs to roughen and become sickle-shaped

Causes

- Genetic inheritance: The disease results from homozygous inheritance of an autosomal recessive gene that produces a defective Hb molecule
- Occurs primarily in persons of African and Mediterranean descent, but it also affects other populations

Pathophysiology

- A change in the gene that encodes the beta chain of Hb results in a defect in Hb (Hb S)
- When hypoxia occurs, Hb S in the RBCs becomes insoluble
- The cells become rigid and rough, forming an elongated sickle shape and impairing circulation (see *Characteristics of sickled cells*)
- Infection, stress, dehydration, and conditions that provoke hypoxia may lead to periodic crisis
- Crises can occur in different forms, including painful crisis, aplastic crisis, and acute sequestration crisis

Key signs and symptoms of sickle cell anemia

- Aching bones
- Jaundice or pallor
- Tachycardia
- Dyspnea

Assessment findings

- Sickle cell anemia
  - Aching bones
  - Chronic fatigue
  - Frequent infections
  - Jaundice or pallor
  - Joint swelling
  - Leg ulcers (especially on ankles)
  - Severe localized and generalized pain
  - Tachycardia
  - Dyspnea
  - Unexplained, painful erections (priapism)
- Sickle cell crisis (general symptoms)
  - Hematuria
  - Irritability
  - Lethargy
  - Pale lips, tongue, palms, and nail beds
  - Severe pain

Key signs and symptoms of sickle cell crisis

- Hematuria
- Pale lips, tongue, and nail beds
- Severe pain

Characteristics of sickled cells

Normal red blood cells (RBCs) and sickled cells vary in shape, life span, oxygen-carrying capacity, and the rate at which they're destroyed. This illustration shows normal and sickled cells and lists the major differences.

NORMAL RBCS
- 120-day life span
- Hemoglobin (Hb) has normal oxygen-carrying capacity
- 12 to 14 g/ml of Hb
- RBCs destroyed at normal rate

SICKLED CELLS
- 30- to 40-day life span
- Hb has decreased oxygen-carrying capacity
- 6 to 9 g/ml of Hb
- RBCs destroyed at accelerated rate

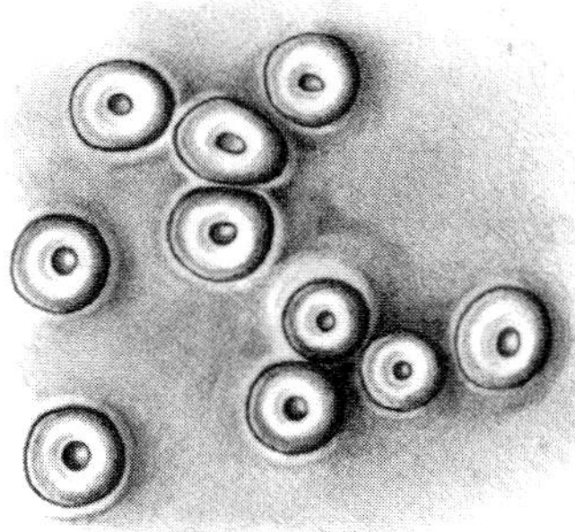

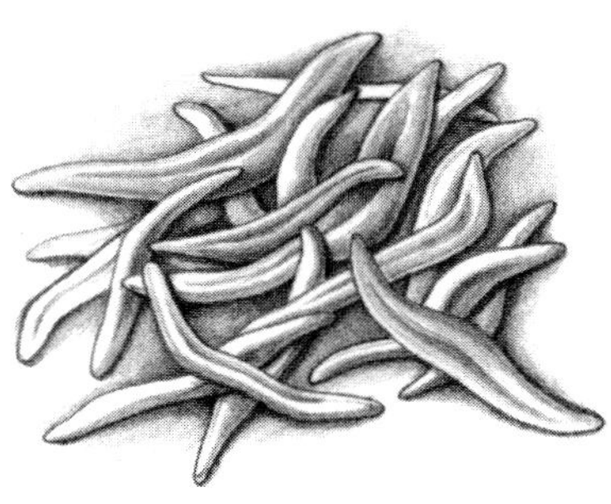

- Painful crisis (vaso-occlusive crisis, which appears periodically after age 5)
  - Dark urine
  - Low-grade fever
  - Severe abdominal, thoracic, muscle, or bone pain
  - Tissue anoxia and necrosis, caused by blood vessel obstruction by tangled sickle cells
  - Worsening jaundice
- Aplastic crisis (generally associated with viral infection)
  - Dyspnea
  - Lethargy and sleepiness
  - Markedly decreased bone marrow activity
  - Pallor
  - Possible coma
  - RBC hemolysis
- Acute sequestration crisis (rare; occurs in infants ages 8 months to 2 years)
  - Hypovolemic shock
  - Lethargy
  - Liver congestion and enlargement
  - Pallor
  - Worsened chronic jaundice

Characteristics of sickled cells
- 30- to 40-day life span
- Hb has decreased oxygen-carrying capacity
- 6 to 9 g/ml of Hb
- RBCs destroyed at accelerated rate

Key signs and symptoms of painful crisis
- Severe abdominal, thoracic, muscle, or bone pain
- Tissue anoxia and necrosis
- Worsening jaundice

Key signs and symptoms of acute sequestration crisis
- Hypovolemic shock
- Liver congestion and enlargement
- Worsened chronic jaundice

Diagnostic test findings

- Hematologic studies: low RBCs, elevated WBCs and platelets, decreased ESR, increased serum iron levels, decreased RBC survival, and reticulocytosis
- Hb electrophoresis: Hb S
- Hb levels: low or normal
- Stained blood smear: shows sickle cells
- Lateral chest X-ray: "Lincoln log" deformity in the vertebrae

Key diagnostic test findings for sickle cell anemia

- Hematologic studies: low RBCs, elevated WBCs and platelets, decreased ESR, increased serum iron levels, decreased RBC survival, and reticulocytosis
- Hb electrophoresis: Hb S

Medical management

- Activity: bed rest during a crisis
- Nutritional supplements: iron, folic acid, and increased fluid intake
- Monitoring: vital signs and I/O
- Laboratory studies: HCT, Hb, RBC, WBC, platelets, ESR, and serum iron levels
- I.V. therapy: saline lock and hydration
- Treatments: warm compresses
- Blood transfusions
- Analgesics: meperidine (Demerol) and morphine
- Analgesic or antipyretic: aspirin and acetaminophen (Tylenol)
- Antineoplastic: hydroxyurea
- Oxygen therapy
- Position: for comfort
- Antibiotics: according to culture and sensitivity reports
- Genetic counseling

Common treatments for sickle cell anemia

- Nutritional supplements: iron, folic acid, and increased fluid intake
- Analgesics
- Oxygen therapy

Nursing interventions

- Maintain the patient's diet
- Encourage increased oral fluid intake
- Administer medications, as prescribed
- Assess cardiovascular, respiratory, neurological, GI, and renal status
- Assess for pain and administer analgesics, as indicated
- Apply warm compresses, as prescribed
- Monitor and record vital signs, I/O, and laboratory studies
- Allay the patient's anxiety
- Individualize home care instructions
  - Avoid restricting circulation
  - Receive childhood immunizations
  - Recognize and promptly treat infections
  - Increase fluid intake
  - Avoid strenuous exercise, vasoconstricting medications, cold temperatures, unpressurized aircraft, high altitude, and other conditions that provoke hypoxia

Key nursing interventions for a patient with sickle cell anemia

- Encourage increased oral fluid intake.
- Assess for pain and administer analgesics, as indicated.
- Apply warm compresses, as prescribed.
- Individualize home care instructions.

Complications

- Retinopathy
- Nephropathy
- Cerebral vessel occlusion
- Hypovolemic shock

- Necrosis
- Infection and gangrene
- Death

- **Surgical interventions**
  - None

NCLEX CHECKS

It's never too soon to begin your NCLEX preparation. Now that you've reviewed this chapter, carefully read each of the following questions and choose the best answer. Then compare your responses to the correct answers.

1. You're caring for a patient with Hodgkin's disease. What symptom is typical of Hodgkin's disease?

- ☐ **A.** A small, hard, irregular, and nontender mass
- ☐ **B.** An enlarged, nontender, firm mass
- ☐ **C.** Pain and swelling at the site
- ☐ **D.** Cat's eye reflex

2. Which of the following is the least important area of home care instruction to include in discussions with a patient with multiple myeloma?

- ☐ **A.** Skeletal system symptoms
- ☐ **B.** Renal system symptoms
- ☐ **C.** Nervous system symptoms
- ☐ **D.** Cardiovascular system symptoms

3. Which substance helps control bleeding when given to a patient with hemophilia B?

- ☐ **A.** Protamine sulfate
- ☐ **B.** Platelet transfusions
- ☐ **C.** Factor IX concentrate
- ☐ **D.** Vitamin K (AquaMEPHYTON)

4. The nurse is reviewing the laboratory report for a patient who underwent a bone marrow biopsy. The finding that would most strongly support a diagnosis of leukemia is the existence of a large number of immature:

- ☐ **A.** lymphocytes.
- ☐ **B.** thrombocytes.
- ☐ **C.** reticulocytes.
- ☐ **D.** leukocytes.

5. The nurse suspects disseminated intravascular coagulation (DIC) in a patient who sustained a pelvic fracture in a motor vehicle accident. Which laboratory test result helps diagnose DIC?

- ☐ **A.** Elevated platelet count
- ☐ **B.** Decreased fibrinogen level
- ☐ **C.** Low fibrin split product level
- ☐ **D.** Decreased partial thromboplastin time (PTT)

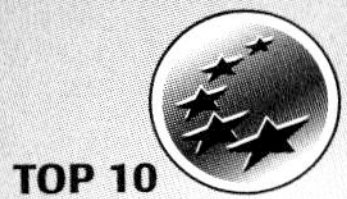

TOP 10

Items to study for your next test on the hematologic and lymphatic systems

1. Facts about RBCs and WBCs
2. ABO blood groups
3. Nursing interventions before and after bone marrow transplant
4. Assessment findings in leukemia
5. Types of lymphomas
6. Diagnostic test findings and medications for treating AIDS
7. How to inject iron solutions
8. How DIC happens
9. Types of hemophilia and their treatments
10. Difference between normal RBCs and sickled RBCs

6. The nurse is planning care for a patient with hemophilia A. A patient with hemophilia A is deficient in which clotting factor?

- ☐ **A.** VII
- ☐ **B.** VIII
- ☐ **C.** IX
- ☐ **D.** X

7. The nurse is preparing to administer iron dextran (DexFerrum) to a patient with iron deficiency anemia. Which of the following is appropriate?

- ☐ **A.** Using a 25G needle
- ☐ **B.** Administering a Z-track injection
- ☐ **C.** Using the same needle to draw up the solution and to administer the injection
- ☐ **D.** Preparing the deltoid site for injection

8. The nurse is administering cyanocobalamin (vitamin B_{12}) to a patient with pernicious anemia, secondary to gastrectomy. Which route should the nurse use to most effectively administer the vitamin?

- ☐ **A.** Topical route
- ☐ **B.** Transdermal route
- ☐ **C.** Enteral route
- ☐ **D.** Parenteral route

9. The nurse is teaching a community group about sickle cell anemia. Sickle cell anemia is most common in patients of which ethnic background?

- ☐ **A.** Asian
- ☐ **B.** Black
- ☐ **C.** Hispanic
- ☐ **D.** White

10. A patient is diagnosed with agranulocytosis. Which food items are prohibited in the patient's diet? (Select all that apply.)

- ☐ **A.** Bacon and sausage
- ☐ **B.** Uncooked celery sticks
- ☐ **C.** Cheese
- ☐ **D.** Raw apple
- ☐ **E.** Cooked carrot sticks

ANSWERS AND RATIONALES

1. CORRECT ANSWER: B

Enlarged, nontender, firm, and painless lymph nodes in the supraclavicular area are the main symptoms of Hodgkin's disease. A small, hard, nontender mass and localized pain and swelling aren't typical symptoms of Hodgkin's disease. A white spot, or cat's eye reflex, is a symptom of retinoblastoma.

2. CORRECT ANSWER: D

Multiple myeloma usually doesn't have a direct effect on the heart. Multiple myeloma usually affects the skeletal, renal, and nervous systems.

3. CORRECT ANSWER: C
Hemophilia B, a congenital bleeding disorder, is caused by a deficiency of factor IX. The treatment for hemophilia B is the administration of factor IX. Vitamin K, protamine sulfate, and platelets are used to stop bleeding, but they aren't specific treatments for hemophilia B.

4. CORRECT ANSWER: D
Leukemia is manifested by an abnormal overproduction of immature leukocytes in the bone marrow. Large numbers of lymphocytes, thrombocytes, and reticulocytes aren't characteristic of leukemia.

5. CORRECT ANSWER: B
DIC involves depletion of such clotting substances as fibrinogen and platelets, which are used for widespread clotting within the vessels. As a result, the patient's fibrinogen level and platelet count are abnormally low. Fibrin split product levels, a by-product of clot lysis, are elevated in DIC. The PTT is elevated because of clotting factor depletion.

6. CORRECT ANSWER: B
Hemophilia A, which affects more than 80% of all hemophilia patients, is caused by a deficiency of clotting factor VIII. A deficiency of the other factors doesn't cause hemophilia A. Hemophilia B results from a deficiency of factor IX.

7. CORRECT ANSWER: B
A Z-track or zig-zag technique should be used to administer an iron injection. This prevents iron from leaking into and irritating the subcutaneous tissue. A 25G needle is used for a subcutaneous injection, not for a deep I.M. injection (such as that needed to administer iron). The needle should be changed after drawing up the iron solution to avoid staining and irritating the tissues. A deep I.M. site, such as the upper outer quadrant of the buttocks, should be used to administer iron. The deltoid site doesn't provide enough muscle mass for an iron injection.

8. CORRECT ANSWER: D
Following a gastrectomy, the patient no longer has the intrinsic factor available to provide vitamin B_{12} in his GI tract. Vitamin B_{12} is administered parenterally (I.M. or deep subcutaneous). Topical and transdermal administration aren't available, and the enteral route is inappropriate in gastrectomy.

9. CORRECT ANSWER: B
Sickle cell anemia, a genetically determined hemolytic anemia, is most common in Blacks. It also occurs in people of Mediterranean descent and, infrequently, in Whites.

10. CORRECT ANSWER: B, D
A patient with agranulocytosis is immunosuppressed and prone to infection from everyday microbes. Uncooked fruits and vegetables contain microbes that may infect the immunocompromised patient. These foods should be prohibited in the patient's diet. Cooked and pasteurized foods are safe.

Glossary
Selected references
Index

Glossary

anemia: reduction in the number and volume of red blood cells, the amount of hemoglobin, or the volume of packed red cells

aneurysm: sac formed by the dilation of the wall of an artery, a vein, or the heart

angiography: radiographic visualization of blood vessels after injection of radiopaque contrast material

anorexia: lack or loss of appetite

ascites: fluid in the peritoneal cavity

ataxia: lack of muscular coordination

auscultation: physical assessment technique by which the examiner listens (usually with a stethoscope) for sounds coming from the heart, lungs, abdomen, or other organs

autoimmune disorder: disorder in which the body launches an immunologic response against itself

bruit: abnormal sound heard over peripheral vessels on auscultation that indicates turbulent blood flow

cardiac output: volume of blood ejected from the heart per minute

crepitation: grating sound produced by bone rubbing against bone

disease: pathologic condition that occurs when the body can't maintain homeostasis

distal: farthest away

dysphagia: difficulty swallowing

dyspnea: difficult, labored breathing

ecchymosis: bruise

embolism: sudden obstruction of a blood vessel by foreign substances or a blood clot

exacerbation: increase in the severity of a disease

fasciculation: involuntary twitching or contraction of the muscle

hematuria: blood in the urine

hemoglobin: iron-containing pigment in red blood cells that carries oxygen from the lungs to the tissues

hemoptysis: expectoration of bloody sputum

hemorrhage: escape of blood from a ruptured vessel

hirsutism: excessive hair growth or unusual distribution of hair

hormone: chemical substance produced in the body that has a specific regulatory effect on the activity of specific cells or organs

hypertension: high arterial blood pressure

hypotension: abnormally low blood pressure

hypoxia: reduction of oxygen in body tissues to below normal levels

idiopathic: disease with no known cause

inspection: critical observation of the patient during which the examiner may use sight, hearing, or smell to make informed observations

insulin: hormone secreted into the blood by the islets of Langerhans of the pancreas; promotes the storage of glucose, among other functions

ischemia: decreased blood supply to a body organ or tissue

jugular vein distention: distended neck veins that may indicate increased central venous pressure

lethargy: slowed responses, sluggish speech, and slowed mental and motor processes in a person oriented to time, place, and person

lichenification: thickening and hardening of the epidermis

lymphadenopathy: enlargement of the lymph nodes

melena: black, tarry stools

murmur: abnormal sound heard on auscultation of the heart; caused by abnormal blood flow through a valve

necrosis: tissue death

oliguria: urine output of less than 30 ml/hour

orthopnea: respiratory distress that's relieved by sitting upright

palpation: physical assessment technique by which the examiner uses the sense of touch to feel pulsations and vibrations or to locate body structures and assess their texture, size, consistency, mobility, and tenderness

pathogen: disease producing agent or microorganism

percussion: physical assessment technique by which the examiner taps on the skin surface with his fingers to assess the size, border, and consistency of internal organs, and to detect and evaluate fluid in a body cavity

peristalsis: intestinal contractions, or waves, that propel food toward the stomach and into and through the intestine

petechiae: multiple, small, hemorrhagic areas on the skin

plasma: liquid part of the blood that carries antibodies and nutrients to tissues and carries wastes away from tissues

platelet: disk-shaped structure in blood that plays a crucial role in blood coagulation

polydipsia: excessive thirst

polyphagia: excessive eating

polyuria: excessive urination

proximal: nearest to

pruritus: severe itching

ptosis: drooping of the eyelid

renal colic: flank pain that radiates to the groin

subluxation: partial dislocation of a joint

thrombosis: development of a thrombus (blood clot)

tophi: clusters of urate crystals surrounded by inflamed tissue; occur in gout

vasopressor: drug that stimulates contraction of the muscular tissue of the capillaries and arteries

virus: microscopic, infectious parasite that contains genetic material and needs a host cell to replicate

Selected references

Bickley, L.S., and Szilagyi, P.G. *Bates' Guide to Physical Examination and History Taking,* 8th ed. Philadelphia: Lippincott Williams & Wilkins, 2003.

Black, J.M., et al. *Medical-Surgical Nursing: Clinical Management for Positive Outcomes,* 6th ed. Philadelphia: W.B. Saunders Co., 2001.

Burns, N., and Grove, S.K. *The Practice of Nursing Research: Conduct, Critique, and Utilization,* 4th ed. Philadelphia: W.B. Saunders Co., 2001.

Connolly, M.A."Chest X-Rays. Completing the Picture," *RN* 64(6):56-62, June 2001.

Craven, R.F., and Hirnle, C.J. *Fundamentals of Nursing: Human Health and Function,* 4th ed. Philadelphia: Lippincott Williams & Wilkins, 2003.

Fischbach, F.T. *A Manual of Laboratory and Diagnostic Tests,* 7th ed. Philadelphia: Lippincott Williams & Wilkins, 2003.

Greggs-McQuilkin, D. "The Specialty of Medical-Surgical Nursing: The Solid Rock, Not the Stepping Stone," *Medsurg Nursing* 12(1):5, 26, February 2003.

Handbook of Medical-Surgical Nursing, 3rd ed. Springhouse, Pa.: Lippincott Williams & Wilkins, 2001.

Holloway, N.M. *Medical-Surgical Care Planning,* 4th ed. Springhouse, Pa.: Lippincott Williams & Wilkins, 2004.

Ignatavicius, D.D., and Workman, M.L. *Medical-Surgical Nursing: Critical Thinking for Collaborative Care,* 4th ed. Philadelphia: W.B. Saunders Co., 2001.

Medical-Surgical Nursing Made Incredibly Easy. Springhouse, Pa.: Lippincott Williams & Wilkins, 2003.

Nurse's 3 Minute Clinical Reference. Springhouse, Pa.: Lippincott Williams & Wilkins, 2003.

Nursing2004 Drug Handbook, 24th ed. Springhouse, Pa.: Lippincott Williams & Wilkins, 2004.

Portable RN: The All-in-One Nursing Reference. Springhouse, Pa.: Lippincott Williams & Wilkins, 2002.

Porth, C.M. *Essentials of Pathophysiology: Concepts of Altered Health.* Philadelphia: Lippincott Williams & Wilkins, 2003.

Professional Guide to Pathophysiology. Springhouse, Pa.: Lippincott Williams & Wilkins, 2003.

Smeltzer, S.C., and Bare, B.G., eds. *Brunner and Suddarth's Textbook of Medical-Surgical Nursing,* 10th ed. Philadelphia: Lippincott Williams & Wilkins, 2003.

Springhouse Review for Medical-Surgical Nursing Certification: An Indispensable Study Guide for the A.N.A. Exam, 3rd ed. Springhouse, Pa.: Lippincott Williams & Wilkins, 2002.

Springhouse Review for NCLEX-RN, 5th ed. Springhouse, Pa.: Lippincott Williams & Wilkins, 2002.

Thomas, S.P. "Anger: The Mismanaged Emotion," *Medsurg Nursing* 12(2):103-10, April 2003.

Yoder, L.H., and Wassum, E. "Medical-Surgical Nurses in the Military," *Medsurg Nursing* 11(4):203, August 2002.

Index

A

i refers to an illustration; t refers to a table.

i refers to an illustration; t refers to a table.

D

E

i refers to an illustration; t refers to a table.

i refers to an illustration; t refers to a table.

i refers to an illustration; t refers to a table.

i refers to an illustration; t refers to a table.

i refers to an illustration; t refers to a table.

S

T

i refers to an illustration; t refers to a table.

i refers to an illustration; t refers to a table.

ABOUT THE CD-ROM

The enclosed CD-ROM is just one more reason why the *Straight A's* series is at the head of its class. The more than 250 additional NCLEX-style questions contained on the CD provide you with another opportunity to review the material and gauge your knowledge. The program allows you to:

- take tests of varying lengths on subject areas of your choice
- learn the rationales for correct and incorrect answers
- print the results of your tests to measure progress over time.

Minimum system requirements

To operate the *Straight A's* CD-ROM, we recommend that you have the following computer equipment:

- Windows 98 or higher
- Pentium 166 or higher
- 64 MB RAM or more
- 8 MB of free hard-disk space
- SVGA monitor with High Color (16-bit)
- CD-ROM drive
- mouse.

Installation

Before installing the CD-ROM, make sure that your monitor is set to High Color (16-bit) and your display area is set to 800 × 600. If it isn't, consult your monitor's user's manual for instructions about changing the display settings. (The display settings are typically found in Start/Settings/Control Panel/Display/Settings tab.)

To run this program, you must install it onto the hard drive of your computer, following these three steps:

1. Start Windows 98 or higher.
2. Place the CD in your CD-ROM drive. After a few moments, the install process will automatically begin. *Note:* If the install process doesn't automatically begin, click the Start menu and select Run. Type *D:\setup.exe* (where *D:* is the letter of your CD-ROM drive) and then click OK.
3. Follow the on-screen instructions for installation.

Technical support

For technical support, call toll-free 1-800-638-3030, Monday through Friday, 8:30 a.m. to 5 p.m. Eastern Time. You may also write to Lippincott Williams & Wilkins Technical Support, 351 W. Camden Street, Baltimore, MD 21201-2436, or e-mail us at techsupp@lww.com.
